DATE DUE

MAR 2 5 2015		
APR 2 0 2015		

Demco, Inc. 38-293

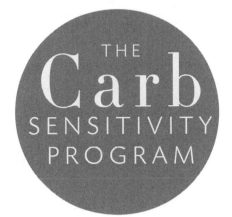

THE
Carb
SENSITIVITY
PROGRAM

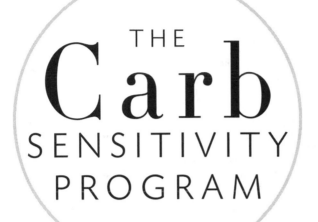

THE
Carb
SENSITIVITY
PROGRAM

DISCOVER WHICH **CARBS** WILL **CURB**
YOUR CRAVINGS, CONTROL YOUR
APPETITE, AND **BANISH BELLY FAT**

NATASHA TURNER, ND

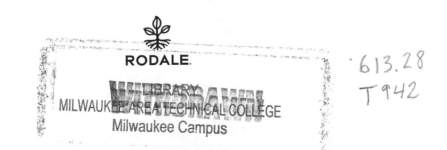

RODALE

First published in Canada by Random House Canada in 2012.

Rodale books may be purchased for business or promotional use or for special sales. For information, please write to: Special Markets Department, Rodale, Inc., 733 Third Avenue, New York, NY 10017

Printed in the United States of America
Rodale Inc. makes every effort to use acid-free ♾, recycled paper ♻.

Book design by Jennifer Lum

Library of Congress Cataloging-in-Publication Data

Turner, Natasha.
  The carb sensitivity program : discover which carbs will curb your cravings, control your appetite, and banish belly fat / Natasha Turner.
      p.   cm.
  Includes bibliographical references and index.
  ISBN 978–1–60961–329–7   hardcover
  1. Low-carbohydrate diet.   2. Reducing diets.   3. Diet therapy.   I. Title.
  RM237.73T87   2012
  613.2'833—dc23   2012006206

Distributed to the trade by Macmillan

2   4   6   8   10   9   7   5   3   1   hardcover

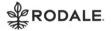

We inspire and enable people to improve their lives and the world around them.
rodalebooks.com

To Uncle Bruce and Aunt Betty,
For your endless generosity of spirit

To Nan and Gramp, Mary and Darrell Rivers,
For showing me unconditional love

And for my Dad,
You taught me to persevere

Introduction   I

PART ONE: CARBS AND YOUR APPETITE, CRAVINGS AND METABOLISM

1. Confessions of a Carboholic Culture   7
2. The Essentials: Understanding Carbs, Insulin and Your Body   24
3. Insulin Spikes and Carb Sensitivity: Why We're Fat,
   Diseased and Aging Quickly   38
4. This Is Your Brain on Carbs   58
5. A Five-Step Prescription for the Carb-Addicted Brain   73

**PART TWO: THE 6-WEEK PRESCRIPTION FOR DETERMINING YOUR
CARB SENSITIVITIES**

6. Rules to Live By: The Dietary Rules Common to
   All Six Phases of the CSP   107
7. The Carb Sensitivity Program—Weekly Meal Plans and
   Permitted Food Lists   134
8. Supportive Supplements for the Six CSP Phases   218

**PART THREE: THE METABOLIC REPAIR PROGRAM: A DEFINITIVE
SYSTEM TO IMPROVE CARBOHYDRATE SENSITIVITY**

9. So You Have a Damaged Metabolism . . .   233
10. Your Metabolic Repair Diet and Metabolic Repair Supplements   260
11. The Metabolic Repair Workout   286

CONTENTS

PART FOUR: TIME-SAVING TIPS FOR THE KITCHEN AND CSP RECIPES

Top Time-Saving Tips for the Kitchen   347

Recipes Permitted in All Phases of the Program   350

Breakfast Recipes   350

Lunch and Dinner Recipes   365

Phase Two Recipes   385

Phase Three Recipes   392

Phase Four Recipes   400

Phase Five Recipes   409

Snack Recipes—Permitted in All Phases   419

APPENDICES

Appendix A: Blood Tests to Assess Metabolic Health
    and Insulin Sensitivity   425

Appendix B: Vegetarian and Vegan Sources of Protein   440

Acknowledgments   443

Resources   446

General Index   450

Recipe Index   463

About the Author   472

INTRODUCTION

Believe in yourself! Have faith in your abilities!
Without a humble but reasonable confidence in your own powers
you cannot be successful or happy.

—NORMAN VINCENT PEALE

Hair loss, incessant carb cravings, followed by the classic "carb coma," an out-of-control appetite, an unwavering obsession with food, hunger that returns soon after eating, belly fat and bulging love handles. Does any of this sound familiar? While you may be nodding your head with recognition, these are actually my own telltale signs of an increased sensitivity to carbs.

I have been managing these symptoms for more than 12 years. And believe it or not, they *intensified* shortly after I began my practice as a naturopathic doctor. There I was, the natural health and nutrition expert, secretly downing chocolate chip cookies and muffins in between patients because I just *had* to have them!

It wasn't until the fall of 1999, when I was diagnosed with polycystic ovarian syndrome (PCOS), that I grasped the common link between my symptoms and my health condition. While I knew PCOS was often associated with an imbalance of insulin (specifically insulin resistance), I did not fully understand how such an imbalance could affect one's metabolism and bodily functions until it happened to me.

At the time, I was prescribed metformin (a diabetes medication often used in PCOS patients to enhance insulin balance) and the birth control pill (to regulate my cycle). But as readers of my previous books already know, I used my own protocols to bring my hormones back into balance—the same process I originally outlined in *The Hormone Diet*. Within just a few weeks, I learned how sticking to my strength-training routine, taking my supplements, getting enough sleep, and choosing the right amount, timing and types of carbs enabled me to be symptom free and to lose my belly fat. It then became my goal to share my personal experiences and help others achieve the same level of health and well-being.

Sounds easy, right? Not always. Like you, I stray off course from time to time. I enjoy dining out. I consume too many carbs in times of stress, frustration or celebration. I get busy and miss workouts. Luckily, the efforts I've made over the years allow me to do these things occasionally, without a return of life-hampering, body-disrupting symptoms.

Knowing this has made me more motivated than ever to constantly seek the best ways to maintain a healthy insulin balance for optimal health and wellness. My research for this book has led me to a definitive conclusion: The long-term health consequences of this state of hormonal disruption are—for lack of a proper medical term—*really scary*. (Even more frightening is the current *worldwide* epidemic of insulin imbalance that you will learn about in Chapter 1.)

From my personal experiences and my years in clinical practice, I know that *optimal insulin balance is the most important factor in living a vibrant, strong and healthy life*. And this book is designed to help you take advantage of all that I've learned so that you can skip past the trial-and-error phase and go right to *results*. If you asked me the three most important things you could do for your health right now, I would give you the following advice: Improve your sleep, discover your current state of carb sensitivity and consume a few essential supplements. How simple does that sound? Surprisingly, though, the effects of implementing these basic suggestions are huge when it comes to restoring and maintaining your insulin balance, achieving your ideal body composition and—perhaps most important—feeling your best for the long term.

The Hormone Diet and *The Supercharged Hormone Diet* both help to restore insulin balance, as well as the levels of many other hormones (including the stress, sex, mood and thyroid hormones). Although both of these plans provide a hormonally balanced program that is personalized according to the reader's food allergies or sensitivities, my clinical practice led me to discover that following these plans alone did not always achieve the desired results. Indeed, a few of my patients failed to continue losing weight, while others had cravings, water retention, high cholesterol, high blood pressure or other symptoms that would not resolve. Clearly, something else was going on, and I had to keep digging to find the solution.

It wasn't long before I had my "aha" moment. *It was all about the carbs!* It is known that carbs have the potential to be food allergens that can trigger inflammation or chronic symptoms such as headaches, digestive upset, dark circles under the eyes, puffiness in the face, fatigue, joint pain, abdominal bloating and more. But here's where it got interesting for me—carbs also generate a metabolic response that is directly linked to the insulin spike their consumption produces. And there I had it: Just like with food allergies, each person's metabolic response to carbs—or what I have termed *carb sensitivity*—is unique.

In Chapter 2, I explain more about how I came to figure out the process presented to you here as The Carb Sensitivity Program (CSP), a 6-week nutrition plan that will help you identify the perfect types of carbohydrates *for you*. You will achieve this by rotating specific carb-based foods in and out of your diet, while carefully monitoring how your body reacts to each new group. You will also follow an exercise program, as well as a supplement regime to aid detoxification and your metabolism. In the pages that follow, each step of the process is outlined for you in a clear and concise way. I have also provided weekly meal plans and recipes to help you get started and stay on track. Everything you need to achieve optimal health is right here.

As I discovered the CSP's true potential to reinvent and revitalize one's state of health, I moved from that original aha moment to a full-fledged "*Eureka!*" My hope is that you too will soon share in my excitement as you come to understand the far-reaching benefits of improved insulin balance.

I want to assure readers of my previous books that my basic philosophy of care has not changed. It is still centered on the importance of balancing all of your hormones, thinking "big picture" when it comes to correctly restoring balance and considering the interrelatedness of the hormones at work in your body. I still believe a process such as the 4-week nutrition prescription in *The Supercharged Hormone Diet,* which helps to identify food allergies or sensitivities as well as restore hormonal balance, must be followed to achieve optimal health. But some of you will need to take the extra step to gain control of erratic or escalating insulin levels. Meanwhile, *all of us* must focus on achieving and sustaining our metabolism and insulin balance—for life. The Carb Sensitivity Program helps with this exact goal.

I believe that everyone will eventually need to complete the CSP because our carb sensitivity—and therefore our tendency to accumulate belly fat and find ourselves at risk for chronic disease—naturally increases with age. Thank goodness there's finally a solution! Besides helping you look your best, I want to help you live your life to the fullest and become your greatest self. You can do this by taking control of what, when and how you eat. I wish you the best as you embark on this plan, which has the potential to change not only your life but also your metabolism. I encourage you to share your feedback, questions and outcome through www.carbsensitivity.com or www.facebook.com/carbsensitivity, where you will also find instructional videos. These sites offer a great opportunity to connect with the carb-sensitive community and to help encourage others. Together, we can achieve perfect balance.

—Dr. Natasha Turner, N.D.

PART ONE

CARBS AND YOUR APPETITE, CRAVINGS AND METABOLISM

Change before you have to.

JACK WELCH

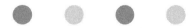

CHAPTER 1

CONFESSIONS OF A CARBOHOLIC CULTURE

You are never too old to set another goal or to dream a new dream.

C. S. LEWIS

We live in a carb-fueled world. Turn on the television any time of the day, and you will be bombarded by tantalizing images of every-thing from high-carb cereals and breakfast sandwiches to fast-food lunches and microwavable dinners. And there's a reason for it. As a society, we *love* our carbs. We eat them to celebrate, to ease the pain of heartbreak, to dampen frustration, to comfort our sorrows or to indulge in a moment of connection. Just recently I saw some-one wearing a T-shirt that read, "I love carbs." Carbs are everywhere: They even have their own clothing line.

This love affair with carbs has been building for a while—about 30 years or more. Pick up the most recent edition of the dietary guidelines for Americans and even here you will find a significant reliance on grains and starches—up to six recommended servings a day! For my age, the recommendation is to have six grain prod-ucts, three cups of dairy, one and a half cups of fruits and two cups of vegetables, and two protein sources a day. While there was a 1600-calorie count included, I can tell you that if I put patients on that diet they could potentially gain a pound a day and have dia-betes by the end of a month! An exaggeration? Perhaps. Nonetheless, as you are about to learn, these government guide-lines are not only painfully outdated but also potentially harmful. For decades now, prominent organizations such as the American

Diabetes Association have been recommending a low-fat, high-carbohydrate diet as a treatment for diabetes. Based on my years of research and clinical experience as a preventive health specialist, I will tell you that this approach cannot and does not work.

If we were to rewind a few centuries—to a time before our taste buds knew of doughnuts, bagels, fortified cereals and the like—we would discover that there were significantly fewer cases of diabetes, and that obesity was a condition of the few, rather than the many. In fact, one could argue that our current obsession with dieting is a direct consequence of this carb addiction that has developed over several generations.

Unfortunately, it seems as if the more we try to fix the problem, the further we get from a real, lasting solution. We frantically try fad diet after fad diet, only to creep back up to our previous weight (or higher!) thanks to cravings, improper sleep habits, daily stresses and our on-the-run lifestyles.

When we examine those diets, it's clear that carbs have replaced fat as the main taboo over the last 10 to 20 years. I cannot count the number of times I have heard someone say, "But I don't eat carbs; I don't know why I'm still overweight." While we have come to understand that carb consumption is linked with weight gain, the majority of us do not realize the many ways that carbs can quietly slip into our diet. Coupled with this confusion is a lack of knowledge regarding the total amount of carbs we can or should consume. Some of us may wonder if we should eat them at all.

So, what's a health-conscious eater to do? Should we join the procarb movement or the anticarb revolution? Surprisingly, the answer has little to do with your taste buds and everything to do with the hormone *insulin* and, more specifically, how your body reacts to the carbohydrates that you *do* consume. The kicker? Each and every body has its own unique response to carbs.

In my previous book *The Hormone Diet,* I presented the following equation for fat loss:

Lasting Fat Loss = Hormonal Balance + (Calories In – Calories Burned)

That equation still works, but what if I told you that I've made an important discovery *within* the scope of "calories in"—a discovery that can help you break through even the most stubborn weight-loss plateau, not to mention banish your risk of diabetes, Alzheimer's, stroke, heart disease and other ailments? Even if you satisfy your cravings with only low-glycemic carbs or religiously follow the latest fitness magazine diet that promises to keep your blood sugar low, you need to remember this: *All carbs = sugar.* In other words, when we look at the calories we are consuming, we must take into account that *all carbs* trigger the release of insulin—a powerful fat-storing hormone.

Insulin is released by the pancreas in proportion to the amount of sugar in the bloodstream (i.e., more sugar = more insulin). While insulin is necessary for the proper functioning of our cells, excess insulin can, over time, predispose you to a condition called *insulin resistance,* which can eventually lead to diabetes and a whole host of health concerns. Sadly, the majority of us have some degree of insulin resistance—and we don't even know it.

In the pages that follow, I will walk you through the ins and outs of insulin, and explain how an excess of this hormone can impact your ability to lose weight and keep it off. But the most important point I want you to absorb—and the reason I wrote this book—is that the consequences of an insulin imbalance are much more dire than the number on your scale or the fit of your clothes. Excess insulin literally causes the slow destruction of bodily tissues and organs, including our bones, muscles, skin, blood vessels, brain, liver and more. And this far-reaching, devastating imbalance is spurred by one basic factor: *the frequency, amount and type of carbohydrates we consistently consume over time, and our body's individual ability to process them.* When our cells become resistant to insulin, we become more sensitive to carbs. The more insulin we have, the fewer carbs we can safely process. And the more carb sensitive we are, the greater the degree of insulin resistance. It's a vicious circle!

Consider this example: Imagine eating a meal consisting of a low-glycemic grain such as quinoa or a sweet potato with your protein and essential fats. Sounds healthy, right? But what if your body dealt with that carbohydrate as though it were a big bowl of chocolate ice cream? No wonder it's so hard to lose weight! If you're having an aha moment right now, read on: The Carb Sensitivity Program (CSP) will reboot your metabolism and fix any faulty communications within your cells so that a good carb, becomes, well, a good carb again. I have discovered that even healthy, low–glycemic index carbs such as beans and sweet potatoes can cause a blood sugar spike and subsequent insulin surge in certain patients—factors that lead to cravings, weight gain and an excessive appetite. In all cases, the carbs that you are sensitive to are the same carbs that spike your insulin. And your metabolic makeup—or degree of insulin resistance—is the determining factor. In the end, it doesn't matter whether the carbs you are consuming are "good" or "bad." What matters is your particular carb sensitivity.

Diabesity: A Modern Plague

Is it really possible that heart disease, stroke, diabetes, osteoporosis, cancer, Alzheimer's disease, inflammatory conditions, muscle tissue loss and disease-causing vitamin and mineral deficiencies may all have one root factor? Or that the early-warning signs of these conditions, such as an expanding waistline, high cholesterol and high blood pressure, can also be traced to the same single underlying cause? The latest scientific research clearly demonstrates that these conditions not only share the same underlying cause—excess insulin—but also require *the same treatment*. The good news? Many of these issues are 100 percent preventable and, in some cases, entirely reversible.

So how prevalent is this insulin imbalance? Dr. Francine Kaufman, a California-based pediatric endocrinologist, has coined the term *diabesity* (diabetes + obesity) to describe a metabolic dysfunction related to insulin imbalance that ranges from mild blood sugar imbalance to full-fledged type 2 diabetes. Obesity, insulin resistance, metabolic syndrome, heart disease and type 2 diabetes have reached epidemic proportions. I dare say there's not a person reading this book who isn't affected by these conditions, either directly or indirectly. Yet as common as these conditions may be, few of us understand how closely related they are.

Diabesity is our modern plague. The Center for Health Reform & Modernization, part of the health care company United Health Group, Inc., warns that *more than half* of all Americans may develop diabetes or prediabetes by 2020, unless they lose weight and become more active. The many conditions that exist under the umbrella of diabesity—from high cholesterol and blood pressure to excess abdominal fat and insulin resistance—affect more than *one billion people worldwide*. As of 2010, more than 100 million Americans (including 50 percent of those over age 65) suffered from diabetes in its various forms and 1.8 million people in Canada had been diagnosed with the disease. Diabesity has been identified as the leading cause of increased risk of heart disease, stroke, dementia, cancer, kidney failure and blindness, to name only a few related ailments.

The vastness of this problem is astronomical. The Centers for Disease Control and Prevention estimates that some 75 million Americans have metabolic syndrome, the clinical condition that manifests as a result of insulin resistance. Even more frightening? Nearly six million are undiagnosed or unaware they have it.

If the epidemic of diabesity among adults isn't concerning enough, the state of our children's health is even more alarming:

- Recent reports from the 2009 *Proceedings of the Nutrition Society* suggest that *one-third* of people born in 2010 will develop diabetes at some point in their lives. Particularly shocking is that many will develop it in childhood. A recent Yale University study indicated that nearly one in four obese kids between the ages of 4 and 18 have prediabetes, or insulin imbalance.

- Each year, kids are getting fatter. Among American children 2 to 5 years of age, more than 10 percent are now obese.
- Research from Harvard shows infant obesity (children under the age of 2) has risen more than 70 percent since 1980.

Clearly, these alarming statistics are not the result of babies eating cake and doughnuts in front of the TV. There is more to the diabesity story than consuming junk food and not exercising enough, as you will learn in Chapter 3. Sadly, it is mom's insulin level during pregnancy that is setting up her child for obesity before he takes his first breath.

According to the November 2010 edition of the *Oxford Journal Online,* the projections for diabetes for 2030 are expected to reach 439 million individuals, or 7.7 percent of the world population. This is nearly 10 times the number of people affected by HIV/AIDS, according to the World Health Organization (WHO). Besides the consequences for individuals, this epidemic has an effect on the world economy. The health-care costs associated with diabetes have been rising steadily over the last decade, reaching $376 billion in 2010 and projected to hit $490 billion by 2030. With numbers like this, you would expect a state of emergency to be declared! And you would think that the world's decision makers would be doing everything in their power to get the word out about the cause of these conditions and how to treat them successfully.

It is urgent that we take steps, including screening, prevention and early management, in an effort to control this evolving epidemic. And that's exactly what the Carb Sensitivity Program aims to do. Specifically, the CSP seeks to explain exactly what those "calories in" should comprise, and the associated impacts on our waistline and our state of health.

The Carb Sensitivity Program

The Carb Sensitivity Program (CSP) is a natural extension of the information presented in my first book, *The Hormone Diet*. The program presented there was the first to support the direct relationship between achieving hormonal balance and lasting weight loss. Through this approach, I was able to demonstrate the extraordinary incidence of hormonal imbalance, and thousands of people came to realize that their common symptoms—such as sleep disruption or cravings—were significant indicators of hormonal disruption. My philosophy was simple: *Balanced hormones = healthy aging and ideal body composition.*

Although this is still the guiding principle for me and my colleagues at Clear Medicine, it's grown into something more. By manipulating and testing how different individuals react to carbohydrates, I have devised a nutrition program that produces quick, consistent and lasting weight-loss results. The CSP recognizes the *main* obstacle to weight loss—*carbohydrate sensitivity caused by insulin imbalance*—and guarantees success where other plans fail. The CSP is unique in that it helps you to discover the perfect types and amounts of carbohydrates to optimize *your* metabolism. You will walk away with a *personalized* plan that sheds body fat, reshapes your body and improves your health. It's a remarkably simple plan, *and it works.*

In my clinical practice, patients on this program have seen extraordinary improvements in their body composition, their overall mood and their digestion, and their blood work. The average weight loss in the first 2 weeks is 5 to 12 pounds, with most patients losing anywhere from 30 to 110 pounds in total, depending on their initial starting point. Incredibly, patients consistently report that their food cravings disappear within just days!

How Can You Tell If You Are Carbohydrate Sensitive (CS)?

Are you wondering if the CSP is for you? Consider this. I hear daily from patients who are perplexed that they are suddenly gaining weight on the *same* diet they have been eating for years and years. Or perhaps they have tried to repeat a successful diet from a few years back, only to discover it no longer has the same effect. Despite their best intentions, these patients are finding that the so-called low-carb, low-fat or low-cal effort just throws them deeper into a state of metabolic imbalance and dietary frustration. Sound familiar? In situations like these, it's not long before you feel like a hamster on a wheel, working hard but getting nowhere fast.

The Carb Sensitivity Program is designed to repair your metabolism and kick-start your fat loss, but in order for it to work, we must set aside the conventional understanding of a carbohydrate as an *essential* source of energy—and replace it with an updated model of thinking that reflects the *needs* of your body today.

When we are CS, our cells do not respond effectively to insulin, which ultimately means the body can no longer burn fat efficiently. But many people are unaware that they are challenged by their carb intake. In fact, the vast majority of us have *different* degrees of sensitivity to carbs, and we don't even realize it. In very basic terms, the degree of your carb sensitivity determines how much fat you are accumulating on your waistline. You can also tell if you are CS by asking yourself these key questions:

- Do you crave carbohydrates?
- Do you have a sweet tooth?
- Do you get sleepy or mental fogginess after meals (i.e., the "carb coma")?
- Do you feel bloated, especially after meals?
- Do you experience water retention or puffiness?
- Do you have a very large appetite or an obsession with food?
- Do you have fat accumulation, especially around your middle?
- Do your feet burn in bed at night?
- Do you have difficulty losing weight?

If you answered yes to any of these questions, a carbohydrate sensitivity may be negatively impacting your metabolism, hormone production and long-term health. This book will help you determine *your* level of carb sensitivity, which will in turn enable you to balance your hormones, improve your energy, ease digestion and lose stubborn belly fat.

The Carb Sensitivity Program will also help you determine which types of carbs you need to *avoid* so that you can keep your insulin at the right level. Remember the guy from the movie *Super Size Me*, who ate a McDonald's-only diet for a full month? Well, his metabolism went completely haywire in fewer than 30 days because of the influence of high-carb, high-fat, fiber-poor, nutrient-deficient foods that caused his insulin level to spike through the roof. Albeit unknowingly, you too may have thrown your metabolism into disarray within the last year or even decades—a situation that may have brought you to the point where your hormonal messengers can no longer send and receive the right signals. In just 6 weeks, the CSP will get you on the path to improved insulin balance. The end result will be a breakthrough in your carb addiction and a welcome end to the yo-yo dieting cycle.

A Dietary Prescription for Metabolic Repair— At Any Age!

There is little argument that the ideal diet for improving a damaged metabolism and insulin resistance should reduce body weight by burning away body fat, while preserving metabolically active muscle tissue. Within the medical field, however, agreement on the design of the specific diet to accomplish these goals is far from unanimous. Some diets recommend more monounsaturated fats, increased complex carbs and high fiber, while others recommend avoiding all forms of carbohydrates. But the vast majority do agree that a high intake of saturated fats and a low intake of fiber are linked to insulin resistance.

Although I believe the macronutrient makeup of a hormonally-balanced diet consists of 35 percent carbs, 35 percent protein, and 30 percent fat, here's where my program differs. I do not believe in a one-size-fits-all approach. The types of carbs that make up the 35 percent must vary, depending on each individual's level of insulin resistance. The more resistant you are to insulin, the lower your diet should be in starchy carbs, such as grains, starchy vegetables, and legumes and the more you should rely on green vegetables and one or two servings of low GI fruits for your carbs. (Now you understand why we should consume fewer carbs as we age: Insulin resistance tends to naturally increase with aging.) There is no doubt that a diet containing excessive amounts of carbohydrates will contribute to insulin resistance. Changing the type and the amount of carbohydrates then offers the potential to reverse insulin resistance and positively impact our metabolism. But the question remains: *Just how many carbs are too many?*

The answer depends largely on the form of the carbs (simple versus complex), our age, our general health status, protein intake, fiber consumption, overall caloric intake, the timing of our meals, vitamin and mineral levels, body composition, activity levels, sleep, stress and even our mood. The Carb Sensitivity Program takes *all* of these variables into account.

Your dietary prescription for metabolic repair will not be based upon slashing calories but rather upon altering the macronutrient makeup of your diet, particularly adjusting the amount and types of carbohydrates and protein you take in. Your fat intake will remain the same, making up approximately 30 percent of your diet. Past studies have shown that a diet higher in healthy (monounsaturated) fats provides an advantage over a low-fat, fiber-rich, high-carbohydrate diet on belly fat loss in type 2 diabetics. Since a smaller waistline (or a decrease in the waist-hip ratio), is closely associated with improved insulin resistance, a diet higher in monounsaturated fat seems to produce a more favorable impact on metabolism. What's more, these changes can occur quickly. Research shows improvement in blood sugar and insulin balance in as little as 15 to 21 days of following a diet high in healthy fat and low in carbs. In contrast, a diet much like that recommended by the US dietary guidelines low in fat and high in carbohydrates appears to *increase* fat gain and, consequently, fuel insulin resistance.

The greatest benefit of the CSP is this: It works! I have seen the results in my clinical practice time and time again, and numerous studies show that diets of similar caloric value, but lower in carbohydrates (e.g., 35 percent versus 45 percent of calories from carbohydrates), provide positive metabolic outcomes. While many diets can result in weight loss, the diet with lower carbohydrates (35 percent in this instance) offers more benefits, including improvements in HDL cholesterol, blood sugar and insulin.

By now, you've probably made a few mental check marks. Perhaps you have checked "yes," with great enthusiasm, to a few questions on the previous quiz and may suspect you are carb sensitive. You've probably realized that you may have some level of metabolic damage. You may even have symptoms of insulin resistance, based not only on the reading on your bathroom scale but also on health conditions you may be experiencing, ranging from high blood pressure and high cholesterol to an ever-expanding accumulation of belly fat.

Researchers at the University of California, San Diego School of Medicine have reported that chronically high insulin may block specific hormones that trigger energy release into the body. In other words, high insulin not only encourages the storage of fat but also inhibits burning body fat for energy. As your ability to effectively use insulin diminishes, you gain more and more weight in an effort to compensate for insulin resistance. Unfortunately, in the majority of the population, these changes are a normal part of aging. I can assure you that the only way to stop this cycle is by eating the right carbohydrates for your metabolism, thereby stabilizing blood sugar and reducing insulin release, and by building more muscle, the largest tissue in the body where insulin does its work.

The Problem with No-Carb and Low-Carb Diets

If you have chosen a great diet, followed it carefully, optimized your workout and *still* aren't getting the results you're looking for, you may need a diet based on your body type and physiological response to carbohydrates. The CSP reduces insulin in your body *by determining how your body processes different carbohydrates as well as by improving your metabolism.*

Here's another important point: If we know our individual blood sugar and insulin response to carbs varies, the recommendation in many current diet plans to remove *all* carbs is clearly unnecessary. This is why an individualized approach is always best—a process that allows you to identify which carbs are okay for you, as well as the types you need to avoid.

Moreover, why cut out carbs for so long? Most low-carb diets recommend complete carb avoidance for 8 to 10 weeks. At the reintroduction point, the risk for gaining back most, if not all, of the weight lost is very high. This reaction is tough to avoid, since a no-carb diet is not sustainable for the majority of us. Eventually our urge to eat carbs overwhelms our desire to keep them away, while our dipping energy levels or fluctuating moods might force us to reach for them—usually late at night standing in front of the fridge or cupboard in a feeding frenzy!

There is a reason people tend to lose *and gain* more weight on a no-carb diet than on any other type of diet. Not only are we unable to stick to a no-carb approach over the long term, but also the majority of us experience bloating, water retention, cravings and rebound weight gain, *plus* another 5 to 10 pounds, once carbs are reintroduced. Why? Since *nothing has been done to improve your tolerance for carbs during the period of avoidance,* your insulin will simply spike again once carbs are back. Ultimately, this approach creates a temporary quick-fix weight-loss solution that fails to address (or, even worse, masks) the true underlying health issues of disrupted communication between the cells and insulin. It is this

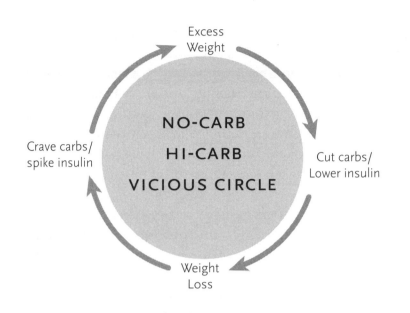

Excess Weight

Crave carbs/ spike insulin

NO-CARB HI-CARB VICIOUS CIRCLE

Cut carbs/ Lower insulin

Weight Loss

powerful relationship—along with the fundamental connection between glucose and insulin—that I want to explore.

From now on, you won't avoid all carbs unnecessarily. Nor will you practice short-term avoidance only to experience the dreaded rebound weight gain later on. Through the CSP, you will discover the perfect type and amount of carbs *for you and your current metabolic state.* You need only remove the carbs to which you're sensitive. Best of all, the Carb Sensitivity Program will help you identify these foods.

You will also be guided through my method to repair your metabolism and *improve* your carb sensitivities, should you discover any. Ultimately, this translates to the possibility of eventually getting more carbs back into your life, without returning to the yo-yo dieting cycle. As an added bonus, this process will also reduce your risk of every single disease associated with aging.

While many diets attempt to define what the "right" type of carbohydrate is, they do not look at identifying the right type of carbohydrate *for the individual.* Carbohydrate tolerance varies widely from one person to another. I also believe the old adage that "a calorie is a calorie" is a myth. Where they come from has a huge impact on the body's reaction. This is particularly true when it comes to calories derived from carbs. Assuming that a meal is balanced with protein, fat and carbs (the three primary sources of calories), a group of people given the exact same plate of food may each respond differently, depending on their individual sensitivity to carbs. The same foods that lead to weight gain in one person could lead to weight loss in another!

Over a period of 6 weeks, you'll discover your body's sensitivity to carbs by swapping certain carbohydrates in your meals and monitoring how your body reacts. Each week you'll introduce a different category of carbohydrates (legumes, grains or starchy vegetables) to your daily diet. No measurements or calculations are required—everything has been laid out in an easy-to-follow plan with straightforward permitted food lists, simple meal plans and tasty recipes.

A Quick Summary of Your Weekly CSP Meal Guide

PHASE	CARBS TO AVOID	PERMITTED CARBS & NOTES ON CS STATUS
Phase 1	No grains, no beans/legumes, no starchy vegetables are permitted this week.	Allowed in all phases: Green/nonstarchy vegetables, one or two low GI fruits
Phase 2	No grains, no beans/legumes. Potential carb sensitivity to starchy vegetables tested during this phase.	Allowed: One serving of starchy vegetables per day. Individuals who gain weight or fail to lose at this stage have high carbohydrate sensitivity and, therefore, a low tolerance for metabolizing carbs. They will do better on a lower carbohydrate diet where the sources of carbs come from green vegetables and low GI fruit intake.

PHASE	CARBS TO AVOID	PERMITTED CARBS & NOTES ON CS STATUS
Phase 3	No grains, no starchy vegetables. Potential carb sensitivity to legumes tested during this phase.	Allowed: One serving of beans/legumes per day. Individuals who gain weight or fail to lose during this week have a moderate carbohydrate sensitivity and a moderate tolerance for metabolizing carbs. They will do better on a diet that includes only 1 serving of a "moderate" amount of carbohydrates per day from starchy vegetables.
Phase 4	No starchy vegetables, no beans/legumes. Potential carb sensitivity to lower carb grains tested during this phase.	Allowed: One serving of low-carb grains per day. This stage, which involves introducing grains, is often the litmus test that uncovers many cases of carb sensitivity (as described in the symptoms listed previously). Individuals who find carb sensitivity here do best on a diet where the sources of carbs are derived from starchy vegetables or legumes.
Phase 5	No starchy vegetables, no beans/legumes. Potential carb sensitivity to higher carb grains and potatoes tested during this phase.	Allowed: One serving of potatoes or certain grains per day. Individuals who have experienced carb sensitivity at this point can tolerate carbohydrates well and may enjoy 1 serving of starchy carbohydrate sources from starchy vegetables, legumes, or low cost carb grains per day without experiencing weight gain.
Phase 6		Individuals who progress to Phase 6 are not carb sensitive. This stage permits the choice of 1 serving of any carbs from the program (starchy vegetables, legumes, low glycemic grains) per day.

If it seems like a lot to take in, don't worry. This process is *very* simple and straightforward. If you carry on losing weight from one week to the next, you should continue with your weekly introduction of carbohydrates. If, however, you gain weight, retain water, or experience cravings, increased hunger or a decrease in energy while consuming a certain category of carbohydrates, your current tolerance has been exceeded. At this point, the carb-introduction process should be halted for 4 weeks. You'll enter into a Metabolic Repair Program, outlined in Part Three, which includes supplements, exercise and lifestyle suggestions designed to *reduce* your CS and *enhance* your sensitivity to insulin so you can eventually enjoy carbs without worrying about side effects such as bloating, cravings, water retention and weight gain.

How to Use This Book

While I recommend that this book be read in full, some of you may be excited to get started right away. If this applies to you, simply move on now to the meal plan and rules set out in Part Two, page 134. Otherwise, I encourage you to read Chapter 2 if you wish to understand more about carbs and the effects of insulin on a normal, healthy body. To learn more about what happens when this relationship goes awry, dive into Chapter 3. Chapter 4 helps you understand the physiological effect carbs have on your brain and how they are addictive. Most of you should definitely read Chapter 5 for basic tips to prevent or solve a strong carb addiction.

Your body's response to each phase of the CSP will determine how to progress through the remainder of the book. If you uncover carb sensitivities and, therefore, a need for metabolic repair, you will be directed to the nutrition, supplement and exercise recommendations in Part Three. Those of you who progress through all six phases without experiencing symptoms of carb sensitivity will complete your CSP process with the nutrition and supplement recommendations outlined in Part Two. The metabolic repair workout in Part Three is also recommended for you; it won't just repair a faulty metabolism, but it will keep a healthy one running on all cylinders.

Now, let's get you started on your journey to lasting weight loss and wellness!

CSP SUCCESS STORY: SANDRA

"Just as I had entered the stage of my life where my career had never been more fulfilling, I felt as if I had lost control of my body. I reluctantly accepted that this must be one of life's trade-offs that no one ever tells you about. I met with Dr. Turner and started the Carb Sensitivity Program. In 3 months I lost 25 pounds and never felt hungry or deprived. I had been worried when she told me that I needed to go off anything that was fermented for a few months—and that wine fell into that category. But once on her program I stopped having cravings and I stopped being hungry—and did I mention I lost 25 pounds!"

SANDRA, 52

STATS	BEFORE	AFTER
Weight	186 lb	161 lb
BMI	29	25

INITIAL CHIEF COMPLAINTS:

1. Weight gain
2. Fatigue
3. Bloating

CHAPTER 2

THE ESSENTIALS: UNDERSTANDING CARBS, INSULIN AND YOUR BODY

A healthy outside starts from the inside.

ROBERT URICH

So you want to shed a few pounds? Eating a "balanced" diet isn't always enough, as evidenced by the myriad of diet books that have popped up over the years, offering countless pages of advice on how to get over the hump and lose that weight. Much has been written about the value of low-carb diets, high-protein diets, complex carbohydrates and the glycemic index (GI). Despite all this information, or perhaps because of it, many of us are left feeling confused about what to eat.

We are also confused about *when* to eat. The old adage about consuming your starchy carbs early in the day is actually not the best approach. You know that infamous 3 o'clock slump? The one that makes you want to reach for coffee and a candy bar? Studies show that consuming too many carbs at breakfast increases cravings and caloric intake later in the day. And too many carbs throughout the day cause insulin spikes that will leave us yawning, sluggish and searching for something more.

No matter what those popular diet books say, cutting out carbs completely is not a good weight-loss strategy. When we eliminate carbs, we take away one of the body's primary fuel sources. This can cause physical stress and elevate levels of the stress hormone cortisol, which can in turn lead to loss of muscle tissue and abdominal fat gain. Without carbs, testosterone plummets, leaving our libido flat and our muscles depleted. At the same time, our happy hormone, serotonin, takes a dip, and we experience cravings, bingeing, depression and sleep disruption. No wonder a no-carb diet is associated with irritability, fatigue and poor performance! It's also unsustainable. Our body naturally puts up a fight when we excessively restrict carbs. Our stress- and appetite-boosting hormones cause us to overeat, and our sinking thyroid hormones put the brakes on our metabolism—certainly not an ideal health and wellness scenario.

Despite their bad rap in recent years, carbs should be a part of our diet. They fuel us with the energy necessary to perform most bodily functions, including muscle and brain activity. But all of this confusion often leaves one wondering: What the heck are carbs anyway? Are they all bad?

Good Carbs, Bad Carbs and Everything In Between

While many of us readily think of bread, pasta, rice, cereals, cookies, cakes, pastries, chips, pretzels and potatoes as the usual suspects when it comes to carb or "starch" sources, most of my patients are surprised to learn that vegetables, fruits and legumes (beans) are also sources of carbs. But by far the sneakiest of all carbs are the sometimes-hidden sugars that make their way into common food items such as syrups, jams, jellies, juices, candies, chocolate milk, flavored yogurts, flavored waters (flat or sparkling), sodas, sauces, energy drinks, energy bars, specialty coffees, granola and granola bars. All carbs, regardless of their form, eventually become sugar (also known as glucose) in our bloodstream. But as we learned in Chapter 1, not all carbs are created equal. Essentially, there are two types of carbs, and what differentiates the two is the rate at which the body converts them into glucose. The so-called "good carbs," or complex carbs, are converted into sugar in much smaller amounts and at a much slower rate than their not-so-good counterparts. Complex carbs contain more fiber than their bad cousins and, as a result, spark less of an insulin release. The "bad" carbs initiate a fast and furious rush of sugar into the bloodstream, a situation that can result in mood swings, cravings, fatigue and even headaches.

We can differentiate good carbs from bad by looking at the glycemic index (GI), which is the measurement of how *quickly* a food ends up as sugar in your bloodstream after consumption. High–GI foods such as white pasta, white rice, potato chips, pastries, cookies, candies, muffins, sodas, bagels and white potatoes are broken down rapidly. These foods are usually also low in fiber. As a result, they cause a huge influx of sugar, followed by *loads* of insulin.

On the other hand, low–GI carbohydrates such as berries, green vegetables and legumes are broken down slowly, allowing sugar to trickle gradually into the bloodstream, thereby limiting insulin release. Low-glycemic carbohydrates typically have a GI of less than 55 and, as mentioned earlier, tend to be higher in fiber. Moderate–GI foods are in the range of 55 to 70; high–GI foods are greater than 70. So remember: Low = Slow = Go for it in most cases—*if* your insulin metabolism is healthy.

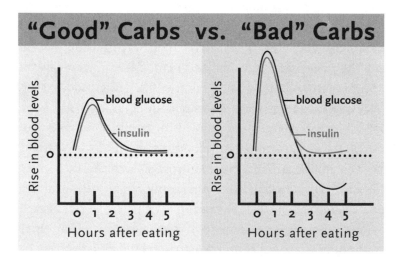

The glycemic load (GL) is a newer measure that builds upon the principles of the glycemic index. GL provides an idea of the total glycemic response to a food or meal (how quickly and how much your blood sugar increases after the item is ingested), and also takes into consideration the amount of carbohydrate per serving. On this scale, a low glycemic load is below 10. While low-glycemic carbohydrates always have a low glycemic load, some foods with a *high glycemic index* actually have a *low glycemic load*. For example, carrots have a high glycemic index, which has prompted most weight-loss diets to recommend avoiding them. But a single serving of carrots actually has a relatively low amount of carbohydrates. As a result, carrots have a low glycemic load, which in fact makes them a *good* choice for those who practise carb-conscious eating habits.

The idea of consuming low-glycemic-load carbohydrates together with lean sources of protein and healthy fats formed the foundation of my first book, *The Hormone Diet*. Step 2—in which I recommended 1 serving of grains or starchy vegetables such as sweet potato, 1 serving of legumes, 2 fruits, unlimited nonstarchy veggies and 1 serving of nuts as the daily sources of carbohydrates—taught readers how to eat for hormonal balance. This way of eating certainly represents a balanced, carb-conscious diet (but by no means a no-carb diet), yet a small percentage of patients failed to continue losing weight following their detox. The question I had to ask was why, especially since all the carbs I recommended were healthy, low–GI carbs. So began my latest research into the net carb.

Net Carbs: Why a Carb Isn't Always a Carb

When you read nutrition labels, you will see that the total amount of carbohydrates is composed mainly of fiber and sugar. *Net carbs* refer to the carbs that will have an impact on your blood sugar and insulin levels—not the total carbs in a serving. It may sound complicated, but discovering a food's net-carb content is actually very simple. Look for the carb total on the label, then simply subtract the fiber. The carbs remaining are the carbs that affect your blood sugar—also called *impact carbs*. Here's an example: A label might say that a serving includes 13 grams of carbohydrates along with 3 grams of fiber. This means the product's net-carb content is 10 grams, not 13.

If all these calculations are making your head spin, don't worry! I've done the work for you. In Chapter 7, you'll find a simple breakdown of permitted food lists for each phase, based on their net-carb content.

NUTRITION FACTS
Serving Size ½ cup (114g)
Servings Per Container: 4

Amount per serving
Calories 90 Calories from Fat 30

	% Daily Value
Total Fat 3g	5%
Saturated Fat 0g	0%
Cholesterol 0mg	0%
Sodium 300 mg	13%
Total Carbohydrate 13g	4%
Dietary Fiber 3g	12%
Sugars 3g	
Protein 3g	

Vitamin A 80%	Vitamin C 60%
Calcium 4%	Iron 4%

*Percent Daily Value is based on a 2,000 calorie diet. Your daily values may be higher on lower depending on your caloric needs.

	Calories	2,000	2,500
Total Fat	less than	65g	80g
Sat. Fat	less than	20g	25g
Cholesterol	less than	300mg	300mg
Sodium	less than	2,400mg	2,400mg
Total Carbohydrate		300g	375g
Dietary Fiber		25g	30g

Calories per gram
Fat 9 • Carbohydrate 4 • Protein 4

Remember: **Net carbs = total carbs – dietary fiber**. In this case, 13g – 3g equals 10g of net carbs. The end number is what impacts your insulin and blood sugar levels.

My investigation into net carbs led to two revelations: First, I was shocked to discover such a wide variation in the net-carb content of healthy, low–GI carbs. For example, I could not believe that sweet potatoes had almost 20 grams more net carbs than summer squash! This would certainly have an impact on one's potential for achieving weight loss while still feeling full, satisfied, healthy, balanced and happy. Second, I realized that each individual's tolerance for carbs varies. I noticed that some people appeared to have an insulin spike even with a small amount of healthy, low–GI carbs, which should have allowed them to avoid the blood sugar spike and subsequent insulin surge that can fuel weight gain.

It is difficult, if not impossible, to predict the blood-glucose reaction of any one person to a certain carbohydrate, even when net-carb content is carefully evaluated. Healthy people who do not have a problem processing glucose will naturally have less of a reaction than those who are prediabetic or beginning to develop a blood sugar and insulin imbalance. Prediabetics still have a blood sugar reading within the normal range but their insulin levels are higher than normal. These are certainly some of the people who respond well to a low-carb or carb-conscious diet.

The Hormonal Effects of Carbs: Carbohydrates, Insulin and Leptin

Now that you know what good carbs, bad carbs and net carbs are, we can delve deeper into how they influence your hormones, your appetite, your body tissues and, ultimately, your ability to lose fat and age gracefully. In the simplest of terms, *consuming the perfect amount of carbs at the proper times and in the right forms helps to promote hormonal balance.* In turn, happy hormones lead to a faster metabolism, improved energy, appetite control and freedom from cravings. Conversely, too many, too few or the wrong types of carbs (high–GI carbs, or even the wrong low–GI carbs for you) at the wrong times can leave you with hormonal imbalances linked to inflammation, accelerated aging, weight gain, cravings, erratic fluctuations in energy, foggy thinking and many other undesirable consequences. All of this is the result of the direct relationship between the carbs you eat and the insulin in your body.

Balanced Insulin Does Your Body Good

Insulin is one of the body's main anabolic hormones. It initiates the building of body proteins, prevents protein breakdown and also promotes the use of sugar as a source of energy. Maintaining the correct amount of insulin in your system offers tremendous benefits. The *right* amount of insulin encourages the growth of your muscles and the refilling of your glycogen stores. You can use these effects to your advantage, especially immediately after exercise—one of the few times when an insulin spike is beneficial.

Let's Take a Sugar Trip

While insulin isn't a common topic of conversation at the dinner table, it is present with your very first bite. Following the course a sugar molecule takes after you eat will reveal insulin's many effects. But let me begin by emphasizing that the following discussion reflects the course of the sugar molecule in a person who is *healthy*—someone with a healthy liver, an adequate amount of muscle, good control over weight and a well-balanced diet without excess caloric intake.

Once glucose is ingested, insulin is released. Immediately, it begins to direct the glucose in your bloodstream to one of three uses:

1. *Immediate use as a fuel source.* In this instance, glucose is burned off right away, particularly by your brain and kidneys. The kidneys take up approximately 10 percent of glucose obtained from dietary sugars and carbs, while up to 20 percent (roughly 120 grams per day) is used by your brain. Unlike fat cells, the brain can't store glucose, so this simple sugar is readily burned up upon use (a process that speeds up during times of stress, such as exams, or even during concentration tasks, such as writing this book). It's no surprise, then, that the brain is extremely sensitive to changing glucose levels, especially considering your brain cells need twice the energy of other cells in your body.

2. *Stored as glycogen in the liver or muscles for later use as an energy source.* The liver, another hungry organ, stores excess glucose as

glycogen, which is tucked away in small quantities both here and in muscle tissue. Your muscles then join in, overpowering your brain and using up to 50 percent of the ingested glucose. Muscles use half the energy immediately and store the rest as glycogen for later. But just as a glass can hold only so much water, the body's capacity to store glycogen is limited. Because most of us consume plenty of carbs daily, our glycogen stores tend to fill up quickly, and this can lead to weight gain. Exercise is one of the best ways to free up more storage space because it causes the body to draw on glycogen for energy. Once the glycogen is used up (for example, when you burn it during a workout), body fat can then be used for fuel.

3. *Stored as fat.* If all of your glycogen storage sites are full and the remaining glucose is not used for energy right away, your body will convert the leftovers to fat, a much longer-term fuel source that is *far more difficult to burn off.* Now you can see why limiting your intake of high-sugar, high-carb foods can be so beneficial. In doing so, you will limit insulin release, which ultimately means less energy will be stored as fat.

In essence then, *insulin is a storage hormone, the one and only hormone that is always telling your body to store energy as fat.* When released in high amounts, *insulin also makes it impossible for us to burn fat.*

There are two main reasons insulin gets released in high amounts. The biggest culprit is usually a diet high in refined sugars or carbs. Over time this leads to the second reason: cells that no longer respond to (*or are resistant to*) insulin's message. The more resistant the body is to insulin's message, the more insulin we need to release to do the same job. And the more insulin we release, the greater the risk for diabetes and other disease conditions. If you want to burn greater amounts of body fat for fuel, you *must* create an insulin-sensitive environment.

Insulin resistance can vary greatly from person to person. Generally, eating more refined, higher-carbohydrate foods evokes a stronger and more rapid insulin reaction. Low-fat or low-protein diets also lead to quicker digestion and faster absorption of carbohydrates into the bloodstream. If we add some fats, fiber and protein to our meals, the process of digestion and entry into the blood is slowed down, which lessens the release of insulin.

Insulin's Many Roles

Insulin is the body's key player when it comes to deciding whether glucose will be burned as fuel for immediate use or stored as fuel for later use. The bad news is that insulin doesn't discriminate between these two activities, and it is the storage of fuel that results in an expanding waistline! Through these two actions, insulin has a profound effect on both the metabolism of fats and carbs as well as the synthesis of proteins and minerals. If our insulin receptors are weak or unable to do their job properly, this ultimately has a widespread and potentially devastating effect on many organs and tissues.

INSULIN REDUCES BLOOD SUGAR

In much the same way as a conductor brings all parts of an orchestra together to create a symphony, insulin ensures harmonious bodily functions by controlling a steady level of glucose. When blood glucose rises above a certain level, insulin is secreted by the pancreas. Any glucose not burned up right away through physical activity is taken out of the bloodstream and stored as muscle glycogen, liver glycogen or body fat. Insulin stops being secreted once our blood sugar falls below a certain range. Without insulin, our cells cannot access the sugar in the bloodstream and will then begin the switch to using an alternate fuel source such as stored body fat.

Our brain is the only exception to this rule, since it requires a constant supply of glucose, available through glycogen stores from our muscle and liver cells. But before you reach for a doughnut as brain fuel, it's important to note that you don't need to *consume* glucose to provide your brain with the glucose it needs to perform. In fact, your liver has the ability to transform the protein and fat you consume into glucose. This is why adequate protein and fat intake is *essential* on a carb-conscious diet.

INSULIN PROMOTES THE FORMATION OF FATS IN THE LIVER WHEN GLYCOGEN STORAGE SITES ARE FULL

Your body can convert only so much glucose to glycogen—your long-term energy source—before your glycogen storage sites reach capacity. Once that happens, any additional sugar taken up by the liver cells will be made into compounds that eventually end up in the bloodstream as triglycerides. When I see excess triglycerides in patients' blood work, it is a key indicator that their carbohydrate–blood sugar–insulin pathway is on overdrive. Right away I know they need to reduce their starchy carb consumption. *Overeating carbohydrates will always lead to fat production and fat storage.* That said, insulin imbalance does not always outwardly manifest as obesity. Sometimes the increase in fat occurs in the liver, where its dangers can remain unseen. Fatty liver may help to explain why many, but not all, obese individuals have insulin imbalances. It also reveals why even slimmer people can be insulin imbalanced and, therefore, at risk of developing type 2 diabetes and cardiovascular disease. Your skinny friend who appears able to chow down on plenty of high-carb foods without the appearance of belly fat may have a different tale to tell on the inside. An ultrasound of that person's liver could show a buildup of toxic fat, or the results of blood work may display a host of abnormalities in liver function.

INSULIN AND YOUR MINERAL BALANCE

As you are now learning, the far-reaching impact of insulin extends well beyond your love handles. Insulin also exerts a powerful effect on your electrolyte and mineral levels. Insulin increases the permeability of many cells to potassium, magnesium and phosphate.

Meanwhile, it causes the retention of sodium, which in turn increases water retention and boosts blood pressure. If you find yourself having to loosen your shoelaces or leave your rings in your jewelry box because you can't slip them on anymore, excess insulin could be exerting its powerful influence. Within the first 2 weeks of the CSP, however, you will find that fluid retention levels drop dramatically or even disappear completely.

The mineral magnesium enhances insulin secretion, which we know facilitates how sugar is processed in the body. Without magnesium, insulin is not able to transfer sugar into cells. When this happens, glucose and insulin build up in the blood, causing various types of tissue damage. If your cells do not respond to insulin properly (as is the case when insulin signaling goes haywire), your cells can't store the magnesium your body needs—it will simply be lost through urination. This in turn causes blood vessels to constrict and blood pressure to increase and further perpetuates the cycle of insulin resistance. It's a catch-22—as much as a decrease in insulin response results in lowered magnesium levels in your cells, magnesium is also necessary for the action and manufacturing of insulin. Many of my patients are magnesium deficient, and I recommend supplementation of this elusive mineral in the majority of cases.

INSULIN, YOUR THYROID AND YOUR METABOLISM

Not surprisingly, all-powerful insulin is one of the first hormones developed in the body. From there, all other hormones are created. This "chief" hormone has a dramatic impact on everything from growth hormone to thyroid hormone. It's estimated that one in 13 people suffers from hypothyroidism, or a deficiency of thyroid hormone, which can increase the risk of obesity, heart disease, insulin imbalance and blood sugar abnormalities. Unfortunately, a large majority of cases are missed because of improper testing or interpretation of blood work. It isn't a coincidence, however, that a growing number of people are being diagnosed with hypothyroidism. The thyroid gland produces one thyroid hormone called T4, which enters the liver and is converted to a more active thyroid hormone, T3. Since insulin controls the majority of what goes on in the liver, a liver that isn't responding to insulin can't convert T4 to T3 very effectively. These patients are at greater risk of suffering with fatigue, weight gain, hair loss, high cholesterol, constipation, dry skin and many other symptoms associated with low thyroid hormone. Interestingly, my patients often experience improved thyroid results on their blood test the moment their insulin balance is restored.

Moving On from Insulin to Leptin

Insulin and leptin are considered the two most important metabolic messengers. While insulin takes charge at the cellular level, deciding whether to burn fat or glucose for energy, leptin controls energy storage and tells the brain how much fat there is on the body and whether to increase its inventory or burn some off.

Clearly, leptin plays a key role in metabolism and the regulation of fatty tissue. The more body fat you have, the higher your leptin levels. When the body is programmed to *respond to leptin properly*, leptin also signals the brain regarding when we are full or when we should continue eating.

Gregory Morton, research assistant and professor of medicine at Harborview Medical Center, University of Washington, has investigated how leptin works on our hypothalamus (the key center of our brain) to influence blood sugar metabolism and the stability of energy in the body. Morton found a direct relationship between insulin, leptin levels and body fat. In fact, his work has shown that a sufficient level of leptin is needed to signal the brain to effectively reduce our food intake, keep body weight down and improve insulin sensitivity.

Because leptin levels naturally increase while we sleep, sleep deprivation can cause a significant drop in leptin. This depletion causes us to feel excessively hungry, which in turn leads to overeating. Besides ensuring we get a good night's sleep, we can improve leptin production and our cellular sensitivity to leptin with regular exercise, sufficient caloric intake (and intake of the right *type* of calories), consumption of healthy unsaturated fats and general weight loss. All of this is covered in the Carb Sensitivity Program.

THE MANY BENEFITS OF JUST THE RIGHT AMOUNT OF LEPTIN
- Lowers body weight
- Lowers percentage of body fat
- Reduces food intake
- Reduces blood sugar
- Reduces insulin
- Increases metabolic rate
- Increases body temperature (in fact, high leptin causes excessive sweating)
- Increases activity level
- Inhibits the synthesis and release of appetite-stimulating chemicals in the brain

Leptin and Your Set Point

We are all familiar with the yo-yo dieting phenomenon—the rise and fall of weight as we go on and off periods of dieting. Science has now determined that leptin plays a role in bringing your body back to its natural "set" point. With extreme weight loss, leptin levels fall and hunger sets in as a very powerful motivator to encourage us to seek out food, eventually bringing our weight back to where we started. At the same time, if our fat stores are increasing too much, extra leptin is produced, which then sends a message to the brain, effectively shutting down the hunger signal and indicating that more should *not* be stored, and excess should be burned. When this occurs and the balance is right, leptin is able to work its magic in regulating fat storage.

Outside the brain, leptin communicates and interacts with several other hormones to influence body weight. Along with insulin, leptin appears to regulate the part of the brain that controls the production of thyroid hormone, the master of our metabolic rate. During a very low calorie diet, *both thyroid hormone and leptin levels fall* as your body's survival mechanism kicks in to preserve body fat. Clearly, an important way to control your overall food intake is to control leptin. As alluring as those "lose 20 pounds in 1 week or less" ads are, a quick starvation diet will eventually lead us right back to where we began.

Let's move on to discuss what happens as we continuously eat the wrong types and amounts of carbs for our metabolism, which gives rise to insulin and leptin imbalance.

CSP SUCCESS STORY: LARRY

"I have been delighted with the Carb Sensitivity Program and lost 11 pounds in the first week. This is the first diet that actually works! I like the personalized nature of the program, and the fact that the program provides me with the understanding of what types of foods I should eat and why. In the end, it has turned out to be not only about losing weight but also being healthy and feeling good."

LARRY, 47

STATS	BEFORE	AFTER
Weight	194 lb	173 lb
Body Fat	22%	17%
BMI	27.4	24.5

INITIAL CHIEF COMPLAINTS:

1. Wanted to have better overall health
2. Excess belly fat

CHAPTER 3

INSULIN SPIKES AND CARB SENSITIVITY: WHY WE'RE FAT, DISEASED AND AGING QUICKLY

It's not what you look at that matters, it's what you see.

HENRY DAVID THOREAU

You've just gained an understanding of the basic actions and effects of insulin in a normal, healthy state. But it is exploring the immediate effects and lasting outcomes of an insulin *imbalance* that will make you realize why the CSP is the perfect way to repair your metabolism for good, as well as increase your ability to eat carbs without experiencing adverse effects such as weight gain or persistent food cravings.

Before we get into a discussion about abnormal insulin, the most important concept to recognize is this:

The more carb sensitive you are, the more prone you are to higher insulin levels due to insulin resistance, and the greater your need for metabolic repair.

The Metabolic Repair Program outlined in Chapters 10 and 11 is designed to improve insulin resistance, thereby reducing excess insulin and diminishing your carb sensitivities. This is my originating principle and the revolutionary approach of the Carb Sensitivity Program.

By now, I hope you realize that insulin plays an essential role in healthy body function *and* that an excess of this hormone absolutely makes you fat. Too much insulin not only encourages your body to store unused glucose as fat but also *blocks* the use of stored fat as an energy source—a double whammy for any waistline. For these reasons, an abnormally high insulin level makes losing fat, especially around the abdomen, next to impossible. It also makes your ability to eat carbs without fueling more weight gain unlikely—a frustrating cycle indeed, since the loss of belly fat is just one piece of what's required to improve insulin sensitivity and reduce your risk of diabetes, heart disease and obesity.

The results of a 2010 study entitled "Insulin Resistance with Aging: Effects of Diet and Exercise," completed by the Baltimore Veterans Affairs Medical Center, provide some much-needed encouragement. The researchers found abnormalities in fat and carbohydrate metabolism (which are also linked to reduced insulin sensitivity) to be common in the obese or diabetic populations. They also discovered that aging is associated with increased insulin abnormalities and increased belly fat. In fact, belly fat was directly linked with high insulin levels. The good news for both middle-aged and older women and men is that the researchers found weight loss through diet and exercise delays the onset of insulin resistance, aids blood sugar balance, increases total body-fat loss and shrinks belly fat.

I am sharing this with you to give you *hope*. No matter what your weight, age or gender, you can see significant improvements with this clinically designed and tested program. Not only will you receive health benefits and functional gains from stronger muscles and improved bloodflow, you just might stop the progression from insulin resistance to type 2 diabetes or heart disease right in its tracks.

Excess Insulin Explained

There are several reasons for excess insulin to be present in the body. As I have mentioned, the biggest culprit is simply consuming too much or the wrong type of carbs. There can, however, be other factors at play:

- Consuming too many nutrient-poor carbohydrates—the type found in processed foods, sugary drinks and soft drinks, foods containing high-fructose corn syrup and packaged low-fat foods.
- Drinking or eating products containing artificial sweeteners. New research has found that people who consume just one diet soft drink a day have a 48 percent increased risk of a heart attack or stroke than those who do not. It appears diet soft drink drinkers consume more salt, fat, sugar and carbs in other food sources, which perpetuates increased insulin release.
- Insufficient protein, fiber or healthy fat intake
- Skipping meals or irregular mealtimes
- Chronic stress, worrying or depression
- Excess alcohol consumption
- Overexercising or other activities that compromise muscle tissue
- Lack of exercise
- Taking steroid-based medications
- Pregnancy
- Poor liver function
- Toxin exposure. Increased exposure to environmental toxins or pollutants has recently been linked to increased belly fat. Estrogen-like compounds such as phlalates and parabens, commonly found in cosmetics and soft plastics, are also associated with increased abdominal fat and weight gain in both men and women.
- Aging

The Short-term Impacts of an Insulin Imbalance: It Brings Your Body Down

Besides turning you into a walking fat-storage facility, excess insulin makes you feel just plain bad. Heart palpitations, sweating, poor concentration, weakness, anxiety, fogginess, fatigue, irritability or impaired thinking are common side effects that may be experienced within the hour following a meal. These symptoms are particularly prevalent in the "crash" you tend to experience following a high-carbohydrate meal or alcohol consumption, both of which can cause irregular peaks and valleys in your insulin level. In essence, you experience an insulin surge and the subsequent fast drop in blood sugar known as *hypoglycemia*. This process can cause you to feel jittery, weak, headachy and irritable—feelings that typically clear as soon as you eat your next meal. Dizziness is also common, along with cravings for something that gives you a boost—such as chocolate, sugar or caffeine.

What's even worse is that our body typically responds to these unpleasant feelings by making us think we are hungry, which in turn causes us to reach for more high-sugar foods and drinks. And then we end up in one vicious cycle of hormonal imbalance, not to mention the dreaded weight gain.

Other common symptoms of an insulin spike are puffiness due to water retention, and abdominal bloating. The water retention may be apparent in your face, especially under your eyes, as well as in your arms and legs. You may notice your rings are tight or that you have dents on your lower legs when you remove your socks. One reason for this, in addition to electrolyte changes, is that for every gram of carbohydrate stored in your muscles or liver as glycogen, 3 to 4 grams of water are stored along with it. You can imagine how a diet dense in carbs might cause substantial water retention. Since insulin also controls sodium uptake in the kidneys and the levels of potassium and magnesium in the body, an excess of this hormone is clearly bad news. The water retention and swelling could leave you looking like that famous little dough boy. He's cute, but he's definitely not anyone's top choice as a physique role model!

Because carbohydrates often trigger a buildup of intestinal gas, abdominal bloating is also common. But let's not confuse water retention and abdominal bloating with the increased fat storage and weight gain that also happens with insulin imbalance. You may notice increased weight in the love handles, bra fat area, triceps, lower body (in women) and belly.

And let's not forget the "carb coma." Sleepiness right after a carb-rich meal is a classic symptom of reduced insulin sensitivity and increased carb sensitivity. A dip in mood and energy is also common, since depression is a frequent consequence of an insulin imbalance. Most patients with high insulin have low levels of serotonin—the "happy" hormone that controls our mood, sleep patterns, self-esteem, ability to make decisions, and cravings and also impacts our digestion (constipation and nausea can be associated with low serotonin). It is also not uncommon to see addictions to smoking, drugs, alcohol or caffeine in insulin-imbalanced individuals.

To make matters worse, too much insulin can cause you to consume more calories. According to Dr. Robert Lustig, a pediatric endocrinologist at University of California San Francisco (UCSF) Children's Hospital, insulin stimulates our appetite by working on the brain in two ways. First, it blocks signals to our brain by interfering with the appetite-suppressing hormone leptin, causing us to eat more and become less active. Second, insulin causes a spike in dopamine, the hormone that signals our brain to seek rewards. Dopamine spurs a desire to eat in order to achieve a pleasurable rush—the same rush we may get from addictive behaviors. No wonder putting down the fork is so tough. We are addicted to food!

Feeling overwhelmed? Don't be! I compiled this list of symptoms in order to develop the Carb Sensitivity Checklist that you will fill out at the end of each CSP phase in Chapter 7. Your answers will determine the next step in your dietary journey. You will either progress to the next phase or be directed to the Metabolic Repair Program in Chapters 10 and 11, which is designed to improve your level of carb sensitivity.

Vitamin C is made in almost all living mammals except humans and a few other species. It is manufactured directly from glucose and actually has a similar structure.

Insulin is known to increase the cellular uptake of vitamin C. But if we know that vitamin C and glucose have similar chemical structure, what happens when glucose levels go up? They compete with one another to enter the cells—and if there is more glucose around, less vitamin C will be allowed in. Surprisingly, it does not take much glucose to create this cellular deficiency. Now we are getting further down into the roots of disease. Be it a common cold or cardiovascular disease, osteoporosis or cancer, the root cause is always at the molecular and cellular level. And you better believe that insulin is going to play a role.

Insulin Imbalance over the Long Haul: Insulin Resistance and Metabolic Syndrome

Clearly, excess insulin can leave us feeling pretty bad in the here and now, but there are much more dire long-term consequences as well. When insulin is present in excess over a period of several months to years, our cells grow accustomed to having so much of it around. As a result, our cellular response to insulin becomes blunted. The pancreas is then called upon to step up its insulin production in an attempt to maintain a normal blood sugar level. This decrease in insulin sensitivity culminates in insulin resistance.

When people are insulin resistant, their muscle, fat and liver cells do not respond properly to insulin. These cells start to demand more insulin to help glucose enter the cells. In turn, the pancreas tries to keep up with this increased demand by producing even more insulin, and a vicious cycle begins. Eventually, the pancreas fails to keep up with the body's need for insulin and excess glucose builds up in the bloodstream, setting the stage for diabetes. Many people with insulin resistance have high levels of both glucose and insulin circulating in their blood at the same time.

NORMAL CELL

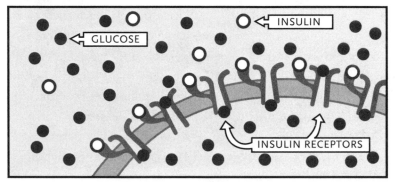

INSULIN-RESISTANT CELL

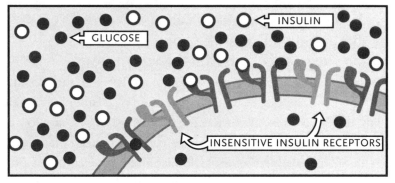

On many of your blood work requisitions from your doctor you will notice an item called fasting blood sugar: This is how doctors check for diabetes. The sugar present in the bloodstream when you wake in a fasting state is an indication of how much sugar your liver manufactured overnight. If your liver cells are becoming insulin resistant, the liver will produce more sugar than it should. Conversely, less sugar in the blood on waking indicates that your liver cells are properly sensitive to insulin's message.

It is currently believed that our liver cells are the first in the body to become insulin resistant. Next come our muscle cells. The wonderful thing about muscle is that it burns both the sugar taken in from our diet and the sugar naturally produced by our liver during the night or in periods of fasting. Once muscles become insulin resistant, less sugar is burned, and blood sugar levels begin to rise. This reality makes strength training a crucial part of the Metabolic Repair Program.

The final tissue to become insulin resistant is our fat cells. As weight increases, so does insulin resistance. It's like throwing gas on a bushfire: more weight gain, more insulin resistance; more insulin resistance, more weight gain. Over time this cycle leads the pancreas to produce more and more insulin, as the cells become used to having so much insulin present so often. A highly functioning pancreas can control blood sugar for a long time by pumping out tons of insulin—but eventually it will not be able to compensate for the increased need. Once production of insulin starts slowing down, or cellular insulin resistance goes up, blood sugar levels follow and diabetes ensues.

Although the symptoms of excess insulin tend to be similar in both men and women, there are some differences. Guys: High insulin typically sparks heightened activity of an aromatase enzyme in your fat cells, which causes more of your masculinizing hormone, testosterone, to be converted into the feminizing hormone estrogen. If this trend continues over the long term, you'll see increased fat deposits in "female" areas, such as your abdomen and even breast tissue, not to mention a negative impact on your sex drive and erectile function. Even scarier is the increase in heart disease risk that is linked to this drop in testosterone too.

Ladies, you are just as vulnerable. The same aromatase enzyme boosts conversion of estrogen to testosterone in women. As a result, high insulin can lead to such lovely effects as increased fat storage in the abdomen, shrinking and sagging breasts, abnormal hair growth, acne and even male-pattern hair loss. Not good!

With long-term insulin imbalance, other physiological changes start to occur in the body. These signs and symptoms characterize a condition called metabolic syndrome, the clinical manifestation of insulin resistance.

According to a joint report from Statistics Canada and the US Centers for Disease Control and Prevention's National Center for Health Statistics, obesity is rising in both countries, with an epidemic of insulin resistance and diabetes sweeping across the nation. The 2011 study found that 34.4 percent of Americans and 24.1 percent of Canadians were obese from 2007 to 2009. Furthermore, the report found the most significant increases in obesity rates in the past 20 years were seen in men aged 60 to 74 and women aged 20 to 39. Among those groups, Canadian obesity rates increased at almost the same rate as those in the United States, which could spell serious problems for those people in the years ahead! It is currently estimated that one-quarter of the world's adult population has full-blown insulin resistance. When we consider the early manifestations of reduced insulin sensitivity, characteristic of carb sensitivity, I expect 75 percent or more of adults have some form of abnormality. This means the same percentage of adults have an issue with carbs. The true magnitude of this problem is almost incomprehensible.

Today, one in four people exhibits one or more of the clinical elements of metabolic syndrome (listed on the following page) by the age of 30, a figure that nearly triples by the age of 65. Even teens are at risk. A study reported in *Circulation: The Journal of the American Heart Association* (April 2005) described obesity and insulin resistance as a menacing tag team that dramatically accelerates cardiovascular risk, even in teenagers.

Diagnosing Insulin Resistance

Before you can address a potential problem, you need to gain a full understanding of your current health picture. While there is not a single test to positively identify the presence of insulin resistance, a collection of clinical assessments will provide the information necessary to make an accurate diagnosis. In the meantime, if you're wondering whether you are insulin resistant or insulin sensitive, take a good look at your waist and pinch your stomach. If you carry excess fat in this area, you very likely have some level of insulin resistance, which also means you are likely carb sensitive. If you're naturally lean, it's safe to say that your insulin sensitivity is in good shape and you can tolerate eating carbs quite readily without weight gain and excess cravings.

A much more in-depth investigation is necessary to definitively determine insulin resistance clinically. A full workup includes blood work, blood pressure readings and, in some cases, additional exams such as an abdominal ultrasound to assess the liver. Should you wish to talk to your health-care provider about this type of investigation, I have outlined all the tests involved in a complete investigation of insulin resistance in Appendix A. According to the current medical definition, metabolic syndrome is diagnosed when *three or more* of the following risk factors are identified:

- Low levels of "good" cholesterol (HDL)
- High levels of "bad" cholesterol (LDL)
- Elevated triglycerides (unsaturated fats)
- Increased waist-to-hip ratio, as fat accumulates around the abdomen and "love handle" areas
- High blood pressure (i.e., above 130/85, according to the National Cholesterol Education Program)
- Elevated fasting blood sugar levels (i.e., greater than 110 mg/dl)
- Increased blood clotting factors and high uric acid

(continued on page 53)

THE RISKS OF METABOLIC SYNDROME
FOR LONG-TERM HEALTH

Beyond obesity and type 2 diabetes, metabolic syndrome is associated with increased risk for the following:

HEART DISEASE

A landmark study published in the *Journal of the American College of Cardiology* (2009) showed exactly what happens in your body—and your heart—when you eat high-carbohydrate foods. Researchers from Tel Aviv University fed healthy volunteers one of four meals: cornflakes with milk, a pure sugar mixture, bran flakes or a placebo. Then they monitored, in real time, what was happening to the patients' arteries. The results were dramatic. Before any of the patients ate, arterial function was essentially the same. After eating, *all except the placebo* group experienced reduced functioning for several hours, which can worsen the effects of heart disease or, in extreme cases, cause a stroke or heart attack. Since the immediate effect of raising your blood sugar is a spike in insulin, this in turn triggers the sympathetic nervous system, which causes arterial spasms or a constriction of the arteries. While that plate of pasta may look great and taste even better, it may just push you over the edge, if you are prone to heart disease.

HIGH BLOOD PRESSURE AND CHOLESTEROL IMBALANCE

Insulin increases the production of a hormone that raises blood pressure (aldosterone) and also spurs a loss of electrolytes (magnesium and potassium), which can cause water retention and arterial narrowing. Combined, these changes lead to high blood pressure.

The majority of my patients are shocked to learn that it is carbs and the influence they have on raising insulin, and not necessarily their fat intake, that leads to high cholesterol. Guess what happens when I drop their carbs and raise their consumption of protein and healthy fats? Upon retesting their blood 3 months later, their total cholesterol, bad cholesterol and good cholesterol are improved most of the time.

STROKE

An October 2010 article in the *Archives of Neurology* showed that insulin resistance appears to be associated with an increased risk of stroke, even in individuals without diabetes. Furthermore, insulin resistance is associated with higher risk for four of the top five leading causes of death in the United States (as reported by the American Heart Association 2003 Heart and Stroke Statistical Update): cancer, heart disease, diabetes and Alzheimer's disease.

CANCER

New research has also uncovered a link between elevated insulin levels and certain types of malignancies, primarily breast, colon and prostate cancer. The connection between insulin resistance, obesity, diabetes and cancer was first reported in 2004 in large population studies by researchers from the WHO's International Agency for Research on Cancer. Cancer researchers now consider that the problem with insulin resistance is that it leads us to secrete more insulin, as well as a related hormone known as insulin-like growth factor (IGF-1), which actually promotes tumor growth. High insulin is also linked to increased risk of recurrence of cancer, so following the CSP could potentially be a lifesaver.

ALZHEIMER'S DISEASE

There is growing evidence that the brain itself can become insulin resistant, which impairs the function of nerves and leads to the buildup of toxic deposits, increasing the risk of dementia, including Alzheimer's disease. Insulin resistance and type 2 diabetes increase the risk of developing plaques in the brain that are associated with Alzheimer's disease, according to new research published in the August 2010 issue of *Neurology*. The study found that people who had abnormal results on three tests of blood sugar control had an increased risk of developing plaques in the brain. Plaques were found in 72 percent of people with insulin resistance and a surprising 62 percent of people with no indication of insulin resistance!

Not surprisingly, then, in those with Alzheimer's disease, the levels of brain insulin and its related receptors are lower. Weakened insulin receptors lead to the loss of electrical signals that are vital for connectivity between brain cells and the ability to learn and retain information. With diabetes, insulin's signals are impaired, and the brain doesn't get the amount of sugar energy that it needs, especially for cognitive function and memory. Chronically high and low levels of glucose directly impact your brain cells and lead to cognitive impairment. In fact, scientists are labeling this brain imbalance as type 3 diabetes. While type 1 and type 2 diabetes occur when the body is unable to produce or use insulin from the pancreas, type 3 refers to lower than normal levels of the newly discovered insulin of the brain. Scientists have known for some time that people with diabetes have up to a 65 percent increased chance of developing Alzheimer's. Think about it—65 percent is a huge number! The incidence of Alzheimer's is currently skyrocketing, and it's certainly no

---

SEASONAL WEIGHT CHANGES LINKED TO METABOLIC SYNDROME

According to researchers from the National Public Health Institute in Finland, the winter blues and the accompanying weight gain increase the risk for metabolic syndrome by as much as 56 percent. To combat these seasonal changes, you can follow the nutrition, supplement and exercise recommendations I have outlined in the Metabolic Repair Program (in Chapter 10) during the winter months. It's certainly the season when carbs seem to be much more alluring.

coincidence the incidence of carb sensitivity is accelerating right along with it.

FATTY LIVER DISEASE

Fatty liver is strongly associated with insulin resistance. New research shows fat accumulation in the liver is one of the primary causes of nonalcoholic fatty liver disease that may increase the risk of cirrhosis, liver cancer or the need for a liver transplant.

SKIN ABNORMALITIES

Abnormalities in the skin that are associated with high insulin include increased formation of skin tags, especially around the neck, and a condition called acanthosis nigricans. Acanthosis nigricans is a darkening and thickening of the skin, particularly in fold areas like around the neck or armpit. Increased wrinkling and accelerated aging also occur with high insulin because of an increase in the abnormal attachment of sugar molecules to collagen (a process called *glycation*) and in free radical stress, which is a known cause of cellular damage and aging.

LOSS OF MUSCLE TISSUE

A study published in the September 2006 edition of *Endocrinology* found that insulin resistance is associated with accelerated muscle protein breakdown and loss of muscle tissue. Remember, we all lose muscle as we age, and we all become more insulin resistant with aging. With the CSP, you can stop muscle loss and improve insulin sensitivity, thereby putting the brakes on aging. Amazing!

REPRODUCTIVE ABNORMALITIES

Infertility and irregular periods and ovulation patterns can often arise as part of a syndrome called polycystic ovarian syndrome (PCOS). In the Introduction I shared with you that I have this condition. PCOS is a hormonal problem that affects young women.

It can be associated with irregular periods or no periods at all, obesity, hair loss, acne and increased growth of body hair. While it has commonly been thought that insulin resistance and obesity increase the risks, new research from a Johns Hopkins Children's Center study shows that it may actually be the pituitary gland's response to high insulin that increases infertility, hormonal imbalance and disrupted ovarian function. Infertility issues also appear to be increasing for both men and women. This could be yet another epidemic related to carb sensitivity.

ANDROGEN IMBALANCE IN WOMEN

The male sex hormones DHEA and testosterone occur naturally in both men's and women's bodies. But high levels of DHEA and testosterone in women are almost always an indication of insulin resistance. This imbalance can lead to hair loss, acne, shrinking breasts, hair growth on the face or deepening of the voice. I have found that these patients respond wonderfully to a long-term carb-conscious approach such as the CSP.

COMPLICATIONS IN PREGNANCY

Researchers at Boston University School of Medicine's Slone Epidemiology Center and Boston University School of Public Health have found that prepregnancy obesity and gestational weight gain are associated with an increased risk of preterm birth. In this study, reported in the February 2011 online version of *Epidemiology*, researchers found obesity and metabolic syndrome were associated with intrauterine infections, systemic inflammation, high cholesterol and triglycerides, and high insulin, all of which can increase the risk of preterm birth. The CSP should also be starting to sound like the perfect plan to enhance fertility—because it is.

CHILDHOOD OBESITY AND INSULIN RESISTANCE

When we look at the food products marketed to kids these days, it's obvious why childhood obesity is flourishing! But research shows that a child's risk of insulin resistance and diabetes may increase long before he or she takes a first bite of junk food. New research presented at the Endocrine Society's 92nd Annual Meeting in San Diego showed that children of mothers with high blood sugar during pregnancy are more likely to have insulin resistance—a risk factor for type 2 diabetes—*even if the child's body weight is normal.* The higher the mother's blood sugar level during pregnancy, the greater her child's resistance to insulin, and the more insulin was found to be secreted into the child's blood after meals.

OSTEOPOROSIS

If you are prone to osteoporosis, you may be shocked to discover that all the calcium in the world won't help you maintain healthy bones if your insulin levels are high. In fact, most of that calcium will be eliminated through your urine or, even worse, will form calcifications in your arteries. In an important feedback loop, insulin signals osteoblasts (cells that produce bone) to activate a hormone called osteocalcin, which in turn promotes glucose metabolism. In those with diabetes or insulin resistance, the process is impaired, thereby heightening the risk for osteoporosis. Add in weight gain caused by insulin resistance, and you have a double whammy that increases your chances of developing brittle, fracture-prone bones. Imagine—many of the supplements I recommend in Part Three to repair your metabolism will also repair your bones!

An insulin imbalance affects more than just the bathroom scale. Take a look at the diagram on the following page to get a sense of the epic consequences of insulin imbalance and, in turn, the many health conditions that can be remedied by the CSP. The CSP will not only help you achieve a slimmer physique, but also lead to a much more positive outcome at your next physical exam!

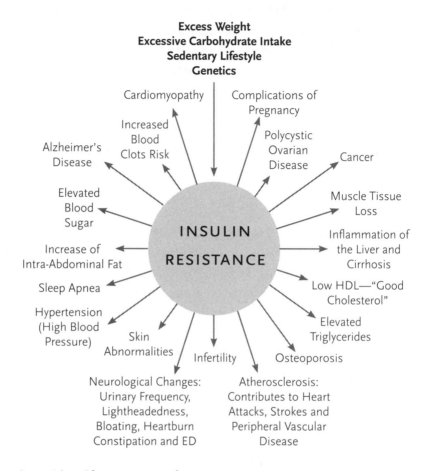

Excess Weight
Excessive Carbohydrate Intake
Sedentary Lifestyle
Genetics

Cardiomyopathy

Complications of Pregnancy

Increased Blood Clots Risk

Alzheimer's Disease

Polycystic Ovarian Disease

Cancer

Elevated Blood Sugar

INSULIN RESISTANCE

Muscle Tissue Loss

Increase of Intra-Abdominal Fat

Inflammation of the Liver and Cirrhosis

Sleep Apnea

Low HDL—"Good Cholesterol"

Hypertension (High Blood Pressure)

Skin Abnormalities

Infertility

Osteoporosis

Elevated Triglycerides

Neurological Changes: Urinary Frequency, Lightheadedness, Bloating, Heartburn Constipation and ED

Atherosclerosis: Contributes to Heart Attacks, Strokes and Peripheral Vascular Disease

Source: Adapted from www.scienceofhunger.com

SKIP THE NICOTINE GUM—GO COLD TURKEY

According to a study published in the journal *Circulation*, long-term use of nicotine-containing chewing gum is associated with insulin resistance and high insulin levels in healthy, nonobese, middle-aged men. If you must use nicotine replacement therapy during smoking cessation, your use should be transient and limited.

Putting Carb Sensitivity, Insulin Resistance and Type 2 Diabetes in Reverse

Decreased cellular sensitivity to insulin's message starts slowly, furtively and silently. And once the process sets in, it is easier to become insulin resistant. The more insulin your body has to produce to keep blood sugar down, the more insulin and leptin resistant you become—unless you take action to reverse the trend.

The right dietary changes and exercise habits can work to reverse insulin resistance, prediabetes and even full-blown type 2 diabetes. While physical activity and weight loss help the body respond better to insulin, changing your eating style is one of the most important steps in reducing insulin. But a standard cookie-cutter diet will *not* work for everyone. Why? Because consumption (or avoidance) of carbohydrates—the foundation of virtually every diet book out there today—is a contributing variable for insulin resistance.

Proper assessment and diagnosis are also important. We need to stop focusing on fasting blood sugar as *the* definitive method of assessing risk for diabetes and blood sugar imbalance. Rather, we need to start zeroing in on insulin. A shocking number of us have elevated insulin that goes unchecked long before diabetes presents itself. This is because most health-care practitioners look for diabetes by testing fasting blood sugar, when fasting blood sugar is, in fact, that *last* thing to go wrong. High insulin after a meal is the *first* thing to go wrong. Testing this value is what successfully allows for early detection—and *prevention*—since insulin resistance can be reversed with the right nutrition, exercise, supplements and stress management.

Recent research led by Dr. Dean Ornish, head of the Preventive Medicine Research Institute in Sausalito, California, found that comprehensive lifestyle changes, including a better diet and more exercise, can lead not only to better body composition but also to dramatic changes at the *genetic* level. In the study, published in *Proceedings of the National Academy of Sciences* (2011), the researchers tracked 30 men with low-risk prostate cancer who decided against conventional medical treatment. The men underwent 3 months of major lifestyle changes, including eating a diet rich in fruits, vegetables, whole grains and legumes; moderate exercise such as walking for 30 minutes a day; and 1 hour of daily stress management methods such as meditation. As expected, they lost weight, lowered their blood pressure and saw other health improvements. But the researchers found more profound changes when they compared prostate biopsies taken before and after the lifestyle changes.

Remarkably, the men had changes in activity in about 500 genes. The activity of disease-preventing genes increased, while a number of disease-promoting genes, including those involved in prostate cancer and breast cancer, shut down. This is just one of many examples that prove *external changes to your lifestyle can alter your health at the cellular level.*

You have now learned that insulin resistance is associated with, or contributes to, virtually *every* chronic disease associated with aging. In fact, many researchers and medical professionals, myself included, view this one variable as the main cause of aging in virtually all life. Combine this with inflammation, free radical stress and high cortisol (due to chronic stress), and I feel you will have identified all of the variables you need to manage if you want to age well. Improving or, at the very least, maintaining insulin sensitivity is *the secret to lasting health and wellness.*

Reading about insulin balance is easy enough, but the reality of managing insulin is mighty tough—especially if you have a carb-addicted mind. Let's move on to discuss the interesting connection between your brain, carbs, your mood and your cravings. Regardless of your level of carb sensitivity, this is information from which we can *all* benefit.

"I thought I was doing everything right, exercising an average of five times a week and making mental notes to avoid all the foods that would add to my weight. I hit an all-time low when an instructor at my gym asked me why I wasn't losing weight and toning up my body in spite of all the exercise I was doing.

"One day a friend handed me a book she was reading, *The Hormone Diet*. I started reading the book immediately, and I felt like Dr. Turner's comments, insight and knowledge were directed towards me. Her book made so much sense! I booked an appointment shortly thereafter and started on a journey to better hormonal health. Dr. Turner is a dynamo of contagious energy who exudes knowledge and compassion every time we meet. She even started me on the next level of her program, called the Carb Sensitivity Program, and the results were amazing! Thank you, Dr. Turner!"

LINDA, 59

STATS	BEFORE	AFTER
Weight	190 lb	168 lb
Body Fat	36%	33%
BMI	30	27

INITIAL CHIEF COMPLAINTS:

1. Weight gain
2. Anxiety
3. Depression
4. Adult acne

CHAPTER 4

THIS IS YOUR BRAIN
ON CARBS

When you reach the end of your rope, tie a knot in it and hang on.

THOMAS JEFFERSON

Make no mistake, carbs are addictive. Many would argue they have just as powerful a pull for some people as cigarettes, drugs or alcohol. You are now familiar with your main metabolic hormones, insulin and leptin, which signal the body to take in food and either store or burn glucose. Insulin and leptin are also two of our big hunger hormones. Understandably, an imbalance results in a major and sometimes uncontrollable boost in appetite.

And if you don't stop the pattern now, it will only get worse. Dr. Zane Andrews, a neuroendocrinologist with Monash University's Department of Physiology, has discovered that key appetite control cells in the human brain degenerate over time, causing increased hunger and weight gain as we age. According to his research, an attack on appetite-suppressing cells creates a serious imbalance between our need to eat and the message to the brain to stop eating. Dr. Andrews found that cells are attacked by free radicals after eating, and the degeneration is more significant following meals rich in carbohydrates and sugars. Moreover, the risk of degeneration is highest if you fall within the 25 to 50 age group. Essentially, the neurons that tell you when to stop eating are being killed off by a dangerous weapon on your plate—carbs!

Gaining Control of Your Appetite

Mounting evidence shows that, besides their ability to boost metabolism, hormones and neurotransmitters (chemical messengers that work within the brain) are involved in appetite control by acting on the *hypothalamus gland,* the part of the brain that governs feelings of hunger and fullness. By collecting and processing information from the digestive system, the internal biological clock, fat cells, stress-controlling mechanisms and other sources within the body, the hypothalamus acts as the master switch that tells us when to eat more and when to put down the fork.

In the midst of the current obesity epidemic, scientists are striving to understand both our struggle to gain control of our appetite and our tendency to overeat. They certainly have their work cut out for them! The chart below outlines just a few of the countless complex factors that influence our need to feed.

FACTORS THAT SPARK THE DESIRE TO EAT	FACTORS THAT QUIET YOUR APPETITE
Sight and smell of food	Out of sight, out of mind
Overweight or obesity	Maintaining a lean body
Exposure to too many foods or tastes at once—buffets and standing in front of the fridge grazing are our downfall	Limiting flavors and varieties of foods in one sitting can help keep appetite in check—avoid buffets or grazing in front of the cupboard or fridge
Cold body temperature	Warm body temperature
Lack of sunlight or bright light exposure	A healthy dose of sunshine or bright light
Internal body clock—we tend to get hungry at similar times each day; appetite increases in the winter	Eating regularly throughout the day and *always* having breakfast
Alcohol consumption	Limiting consumption of alcohol to one glass of wine after your meal
Dehydration	Staying well hydrated
Jet lag, sleep deprivation and shift work	Sufficient, good-quality sleep

FACTORS THAT SPARK THE DESIRE TO EAT (continued)	FACTORS THAT QUIET YOUR APPETITE (continued)
High intake of carbohydrates and lack of fiber and fats that help us feel full and satisfied	Consuming a mix of protein, carbohydrates and healthy fats at each meal and snack
Brain chemistry imbalance (low serotonin and dopamine)	Balanced brain chemistry (sufficient serotonin and dopamine)
High-fructose corn syrup (HFCS) and artificial sweeteners	Avoiding processed carbohydrates, artificial sweeteners, fructose and HFCS
Emotional causes: stress, anxiety, depression, loneliness, boredom	Managing stress and feeling satisfied (emotionally, sexually and otherwise)
A compromised digestive system	A healthy digestive system

GUT HORMONES THAT HELP YOU FEEL FULL

Hormones are the driving force behind your appetite control or desire to eat in response to the factors listed in the previous chart. For instance, your empty stomach releases grehlin, which then travels to your brain and stimulates the desire to eat. After you consume food, your satiety center is stimulated by hormones (particularly CCK and PYY) that are released from your stomach and intestines as they stretch when filled with food, or when fat and protein are present. Here's a quick rundown of some of the hormones that work to make you feel full.

CHOLEYSTOKININ (CCK)

CCK causes the pancreas to produce enzymes that break down protein, carbohydrates and fats. It also causes the gallbladder to release bile into the small intestine. CCK is released when we eat fats, and it is part of the reason fats make us feel full and satisfied. It is also why low-fat diets are not sustainable, since our appetite naturally becomes uncontrollable. High-fiber meals also promote CCK release, but the effects of CCK on appetite are not long acting. If the stretching of your stomach causes this satiety signal to be released, then filling your stomach with plenty of high-fiber, high-water-content foods rather than small amounts of rich, calorie-dense foods (such as muffins) certainly makes sense.

PEPTIDE YY (PYY)

Peptide YY is produced lower in the gastrointestinal tract in response to meals. It packs an appetite-inhibiting punch, slowing the digestive process to cause us to feel full for longer. Protein consumption causes the release of PYY, so eating protein regularly throughout the day will keep your appetite under control. This is also the reason you should eat your protein first at mealtime.

ENTEROSTATIN

Also produced by the GI tract, enterostatin reduces our perception of hunger and appears to cut our intake of fats.

BOMBESIN AND GASTIN INHIBITORY PEPTIDE (GIP)

Bombesin and gastrin inhibitory peptide (also known as gastrin-insulin peptide) reduce food intake in obese and lean people. In fact, studies show animals lacking the bombesin receptor become obese. These two hormones are released in conjunction with PYY to calm our appetite and digestion. GIP also stimulates the release of insulin from the pancreas.

OXYNTOMODULIN (OXM)

Oxyntomodulin is released from the endocrine intestinal cells. It inhibits the release of our stress and appetite-stimulating neuropeptide NPY. Therefore, OXM induces a feeling of fullness by shutting down the feeding centers in our brain.

SEROTONIN

Serotonin is a neurotransmitter that influences mood. It has also been implicated in the control of how much food we eat during a sitting and how often we feel the need to eat. The mechanism for this control lies within the serotonin receptors in our central nervous system. These receptors are sensitive to circulating levels of tryptophan (the precursor to serotonin), macronutrients and CCK, which control our sensation of fullness.

Serotonin receptors in the hypothalamus also inhibit NPY, that potent stimulator of hunger and food intake. Serotonin is a part of an integrated network for short-acting appetite control, while leptin is a hormonal indicator of long-term fat and energy reserves. In other words, serotonin satisfies our appetite in the here and now, while leptin is the long-term driving force that keeps it in check.

Your Appetite and Your Carb Sensitivity

Many people struggle with overeating because they never feel full. For them, food can bring both pleasure and pain. There is little doubt that these people are CS. As you now know, CS people tend to sustain a higher insulin level in the blood and a coinciding decreased sensitivity of insulin within the cells. This causes the body to stop responding to insulin's message that caloric intake is sufficient. With the insulin response dulled, the CS body will continue to grab every calorie it can and deposit it as fat. Within this scenario, no matter how little you eat, you will gradually gain weight. At the same time, your cells cannot absorb the glucose they need, so they signal your brain that you need more carbohydrates or sugars. The result is persistent cravings for calorie-dense foods. Yikes!

CS people face very real chemical and hormonal changes upon eating carbohydrates. For them, carb consumption will increase hunger and decrease the sense of fullness that non–CS people would feel. For these people, carb consumption *actually produces a compulsion to eat,* often at the least opportune times for calorie burning, such as late at night. Eating carbs initially produces a pleasurable feeling, followed by an uneasy sensation, weariness and an urge to snack more.

CS people actually become hungrier with each carb-rich meal or snack. For CS people, the carbohydrate-insulin-serotonin connection has malfunctioned. Remember, serotonin is responsible for helping us feel full. As a result, for those whose serotonin levels do not rise sufficiently, the feeling of "being satisfied" is never achieved. This leads the CS person to overeat and begins a cycle of craving more carbohydrates. The constant "needing something more" feeling can never quite be curbed. The production of insulin continues to rise with the further consumption of carbohydrates . . . and the cycle rages on.

Because larger quantities of carbs may be consumed more frequently without any increase in satisfaction, CS people need to eat in a way that *stops* the cycle of excess insulin production and, over time, improves insulin sensitivity. When the *right types* and *amounts* of carbs are eaten—tailored to the individual's metabolic profile— less insulin will be produced. The body's tendency to store excess calories in the fat cells will decrease and its ability to break down stored fat will improve.

THE CARB-ADDICTED BRAIN

While we know that muscle and fat cells can become insulin resistant, it was previously thought that the brain was not sensitive to this omnipotent hormone. However, it has recently been discovered that insulin receptors exist throughout the brain, especially in regions that control appetite, food intake and, in turn, body composition. In those who are insulin sensitive, a rise in insulin after a meal promotes satiety by increasing glucose and subsequently boosting the metabolic activity in regions of the brain that control appetite.

In those who are insulin resistant, the insulin boost experienced after a meal no longer results in a significant sense of satiety. The effects of this communication breakdown extend past the amount of food on your plate to impact weight gain, obesity, type 2 diabetes and even fertility, according to research completed by scientists at the Joslin Diabetes Center alongside researchers in Germany. Using genetically altered laboratory mice, the researchers found that the mice in which insulin action was blocked gained weight at a considerably higher rate than their counterparts, developed insulin resistance in other tissues of the body and exhibited a 50 percent decrease in fertility. The mice also showed increased levels of the hormone leptin, which helps the body regulate fat.

Dopamine and Carb Addiction

So it's clear that excess insulin stimulates our appetite and heightens our cravings for carbs. Yet the simple act of eating carbs serves to trigger only more insulin production—yet another vicious circle. Besides insulin, however, other hormones can also drive us to reach for carbs. Dr. Mehmet Oz recently did a segment on his popular daytime television show entitled "Carbs: The Cocaine for the Brain." A powerful title, but he just might be right in suggesting that carbs could be the most addictive substance of all, consumed by virtually everyone on a daily basis. Imagine—bread, pasta, fries, potato chips and other unhealthy carbohydrates could be even more addictive than cocaine!

As with other drug addictions, the body will need more and more carbs over time in order to get the same "fix." And if you try to quit carbs cold turkey, you may go through a very noticeable withdrawal. In fact, in experiments involving both animals and humans, the consequences of suddenly stopping a high-carbohydrate diet appear to mimic the mental and physical symptoms of drug withdrawal. These symptoms included headaches, moodiness, tension, restlessness, anxiety and depression, and a severe mental preoccupation with getting more carbohydrates.

According to data published in *Obesity Research* (November 1995) from Princeton University, "food addiction" evolves as a result of changes in brain pathways. Sugar and carbs cause the release of the hormone *dopamine* in the brain—the same response activated by addictive drugs. These chemical adaptations cause changes in dopamine release over time. In this particular study, rats actually became sugar dependent, paving the way for theories that carbs can be physiologically addictive. No wonder we find cutting carbs and losing weight so hard!

The primary effect of excess carb consumption includes a dopamine rush—the same mood hormone released with other addictive behaviors, such as out-of-control gambling, sex addiction, drug and alcohol abuse, and smoking. Now we can place sugar and carbs into the same category. You can even see the similarities by examining the behaviors of recovering alcoholics—those daily drinks are often replaced with heaps of coffee, endless amounts of candy, and chain smoking.

Serotonin and Carb Addiction

Though serotonin is typically recognized as a brain chemical, most of this neurotransmitter is produced in our digestive tract. Serotonin exerts a powerful influence over mood, emotions, memory, cravings (especially for carbohydrates), self-esteem, pain tolerance, sleep habits, appetite, digestion and body temperature regulation. Wow! When we're depressed or down, we naturally crave sugars and starches to stimulate the production of serotonin. Also, when we're cold or surrounded by darkness, serotonin levels drop. There is a real reason for that dreaded winter weight gain after all!

Serotonin is often thought of as our "happy hormone," especially because its production increases when we're exposed to natural sunlight and when we focus on one thing, rather than multitasking. Production of serotonin is also closely linked to availability of vitamin B6 and the amino acid tryptophan. So if our diet lacks sufficient protein or vitamins, we run a greater risk of developing a serotonin deficiency. We may experience a dip in serotonin in relation to physiological causes, dieting, digestive disorders and also stress, since high levels of the stress hormone cortisol rob us of serotonin.

The World Health Organization (WHO) has projected depression and anxiety will soon be the number-one disability experienced by adults. Both depression and anxiety are linked to elevated cortisol, coupled with an imbalance of our "feel good" hormones, including serotonin, dopamine and noradrenaline (all of which, by the way, also affect appetite).

Plenty of sunlight; a healthful diet rich in protein, minerals and vitamins; focusing on one task at a time; regular exercise; and good sleep all come together to support serotonin. When we measure our current lifestyle against all the elements necessary for the body's natural production of serotonin, the wide-ranging epidemic of low serotonin is not surprising. Add in *chronic stress and multitasking*— two of the main causes of serotonin depletion—and it's a wonder any one of us has been left unaffected by low serotonin. Ongoing stress, just like depression, can deplete our serotonin reserves, leading to intense food cravings, particularly for the sugar and refined carbohydrates that tend to mimic the soothing effects of serotonin. Persistently low serotonin leads to sagging energy, bouts of depression, worrying and dwelling, low self-esteem, difficulty making decisions, early-morning waking and compulsive eating.

Researchers from Tufts University have provided scientific support for the close link between anxiety disorders, depression and higher risk of obesity. A study published in the March 2006 issue of the *Archives of Pediatrics and Adolescent Medicine* discusses the involvement of serotonin in both mood and appetite regulation. The data show that patients suffering from depression (and, therefore, low serotonin) often turn to food, particularly carbohydrates, to temporarily boost their levels.

What's more, according to a research paper entitled *Brain Serotonin, Carbohydrate-craving, Obesity and Depression* from the Massachusetts Institute of Technology, serotonin-releasing brain neurons are unique in that the amount of serotonin they release is dependent on food intake. Carbohydrate consumption increases serotonin release, while protein intake does not. Researchers found that many patients *learn* to overeat carbohydrates, particularly snack foods rich in carbohydrates and fats, to make themselves feel better.

Clearly this tendency to use certain carb-rich foods as though they were drugs is a frequent cause of weight gain. It is also an underlying factor in patients who gain fat when exposed to stress, in women with premenstrual syndrome, in patients with "winter depression" and in those attempting to give up smoking. Regardless of the cause of your stress, it doesn't take much before it causes you to abandon your diet and reach for the comforts in the cupboard.

By now you get that excess carb consumption can cause weight gain and insulin resistance. Although antidepressant medications such as selective serotonin reuptake inhibitors (SSRIs) are effective in raising serotonin in the short term, some evidence suggests these medications actually deplete serotonin over the long haul. Furthermore, weight gain is one of the most common side effects of antidepressant drugs, possibly due to an adverse effect on insulin sensitivity. I recently found a study that showed poorer glucose control in diabetics taking these medications because of an increase in insulin resistance. Yet another vicious circle.

Serotonin has also been proven to interact closely with leptin, the hormone responsible for appetite control. A 2007 study conducted by researchers at Cambridge University and published in *Expert Reviews of Molecular Medicine* showed serotonin to be an important regulator of energy balance. The findings revealed that serotonin acts on specific receptors in the brain, in connection with leptin, to affect how much we eat.

In light of the clear link between obesity and depressed levels of serotonin and dopamine, the likelihood that many overweight and obese patients suffer from an imbalance of these hormones cannot be ignored. To successfully regulate appetite control and weight loss, therefore, brain chemistry must be addressed along with blood sugar and insulin balance. The catch is that insulin resistance, often associated with obesity, also blocks the activity of serotonin in the brain. Therefore, in order to affect your body's response to insulin (and ultimately, the number on your scales), serotonin levels must be improved, which will aid in breaking free from carb addiction.

Cortisol, Carbs and Cravings

In a society where we are constantly on the go, and an abundance of foodstuffs is readily available to us 24/7, we eat for many reasons other than hunger. The triggers that make us reach for food are wide ranging: the stress of sleep deprivation, lack of sunlight, cold temperatures, the angst of a data-eating computer virus (which I experienced while writing this book!), marital strife, work stress or caring for a sick relative. Distress triggers can also arise from the hormonal changes of PMS, menopause, chronic pain or exhaustion from overworking or overexercising.

According to Professor of Physiology Mary Dallman at the University of California, who studies the effects of stress on appetite and obesity, two predominant endocrine hormones, cortisol and insulin, heavily influence caloric intake by acting on the brain. The stress hormone cortisol, in particular, activates a strong response in the brain to match our perceived stress with a desire to eat *comfort foods*—the tasty treats we associate with pleasant experiences, often from childhood. Unfortunately, consuming comfort foods, which are typically high in carbohydrates and fat, can cause a resulting spike in our insulin level, leading to the accumulation of belly fat.

Another stress hormone called neuropeptide Y (NPY) also plays an important role in controlling your eating habits by working in your brain. Once released, NPY decreases your metabolic rate, causes more belly fat storage and also fuels your appetite for sugary foods and carbohydrates—a triple whammy for your waistline and your fat-loss efforts.

So many side effects of stress conspire to make you fat! Together, high cortisol and elevated NPY impact your metabolism, appetite and body composition in the following nasty ways:

- Cortisol depresses your metabolic rate by interfering with thyroid hormone.
- Cortisol and NPY fuel your desire for fatty foods and carbohydrates.
- Cortisol and NPY boost abdominal fat storage.
- Cortisol depletes your happy hormone, serotonin, causing depression and more carbohydrate cravings.
- Cortisol can cause blood sugar imbalance, resulting in hypoglycemia and symptoms of shakiness, irritability, fatigue and headaches between meals.
- Cortisol causes you to eat more than you need to by stimulating appetite-boosting NPY and blocking appetite-suppressing leptin.
- Cortisol saps testosterone, which can result in languishing libido and a host of serious health risks.
- Cortisol eats away muscle and slows repair of metabolically active muscle cells.
- Excess cortisol leads to sleep disruption, a known cause of weight gain.
- Cortisol blunts the growth hormone that helps build metabolically active muscle, aids tissue rejuvenation and slows the effects of aging.
- Cortisol and NPY both decrease cellular sensitivity to insulin, resulting in elevated insulin levels, insulin resistance and accumulation of abdominal fat.

Through a complicated network of hormonal interactions, prolonged stress results in a raging appetite, metabolic decline, loads of belly fat and a loss of hard-won, metabolically active muscle tissue. In other words, stress makes us soft, flabby and much older than we truly are!

Since symptoms of stress vary widely, pinpointing whether or not it's the main culprit behind your emotional eating or "carboholic" nature can be difficult. The classic symptoms of stress, however, include a tendency to wake between 2 and 4 a.m., headaches, salt cravings, digestive concerns, anxiety, muscle tension and more. You can assess your cortisol using a salivary cortisol profile test that collects saliva at four different points during the day (see Resources, page 446). When properly balanced, your cortisol should be highest at around 6 a.m. and lowest at night.

Identifying the Problem: Are You a Carb Addict?

There's no doubt that the more carb sensitive you are, the more prone you are to carb addiction. And addiction to carbs is certainly a reflection of an insulin imbalance, specifically reduced insulin sensitivity, which raises insulin. But regardless of your current state of carb sensitivity, my bet is that 99 percent of you could use some help to deal with an appetite stuck in overdrive, carb cravings or stress-related eating. Many of you may even consider yourself a full-blown carb addict, in need of an intervention to break your food obsession. Some sources say 75 to 85 percent of overweight adults identify themselves as carbohydrate addicts. Since at least 60 to 70 percent of adults are in fact overweight, this is a problem that is affecting a large portion of our population.

Let's begin by distinguishing between a craving and an addiction. While a craving denotes something you feel you want once in a while, an addiction reflects a *need* to have carbs to allow you to feel "normal." With a carb addiction, just like any other drug addiction, you may also eventually notice that you need more and more to get the same results or that you have withdrawal symptoms when you don't get your carbs. Do you think you could be carb addicted? Ask yourself if any of these statements or questions apply to you:

    1. I feel I *have* to eat carbs in the morning. According to psychotherapist Dr. Mike Dow, the desire to eat "bad" carbs within 1 hour

of waking is a strong sign that you are a carb addict. (This same assessment tool is used to diagnose drug addictions and alcoholism.)

2. I get tired or feel foggy in the afternoon.
3. I find myself searching for a sugar, starch or caffeine fix in the afternoon.
4. I have a hard time stopping once I start eating my favorite carb foods (starches, sweets, snacks).
5. When I feel stressed, my first response is to want to eat something. I use foods to fill an emotional need.
6. I can't live without my favorite carb foods.
7. I have a tendency to binge.
8. I frequently crave high-carb foods (sweets, pasta, bread, etc.).
9. I am a compulsive eater. I wish I could control my eating.
10. I am overweight, even though I feel I don't really eat that much.
11. I experience carbohydrate withdrawal symptoms including headaches, irritability, mood swings, trouble sleeping and anxiety.

If you answered yes to any of these questions, you likely have a carb addiction. Breaking this addiction will be part of the key to curbing your sensitivity to carbs, as well as to lasting weight loss and hormonal balance. If you are indeed a carb addict, the CSP is the perfect plan for you. The CSP will allow you to focus on attaining your carbs from nonstarchy vegetables, nuts and small amounts of low-glycemic fruit. Minimizing your grain and sugar intake, as I prescribe in the first 3 weeks of the program, will certainly help to break the cycle of addiction. In fact, most patients tell me their cravings and obsessions with food are gone within just 3 to 4 days of following this plan.

Working together, the endocrine, nervous and digestive systems can either help or hamper your appetite control. Once you understand these complex systems and get them communicating optimally with each other, you will be well on your way to feeling balanced and achieving lifelong health. Although the nutrition program of the CSP will solve a majority of carb-addicted cases, you can set the foundation for guaranteed success by beginning with the five steps to restore balance in the carb-addicted brain, found in the next chapter.

CSP SUCCESS STORY: DONNA

"I was approaching 50, tired, finding it more difficult to keep the pounds off, having more aches and pains and fearful of becoming a diabetic. I knew my hormones were playing a part in my wellness and felt a more holistic approach made sense. I stumbled across Dr. Turner on a TV show talking about the effects of carbs on hormone balance and overall health. With Dr. Turner's expertise and gentle ways, I have learned so much more about carbs than I thought possible. I am 28 pounds lighter, more energetic and more flexible. How lucky am I to have experienced the Carb Sensitivity Program!"

DONNA, 50

STATS	BEFORE	AFTER
Weight	162 lb	134 lb
BMI	30.6	25.4

INITIAL CHIEF COMPLAINTS:

1. Weight gain
2. Belly fat
3. Joint and shoulder pain

CHAPTER 5

A FIVE-STEP PRESCRIPTION
FOR THE CARB-ADDICTED BRAIN

You can't build a reputation on what you are going to do.

HENRY FORD

A grumbling stomach, carb cravings and a surging appetite are among the major issues that lead people to *regain* their weight after completing a standard diet. Now that the questionnaire (pages 70–71) in the last chapter has helped you to determine whether you have a carb addiction, the suggestions presented here will help you restore healthy brain chemistry and free yourself from your carb obsession.

The recurring cycle of restraint → cravings → resisting cravings → stronger cravings → giving into cravings is common to every type of addiction, from cigarettes to alcohol to cocaine and, as you now know, to carbohydrates. For most of us, the only way to break this vicious cycle is to reduce the intensity of the cravings. Unfortunately, frequent relapses and bingeing are as common for those trying to kick carbs as they are for any other recovering addict.

With some rare exceptions, most addicts cannot win the battle without some assistance. The majority of us simply do not have long-term control of our carbohydrate cravings. As we discussed in Chapter 4, this inability to keep cravings in check is not a matter of willpower—it is physiologically driven. Compulsive eating, emotional tension, reduced numbers of dopamine "pleasure" receptors, stress, low serotonin and our genetic makeup are just a few of the factors that fuel our brain-biochemistry-based cravings for carbohydrates. It makes sense, then, that the treatment for carb addiction should focus on the area of the brain that is influenced by the hormones involved in appetite control—the hypothalamus. This is where the problem actually arises.

You will recall that several hormones affect the appetite-regulation system in the brain. At least four major factors contribute to our strong urge to consume carbs:

1. *Excess stress hormone.* Stress hormones such as cortisol and neuropeptide Y stimulate the hypothalamus to increase appetite, specifically for carbohydrates. Both are released when we are anxious, sleep deprived, dehydrated or under any other kind of stress. The hormone grehlin, released from the stomach, also stimulates appetite by acting on the hypothalamus. Grehlin also increases during sleep deprivation and calorie restriction.

2. *Low serotonin.* A chemical imbalance involving low serotonin may cause irresistible urges to eat carbs too often or at inopportune times (like that late-night binge episode we have all experienced). This imbalance is often linked with depression and anxiety.

3. *Norepinephrine imbalance.* Problems in another area of the brain can increase emotion-induced overeating of carbohydrates, particularly when we are tired, bored, tense, depressed or nervous. This type of overeating usually involves the hormone norepinephrine, which is similar to the stress hormone adrenaline. Many of the same treatments that aid a dopamine and stress imbalance also help to balance this hormone.

4. *Low dopamine.* When we eat (or overeat) simply because we are seeking a boost of pleasure or a "fix," a deficiency of dopamine is usually involved.

No matter how strong willed you think you are, struggling against cravings that begin in the brain is a losing proposition. That is why a plan designed to reduce the brain's craving-inducing, appetite-enhancing activity is the best and most effective approach. In addition to the dietary program you will embark upon in Chapter 6, you can choose to implement specific appetite-controlling behaviors, lifestyle suggestions and supplements that can provide additional help, especially in the first few weeks of your diet, until the brain pathways involved in your carb cravings are subdued.

A Five-Step Prescription to Beat Your Carb Addiction

If you suspect an addiction to carbs, the following lifestyle, dietary and supplement suggestions will help you to restore balance, cut cravings, improve your mood, reduce stress, and help to break the carb-addiction cycle. Should you decide to use one or more of my supplement suggestions in Step 5, you should do so for at least 1 to 3 consecutive months to allow optimal effectiveness.

Step 1: Sleep Well and Manage Stress

SLEEP

These days, quality sleep seems to fall to the bottom of our priority list. But besides leaving you feeling less than your best, poor sleep interferes with your blood sugar and insulin balance, hormonal balance, appetite control and fat loss, *even* when your diet and exercise routines are right on track. Lack of sleep also contributes to an increased amount of inflammation in the body, which, as you will learn in Chapter 9, is a major contributing factor to metabolic disruption, diabetes and obesity.

Even a short-term sleep debt can cause metabolic disruption. After only a few nights of sleep deprivation, glucose tolerance tests make otherwise healthy people appear prediabetic. Specifically, regulating blood sugar after a high-carbohydrate meal can take up to 40 percent longer than normal!

A recent study published in the *Lancet* also showed that sleep deprivation causes stress hormones to rise in the evening and heightens the stress response during waking hours. Another study, published in the *Journal of Endocrinology and Metabolism* in 2001, was one of the first to show that chronic insomnia leads to high cortisol and hyperactivity of the brain's stress-response pathway.

As you know, high cortisol fuels appetite and increases our cravings, particularly for sugary and carb-laden treats, even when we have eaten enough. Overeating calorie-rich, nutrient-poor foodstuffs then causes our blood sugar to spike, our insulin to soar and, eventually, unwanted fat to collect around the abdomen.

Not only does poor sleep pack on pounds, but good sleep actually helps you to lose weight by influencing the hormones that control your appetite and increase your metabolism. A 2004 study at the University of Chicago was the first to show sleep as a major regulator of appetite-controlling hormones and also to link the extent of hormonal variations with the degree of hunger change. More specifically, researchers found *appetite-enhancing ghrelin increased* by 28 percent, while *appetite-curbing leptin decreased* by 18 percent, among subjects who were sleep deprived. Appetite was not the only factor found to increase with lack of sleep. The desire for high-calorie, high-sugar foods also jumped with insufficient slumber. So we not only eat more, but more of the wrong choices.

In the same year, researchers at the Stanford School of Medicine found that subjects who had only 5 hours of sleep per night had less leptin, more ghrelin and experienced an increase in their BMI, *regardless of diet and exercise.* Let's face it: No one feels good after endless nights of tossing, turning or staring at the ceiling.

It's clear that good sleep is vital for prevention of cravings, but many factors can interfere with your slumber, some of which may surprise you. Follow these rules to promote healthy rest and to gain the most benefit from your sleep:

- Sleep in complete darkness. Even a small amount of light can hamper your sleep.
- Sleep nude (or at least with loose-fitting nightclothes). Avoid sleeping in tight undergarments (bras, girdles, briefs, etc.).

Tight clothing increases body temperature and interferes with the release of melatonin, a hormone essential to the regulation of sleep-wake patterns.

- Establish regular sleeping hours. Try to get up each morning and go to bed every night at roughly the same time. Believe it or not, oversleeping can be as detrimental as sleep deprivation. How energized and alert you feel each day is an important indication of how much sleep is right for you.

- Get to bed by 11 p.m. Since the invention of electricity (not to mention television and computers), we have begun staying up later and later. This change has resulted in a largely sleep-deprived society. Our stress glands—the adrenals—recharge or recover most between 10 p.m. and 2 a.m. Going to bed before 11 p.m. (10 p.m. is even better), therefore, is optimal for rebuilding your adrenal reserves. I know this can be a difficult change to implement if you are a night owl, so I recommend to my patients that they start going to bed 15 minutes earlier each week until they reach their new target time.

- Sleep 7 ½ to 9 hours a night. The American Cancer Association has found higher incidences of cancer in individuals who consistently sleep fewer than 6 hours or more than 9 hours nightly. Oversleeping should also be a red flag. Consistently needing more than 9 hours of sleep warrants a visit to your doctor for further investigation, as this may indicate an underlying medical condition such as hypothyroidism, depression or a deficiency of iron, folic acid or vitamin B12. Some of us simply require more or less sleep than others. If you awaken without an alarm and feel rested, you're likely getting the right amount of sleep for you.

- See the light first thing in the morning. Daylight and morning sounds are key signals that help awaken your brain. Turning on the lights or opening the blinds is the proper way to reset your body clock and ensure that your melatonin level drops back to "awake" mode until the evening. Exposure to morning light has been proven to be one of the simplest ways to increase your energy for the entire day. It's also been shown to boost testosterone in men and fertility in women by stimulating luteinizing hormone release from the pituitary gland. Enhance this action further by exposing yourself to sunlight and by getting outside during the day. I can't say enough about the benefits of getting outside, even for 10 to 20 minutes, in the morning light.

- Keep household lighting dim from dinnertime until you go to sleep. Believe it or not, this simple step not only prepares your body and hormones for sleep but also helps your digestion, according to studies.

- Be aware of electromagnetic fields (EMFs) in your bedroom. EMFs are emitted from digital alarm clocks and other electrical devices and can disrupt the pineal gland and the production of melatonin and serotonin. They may have additional negative effects including an increased risk of cancer. If you must use electrical items, try to keep them as far away from the bed as possible—at least 3 feet.

- Use your bed for sleeping and sex only. If you have kids, you know how easily your bedroom can become Grand Central Station. But you should definitely avoid engaging in any other activities in bed, as you may start to associate the bedroom with sleep-robbing chores and tasks rather than relaxing sleep and intimacy with your partner. Above all, *never* work or eat in bed.

- Create a serene space. In my last two homes, I painted the bedroom in calming, dark earthy tones. Shades like these help make the bedroom a relaxing place. Choose bedroom colors and furnishings that make you feel calm and happy. Over the years I've also realized that clutter is a state of mind. Keeping your bedroom neat and clutter free can be challenging, especially if you live in a small space. Just remember, the bedroom's primary purpose is for sleep and sex. You'll be amazed how much better both will be if you keep your bedside tables and dresser tops clear of clutter.

- Choose comfortable, soothing bedding. Several companies now offer organic cotton bed linens that are free of harmful dyes and toxins. These can be a great investment if you have sensitive skin or simply care about the impact of heavy pesticide use on the environment. Personally, I find all-white bedding very soothing and welcoming after a long day of sensory overload. Whatever your taste dictates, select bedding that pleases your eye and feels good on your skin. You should also make sure your bedding keeps you warm but doesn't overheat you. In the winter, you may wish to use a duvet, while a thin blanket with a sheet might suffice for summer. Small changes like these will help create a calming, comfortable environment conducive to restful sleep.

- Keep your bedroom cool but not cold. No matter how chilly the weather gets outside, your bedroom temperature should be no warmer than 70°F for sleeping. Remember, our body needs to cool slightly at night to ensure the proper release of melatonin. However, make sure your air conditioner is not blasting all night long in the summertime. Research shows air-conditioning can cause weight gain. We naturally burn fewer calories when we're not working to keep cool, and our appetites tend to decrease when we are warmer.

- Avoid using a loud alarm clock. Waking up suddenly to the blaring wail of an alarm clock can be a shock to your body. You'll find you feel groggier when you are roused in the middle of a sleep cycle. Getting enough sleep on a regular basis should make your alarm clock unnecessary. In fact, sleeping through an alarm or relying on an alarm daily may indicate that you are sleep deprived. If you do use an alarm, you should awaken just before it goes off. If you must use one, I recommend the Bose alarm. It starts off at a moderate volume and slowly gets louder, so you aren't jarred out of your sleep. You can also investigate a sunrise alarm, an alarm clock with a built-in natural light bulb that simulates a sunrise. This method of waking has the clinically proven added bonus of increasing your mood, mental focus and energy throughout the day.

- If you go to the bathroom during the night, keep the lights off. Even brief exposure to light can shut down the melatonin production that's so crucial for good sleep. If you absolutely must use a light in the loo, try a flashlight or night light instead of the bright overhead light. Another option is to use a dimmer switch or a night-light fitted with a red bulb, since red light exposure at night appears to have less of a negative impact.

NATURAL SLEEP AND SLEEP AIDS

If you find you need additional remedies to help improve your sleep, try one or more of these:

- **Clear Balance—Stress Modifying Formula.** This contains Relora, my favorite choice for chronic stress and sleep disruption. And boy does it work. A mixture of the herbal extracts *Magnolia officinalis* and *Phellodendron amurense*, Relora is medically proven to reduce stress and anxiety. It's often the best option for patients who tend to wake up throughout the night, for highly stressed individuals and for menopausal women with hot flashes that cause sleep disruption. Relora can significantly reduce cortisol and raise the antiaging, antistress hormone DHEA within only 2 weeks of use. Take 2 capsules before bed and 1 in the morning to ease the effects of stress and improve your rest.
- **Magnesium glycinate.** I once had a patient question whether I had given him a drug because this simple mineral worked

so well for his sleep! Magnesium calms your nervous system, induces relaxation, reduces blood pressure, decreases cravings, soothes PMS tension, increases energy during the day, and treats and prevents constipation and muscle cramps. As an added bonus, it also reduces sugar cravings and aids insulin sensitivity. It's truly one of nature's "wonder drugs." Take 200 to 800 mg at night. Begin at 200 mg and keep increasing the dosage until you reach bowel tolerance (i.e., the point at which you develop loose stools).

- **Ashwagandha.** Ayurvedic practitioners use this dietary supplement to enhance mental and physical performance, improve learning ability, and decrease stress and fatigue. Ashwagandha is a general tonic that can be used in stressful situations, especially for insomnia, restlessness or when you are feeling overworked. Studies have indicated that ashwagandha offers anti-inflammatory, anticancer, antistress, antioxidant, and immune-modulating and rejuvenating properties. The typical dosage is 500 to 1,000 mg twice daily. Capsules should be standardized to 1.5 percent withanolides per dose. My favorite brand is AOR.

- **GABA.** Gamma-aminobutyric acid (GABA) is an inhibitory neurotransmitter, a brain chemical that has a calming effect. It's well suited for individuals who experience anxiety, muscle tension or pain. Take 500 to 1,000 mg before bed. Alternatively, take GABA 10 to 20 minutes before your evening meal. The standard dose of 500 mg twice daily can be increased to a maximum of three times daily, if needed, but this dosage should not be exceeded. You can also consider Clear Calm—GABA Enhancing Formula.

- **5-HTP.** A derivative of tryptophan that also contributes to the creation of serotonin, 5-HTP has been found to be more effective than tryptophan in treating sleep loss related to depression, anxiety and fibromyalgia. 5-HTP appears to increase REM sleep. It also decreases the amount of time required to fall asleep, as well as the number of nighttime awakenings. And remember, the higher your serotonin, the less your risk of carb cravings. Take 50 to 400 mg a day, divided into doses throughout the day and before bed. Clear Mood—Serotonin Support Formula works very well because I have included the vitamin cofactors needed for the production of serotonin along with 75 mg of 5-HTP per capsule.

- **Melatonin.** This hormone decreases as we age, as well as during times of stress and depression. Take 0.5 to 3 mg at bedtime. Try opening up the capsules and pouring the contents under your tongue. You can also purchase melatonin in sublingual form for fast absorption. Supplements tend to be effective for insomnia only when melatonin levels are low, so if you find it doesn't work for you, this could be the reason.

Many of these products are available through www.carbsensitivity.com.

SUBDUE STRESS

Even when we know what and how much we are supposed to be eating, emotional factors and stress greatly influence our food choices and consumption. Eating can be a very pleasurable, often social, experience closely tied to feelings and emotions. Many of us use food for comfort, or to cope with stressful, upsetting situations, especially when we have not developed more effective coping strategies. We also eat when we're bored, feel like celebrating, want to boost our spirits or avoid dealing with anxiety, fear, anger and resentment. In the very short term, food can make us feel good. But over the long haul, stress-related eating can leave us with feelings of guilt and regret, not to mention excess pounds. You can, however, use meditation, massage and laughter to reduce stress-related eating.

- *Meditation.* Meditation has amazing effects on your hormones. It lowers the stress hormones cortisol and adrenaline and raises antiaging, antistress hormones DHEA and serotonin. The only requirement is discipline and the ability to comfortably spend a few moments alone without distractions. Once you incorporate it into your daily routine, you'll find the journey to enlightenment is accompanied by endless physical, emotional and spiritual benefits.

HOW TO MEDITATE IN FIVE SIMPLE STEPS

1. **Get comfortable.** Sit or lie in a comfortable, quiet place where you will not be interrupted or distracted. You may want to designate a space at home for this.

2. **Clear your mind.** Close your eyes, rest and *do nothing.*

3. **Concentrate on your breath.** Focus on the sound of your breathing and how it feels flowing in and out of the edge of your nostrils. I find it useful to imagine my breath washing in and out like waves on the beach. You can also pick a word or a phrase that is soothing or meaningful to you. One patient of mine, an extremely tense 85-year-old man with high blood pressure, picked the word *quiet*, which I thought was a great choice. Repeat the word or phrase to yourself each time you exhale.

4. **Practice body awareness.** Check for tension, especially in your jaw, scalp, forehead, shoulders, lower back and hips—all the way down to your toes—by consciously examining each body part. Relax the areas that feel tight, as you continue breathing.

5. **Stay in tune with your breathing or the repetition of your word or phrase.** You'll be amazed at how often thoughts start creeping into your mind. Just acknowledge them and return your focus to your breathing. With practice, the amount of time you'll be able to sit without your mind

wandering will lengthen, and you may even find that
solutions you've been searching for will appear.

Some forms of meditation may involve physical, repetitive
motions such as running or cycling. If you want to meditate
while engaging in these activities, practice staying focused on
your breathing and allow your thoughts to flow freely. This form
of meditation is very helpful for people who have a difficult time
sitting still.

- *Massage.* More than just an enjoyable indulgence, massage
  offers a host of health benefits that can help our weight-loss
  efforts. A study from the *International Journal of Neuroscience*
  (October 2005) found that massage increases endorphin
  release, which is excellent for treating pain, depression and
  anxiety. Massage helps ease activity in the sympathetic
  nervous system (responsible for our fight-or-flight response)
  and increases our parasympathetic response (which induces
  us to rest and relax).

  Moreover, we know that the cortisol and adrenalin we
  produce when we're under stress are destructive to our body
  tissues, immune system and adrenal glands when they are
  present in high amounts for long periods of time. One of the
  functions of the liver is to break down stress hormones and sex
  hormones. Massage, which assists the bloodflow and lymphatic
  delivery of hormonal waste to the liver, expedites this breakdown process, thereby helping to relieve stress in the body.

  Remember: Anything that reduces our sympathetic
  nervous system's responses can help propel weight loss, ease
  water retention and boost appetite control. So beyond simply
  feeling good while you are on the table, massage has definite
  physiological benefits.

- *Laughter.* I once prescribed watching the movie *Planes, Trains and Automobiles* to a 65-year-old woman who was constantly worried about her health. I also told a diabetic man of 35, "Don't come back here unless you've done something *fun.*" I kid you not.

  Research shows that a good chuckle can relieve stress and improve health. Professor Lee S. Berk of Loma Linda University in California has found that the mere anticipation of laughter has significant positive hormonal effects. In a recent study, one group of subjects was told they were about to watch a funny movie, while the second group was told that they would be reading magazines for 1 hour. When tested, those who were told about the movie had 27 percent more beta-endorphins and 87 percent more human growth hormone. In previous studies, Berk found that laughter reduced cortisol and adrenaline and enhanced the immune system for 12 to 24 hours. So, watch funny movies and make time for laughter in your life—or just think about doing it!

FEEDING YOUR FEELINGS:
HOW TO CONTROL EMOTIONAL EATING

It's not surprising that emotional eating has little to do with your actual hunger; it is directly related to emotional triggers. Our emotions can have a powerful influence on our actions, especially eating. But the fact that you have picked up this book shows that you are ready to replace old, unhelpful patterns and replace them with healthier steps. According to Natalie Shay, a Clear Medicine expert specializing in stress, emotional eating and psychotherapy, the three most important ways to stop emotional eating are to do the following:

1. Become aware of your true hunger signals.
2. Become aware of exactly which emotions drive your eating.

3. Learn to stop punishing yourself every time you eat something that you are trying to avoid.

Natalie recommends that you begin your healing journey by creating a hunger scale from 1 to 10, with 1 representing when you feel so starved you can't think straight, and 10 representing when you feel so full you can't move. Spend the first part of your program writing down your hunger levels before and after each meal. Try to stay between 4 and 6.

Next, notice which emotions you experience at each meal, before and after you eat. Are you bored? Sad? Angry? Lonely? Try to be honest with yourself without being hard on yourself. Remember, building self-awareness is a huge first step!

Finally, try to be aware of the negative messages you impart to yourself and make a commitment to no longer beat yourself up. The easiest way to start this challenging task is to spend a week writing down any negative thoughts about yourself in a notebook. Throughout this process, you need to be patient—and honest.

Each of these exercises should take no more than about 5 minutes. The key is to write down exactly how you are feeling at the moment, without thinking about it or editing yourself. Remember, although food feels like your enemy at times, you have brought it into your life as a coping mechanism. It has actually helped you to get to where you are today. Once you become aware of your actions, you will see how simple it is to break old patterns and to free yourself from emotional eating.

Step 2: Keep Your Digestive Tract Working and Use My Specific Diet Tips to Curb Cravings

MAINTAIN A HEALTHY DIGESTIVE TRACT

If you find that you have persistent gas and bloating, even after following the CSP meal plan and using supplements to support detoxification of the digestive system (suggested in Chapter 8 as part of the basic CSP supplements) for at least 5 days, taking a digestive enzyme with your meals is the next logical step. Look for one that contains a mixture of enzymes for breaking down protein, carbohydrates and fats (proteases, amylases and lipases, respectively). My favorite choices are Ultrazyme from Douglas Labs, Digestive Enzyme Ultra from Pure Encaps or Digest Plus from Genestra. Udo's Enzymes are also a viable option available at most health-food stores.

GET YOUR FILL OF FIBER

Dr. Robert Lustig, a pediatric endocrinologist at University of California San Francisco (UCSF) Children's Hospital, presented a comprehensive review of obesity research published in the August 2006 edition of the journal *Nature Clinical Practice Endocrinology & Metabolism*. In the study, he determined a key reason for the epidemic of pediatric obesity—now the most commonly diagnosed childhood ailment—is that high-calorie, low-fiber Western diets promote hormonal imbalances that encourage children (and adults!) to overeat. He wrote:

> Our current Western food environment has become highly "insulinogenic," as demonstrated by its increased energy density, high-fat content, high glycaemic index, increased fructose composition, decreased fiber, and decreased dairy content. In particular, fructose (too much) and fiber (not enough) appear to be cornerstones of the obesity epidemic through their effects on insulin.

Changes in food processing over the past 30 years, particularly the removal of fiber and addition of sugar to a wide variety of foods, have created an environment in which our foods are essentially addictive. As Dr. Lustig notes, both excess sugar and insufficient fiber promote insulin production and suppression of leptin activity in the brain. Getting enough fiber every day can be tough, but I have included several tips in Chapter 6 that can help you up your fiber intake.

SKIP ARTIFICIAL SWEETENERS

The past 25 years have seen a dramatic increase in the consumption of artificially sweetened foods, including those containing sucralose, aspartame, saccharin, etc. Yet the incidence of overweight and obesity has also increased markedly during this period. Despite the superficial logic that consuming fewer calories will lead to weight loss, the evidence is very clear that using artificial sweeteners can, paradoxically, *cause weight gain.*

Most of us are aware of research showing the links between specific artificial sweeteners such as aspartame and saccharin and cancer. But all artificial sweeteners are also known to cause increased cravings and weight gain and may subsequently contribute to insulin resistance. According to a study by researchers at the University of Texas San Antonio, middle-aged adults who drink diet soft drinks drastically increase their risk of gaining weight later on. The study monitored the weight and soda-drinking habits of more than 600 normal-weight subjects aged 25 to 64. When researchers followed up with the participants after 8 years, they discovered those who consumed one diet soda a day were *65 percent more likely to be overweight than those who drank none.* Drinking two or more low- or no-calorie soft drinks daily raised the odds of becoming obese or overweight even higher. The real shocker? Participants who drank diet soda had a *greater chance of becoming overweight than those who drank regular soda!*

Artificial sweeteners appear to be a double-edged dieting sword. They do not allow for the leptin release that normally happens when we eat the sugars that signal the brain that our hunger is satisfied. At the same time, even though artificial sweeteners do not cause our blood sugar to rise, our body still responds as though there is sugar in our bloodstream by secreting insulin. Between the low leptin and high insulin, our appetite and cravings go haywire. Knowing that high insulin is a stepping-stone to type 2 diabetes and obesity, we cannot overlook the connection to the number of diabetic, prediabetic and overweight people who use these types of products.

Apparently, the taste and feel of food in our mouth influences our learned ability to match our caloric intake with our caloric need. For instance, we learn very early on that both sweet tastes and dense, thick foods signal high calorie content. Our innate ability to control how much we eat (and, therefore, our body weight) may be weakened when this natural link is impaired by consuming products that contain artificial sweeteners. These foods and drinks prompt us to eat more because they often have a thinner consistency and texture than regular, sugar-sweetened foods. You may have noticed this textural difference in the past when drinking diet versus regular soda or eating yogurt sweetened with artificial sweeteners.

AVOID HAVING "ONE TOO MANY"

Many of us like to enjoy a refreshing cocktail or glass of wine once in a while, but we need to approach these drinks with caution. Alcohol is a known appetite stimulant and frequently causes us to overeat because it also lowers our inhibitions. Just a few drinks, especially those mixed with sugary fruit drinks or soda, can cause a serious insulin spike, resulting in hypoglycemia (low blood sugar). Even the healthiest among us can experience low blood sugar with alcohol consumption.

Even a little bit of alcohol (i.e., more than 2 to 3 glasses per week for women, or 4 to 5 for men) lowers leptin and raises cortisol. This double whammy leads to disturbed sleep, night waking and those signature next-day cravings for greasy hangover foods. Over time, chronic overuse of alcohol can reduce the body's responsiveness to insulin and cause sensitivity to sugar in both healthy individuals and alcoholics with liver cirrhosis. In fact, a high percentage of those with alcoholic liver disease are glucose intolerant or diabetic.

DO A DAILY DOSE OF OLIVE OIL

A diet rich in olive oil not only aids appetite control and prevents belly fat accumulation, but also guards against the insulin resistance and drop in adiponectin typically seen in people who eat a high-carbohydrate diet. Adiponectin is a chemical mediator naturally produced in our fat cells. It is known to increase fat burning and insulin sensitivity. Adiponectin levels are lower in individuals with obesity, insulin resistance and inflammation. Patients with coronary heart disease also have lower adiponectin levels, which suggests that it offers protective benefits against arterial disease. According to a study in the *Journal of the American College of Nutrition* (October 2007), consuming olive oil at breakfast is especially effective in this regard. For these reasons, I formulated a supplement called Glyci-Med Forte that's rich in olive and avocado oils for use at breakfast. The majority of people using this supplement find it aids appetite control, reduces cravings and boosts belly fat loss. But the *British Journal of Nutrition* (December 2003) revealed another amazing tidbit about olive oil: Besides helping us lose weight, balance our hormones, reduce inflammation and keep insulin under control, olive oil also breaks down the fat cells we already have!

ENJOY APPETIZERS AND EAT SLOWLY

It takes time for hormonal messages to reach the feeding centers of your brain, so the idea of whetting your appetite with a few hors d'oeuvres before a meal may have a solid scientific basis. According to a study in the October 2006 issue of the journal *Cell Metabolism,* researchers found that the very first bites of food sparked brain activity in the hunger centers of rats trained to stick to a strict feeding regimen. The findings also revealed that the brain center responsible for telling us when we are full or satisfied appears to turn on *as soon as food hits our stomach*, rather than when we actually sense that full feeling. Enjoying a healthy appetizer beforehand and eating slowly throughout the meal are two basic habits that can help you avoid consuming too much in one sitting. If you tend to eat quickly, why not use chopsticks instead of utensils, count the number of times you chew, or simply practice putting down the fork between bites?

REMEMBER THAT TIMING IS EVERYTHING

You skip breakfast because you just don't feel like eating. You're not hungry at lunch so you grab a muffin. By the end of the day, you have consumed very few calories. Then, at 8 p.m., when most people are finished eating for the day, you're standing in front of the fridge gobbling everything in sight. Believe it or not, your hormones (and your body overall) function at their best when you keep to a consistent eating schedule. By eating smaller meals more frequently (i.e., approximately every 3 hours), you will also help maintain a steady level of blood sugar. A 1968 study published in the *Journal of Personality and Social Psychology* manipulated "dinnertime" for 22 obese and 24 healthy-weight individuals to determine whether eating behavior changed when standard mealtimes were altered. They found that the obese group ate more when they thought they were eating *after* their regular dinner hour than they did when they thought that they were eating *before*.

Moreover, skipping a meal entirely causes blood sugar imbalance and raises cortisol levels, which in turn has a host of negative consequences from increasing belly fat to disrupting insulin receptors. When cortisol is too high, we can have difficulty falling asleep or experience frequent waking throughout the night, especially between 2 and 4 a.m. To avoid this unhealthy situation, aim to eat within 1 hour of rising and then every 3 to 4 hours during the day. Stop eating approximately 2 to 3 hours before bedtime. This practice will stabilize blood sugar, reduce stress, eliminate sugar cravings and maintain your energy level. Eating at the same times every day will also help to lower excess insulin and reduce the chance that you will overeat later in the day.

> **THE RIGHT TYPES OF FAT WILL KEEP YOU SLIM**
> Saturated fats such as those in red meats and full-fat dairy products increase our urge to eat by reducing our appetite-suppressing hormones leptin and CCK. It's best to limit your intake of these types of fats and choose healthy options such as avocado, olives, olive oil, walnuts and almonds instead. This will keep your appetite under control and cravings in check.

ALWAYS BALANCE CARBOHYDRATES, FATS AND PROTEIN

By now, you should understand what happens when you eat carbs. Your digestive system breaks them down into sugar, and your pancreas then releases a rush of insulin to move the sugar from your bloodstream into your cells. Carbohydrates also trigger the production of serotonin, which creates an accompanying "serotonin high" for a brief period until the serotonin is depleted and our blood sugars come crashing down. That crash makes us crave more carbs, and the destructive cycle continues. These cyclical insulin highs and lows perpetuate further hormonal imbalances, including decreased leptin, sex-hormone imbalance and cortisol imbalance.

Eating too many carbs in isolation (or the wrong types of carbs) is like letting your car race down the road at lightning speed—it won't take long to crash and burn. In the case of carbs, you will find yourself quickly reaching for your next meal or snack. By consuming protein and fat together with carbohydrates, however, we can effectively put the brakes on the sugar entering our bloodstream. Sugar then cruises into our bloodstream in a slow and controlled manner, providing us with consistent energy for a longer period of time and preventing the insulin spike that occurs when we eat carbs alone. This glycemically balanced technique, combined with eating often and eating enough, is a guiding principle behind the CSP nutrition plan.

Step 3: Keep Warm and Soak Up Some Sun

BODY TEMPERATURE

It's hard to believe, I know, but climate control can make us fatter. In a study published in the June 2006 edition of the *International Journal of Obesity,* University of Alabama at Birmingham, Dr. David Allison suggested that air-conditioning is one of 10 factors that may play an important role in today's weight crisis. Dr. Allison showed a fascinating link between the proliferation of air-conditioning in the southern United States and the higher prevalence of obesity in this region.

Changes in temperature, either up or down, can be perceived by your body as a stressor to which it must respond. This response requires energy and also influences our hormonal balance. For instance, when our body temperature drops, our sympathetic nervous system releases adrenaline, our blood vessels constrict to prevent heat loss, and we may start to shiver. When we are hot, more bloodflow is directed toward our skin to allow heat to escape. Sympathetic stimulation causes us to start sweating, which also requires calories. In fact, I found one study showing that women who lived in a constant 80-degree climate burned almost 250 more calories a day at rest than women in a 70-degree environment.

Beyond the caloric expenditure involved in maintaining a constant core temperature, heat can help to control our weight by suppressing our appetite. An all-you-can-eat buffet certainly loses its appeal when we're hot. But people living with constant climate control often fail to feel the heat. Now, don't go cranking up your thermostat just yet. Heat does not work for long-term weight control. When we're constantly warm, less thyroid hormone is required to generate heat via our metabolism.

Our temperature also closely affects our sleep quality, since we need to cool down slightly in order to properly activate the release of sleep-enhancing melatonin. We also know that sleep quality directly influences our body composition. As we age, our natural ability to maintain and control our body temperature becomes less reliable. Could poor temperature control—and its many repercussions— be yet another reason for weight gain and hormonal imbalance as we age? I think so.

The vast majority of my patients report experiencing far more restful nights after they get started on the Carb Sensitivity Program. I believe these improvements are brought about by consistently balancing blood sugar, which helps to stabilize stress hormones (remember, skipped and unbalanced meals raise cortisol). I am still certain that blood sugar balance plays a role, but I have also found a study in the *Journal of Biorhythms* (2002) that links melatonin production to the carbohydrate content of evening meals. After only 3 days of consuming excessively carbohydrate-rich meals in the evening, salivary melatonin levels were reduced in otherwise healthy men. Less melatonin release, as we know, can cause sleep disruption, and sleep disruption means more cravings for carbs.

Without realizing it, I was encouraging better melatonin release in my patients by recommending that they consume carb-conscious dinners. What's the link? Body temperature rises when we eat carbohydrates and stays elevated for about 8 hours after consumption. The warmer we are, the less melatonin is released during sleep.

Alcohol also increases our nighttime temperature, which could be another reason (besides its impact on our blood sugar and stress hormones) for its sleep-disrupting effects. Researchers from France suggest this may also explain some clinical signs observed in alcoholic patients, including sleep and mood disorders. They go on to say that the negative effects of jet lag, shift work and aging—all of which are known to alter our body temperature by influencing our hormones—can be aggravated by alcohol. These factors can, therefore, affect our waistline too.

Most of us love the feeling of warm summer sun on our skin, but exposure to sunlight can also significantly improve our weight-loss efforts. When the skin is exposed to sunlight, the production of melanocortin is triggered. This powerful hormone suppresses the appetite centers, which speeds up metabolism and promotes fat loss. Melanocortin also stimulates thyroid hormone production and appears to be an important mediator for both leptin and insulin. Beyond the science of it, sunlight is a great mood booster, and when we are happy, we are less likely to turn to food to counteract plummeting serotonin levels. All awesome news for me, as a self-confessed sun bunny!

We also produce vitamin D when our skin is exposed to the ultraviolet B (UVB) rays in bright sunlight. Rising vitamin D levels activate the production of leptin, which signals the brain when the stomach is full. As we learned in previous chapters, depleted leptin levels interfere with normal appetite control. A study led by Dr. Helen MacDonald, from Aberdeen University's Department of Medicine and Therapeutics, found that adequate levels of sunlight can significantly reduce obesity. Her research team monitored more than 3,100 postmenopausal women living in northeast Scotland over a 2-year period. They discovered that women who had the *highest BMI* had the *lowest amounts of vitamin D* in their blood. Similarly, researchers at Tufts University in Massachusetts showed that obesity increases a person's chances of having low vitamin D levels. A possible explanation is that body fat absorbs available vitamin D so that it is not readily available for use by the body. All the more reason to embark on the CSP—with safe sun practices in mind and vitamin D supplements in hand.

Step 4: Enjoy Regular Sex

Believe it or not, satisfying your sexual appetite can help quell your growling stomach and your need to nibble on candy too. Our libido (that's scientific lingo for sex drive) is determined by a set of complex physiological processes that involve delicate interactions between our brain, body and hormones. For instance, an appetite-suppressing compound in the brain also controls our sexual arousal by stimulating the release of oxytocin. Also involved in sexual responsiveness and orgasm, the hormone oxytocin counteracts stress and depression by combatting the harmful effects of cortisol.

Besides being a natural stress-buster, oxytocin helps prevent normal stomach hunger from going out of control in your brain. According to a paper published in the journal *Progress in Brain Research* (2008), oxytocin causes a fundamental shift in motivational behavior, switching our physiological drive to find and consume food to the desire to reproduce.

Apart from sex, you can also boost your oxytocin levels by getting a massage, spending time with a good friend or hugging someone you care about. Sex also provides a nice dose of dopamine, which increases steadily to the point of orgasm and then declines, also helping to curb our need to feed. Apparently, the dopamine pathways in the brain involved in stimulating desire for both sex and food are shut down by the hormones released immediately after we have an orgasm. Can you imagine better news for appetite and craving control?

Step 5: Use Supplements to Balance Brain Chemistry and Beat Stress

Supplements can provide immeasurable help in reducing cravings and reining in appetite-boosting hormones, especially in the first few months of your diet, or until the brain pathways involved in carb cravings and addiction are subdued. If you suspect you have an addiction to carbs or a tendency toward emotional eating, the following supplements will help you to restore balance, cut cravings, improve your mood, reduce stress and help break the cycle of carbohydrate addiction. I recommend trying one to two of the recommended formulations below for a minimum of 1 to 2 consecutive months in order to accurately judge its effectiveness on your brain chemistry.

If you are unsure of the hormone that you need to balance with the help of supplements, take the following quiz. Give yourself one point for every symptom that you check off. A high score on a particular group of symptoms or risk factors may indicate that this hormonal imbalance is contributing to your carb addiction.

HORMONAL IMBALANCE: LOW GABA

☐ PMS characterized by breast tenderness, water retention, bloating, anxiety, sleep disruptions or headaches
☐ Feeling wired at night
☐ Aches and pains or increased muscle tension
☐ Irritability, tension or anxiety
☐ Difficulty falling asleep
☐ Irritable bowel
☐ Frequent gas and bloating

TOTAL _____ (Warning score: > 4 points)

TREATMENT OPTIONS FOR LOW GABA:

1. GABA. Ideal for individuals who experience anxiety, muscle tension or pain. Take 500 to 1,000 mg before bed. Alternatively, you can take GABA 10 to 20 minutes before your evening meal for appropriate absorption. The standard dose of 200 mg three times daily can be increased to a maximum of 450 mg three times daily, if needed, but this dosage should not be exceeded.
2. Clear Calm—GABA Enhancing Formula (Clear Medicine). Clear Calm is an effective blend of critical amino acids and nutrients that provide support for a calmer mind. It includes inositol, which contributes to muscular and nerve function, and GABA, which regulates growth hormone synthesis, sleep cycles and body temperature. Another ingredient, glycine, plays an

important role in the activity of certain neurotransmitters. Take 1 to 3 capsules before bedtime.

3. Taurine. This amino acid plays a major role in the brain as an inhibitory neurotransmitter. Similar in structure and function to GABA, taurine provides an antianxiety effect that helps calm or stabilize an excited brain. Taurine also decreases carbohydrate cravings and aids the release of insulin. Further, it supports healthy fat metabolism in the liver and is a potent antioxidant. Taurine is also effective for treating migraines, insomnia, agitation, restlessness, irritability, alcoholism, obsessions, depression and even hypomania/mania (the "high" phase of bipolar disorder or manic depression). In a study on diabetic rats, published in the *American Journal of Clinical Nutrition* (January 2000), taurine significantly decreased both weight and blood sugar in animal subjects. A study published in *Biochemistry* (October 2008) revealed that taurine administered to diabetic rabbits resulted in a 30 percent decrease in blood sugar levels. While taurine's impact on insulin resistance in humans needs further study, these animal studies are promising. Take 500 to 1,000 mg a day, without food. Taking your last dose before bed is often most helpful.

HORMONAL IMBALANCE: LOW SEROTONIN

☐ PMS characterized by hypoglycemia, sugar cravings and/or depression
☐ Feeling wired at night
☐ Lack of sweating
☐ Poor memory
☐ Loss of libido
☐ Depression, anxiety, irritability or seasonal affective disorder
☐ Loss of motivation or competitive edge
☐ Low self-esteem
☐ Inability to make decisions

- [ ] Obsessive-compulsive disorder
- [ ] Bulimia or binge eating
- [ ] Fibromyalgia
- [ ] Increased pain or poor pain tolerance
- [ ] Headaches or migraines
- [ ] Cravings for sweets or carbohydrates
- [ ] Constant hunger or increased appetite
- [ ] Inability to sleep in no matter how late going to bed
- [ ] Irritable bowel
- [ ] Constipation
- [ ] Nausea
- [ ] Use of corticosteroids

TOTAL _____ (Warning score: > 5 points)

TREATMENT OPTIONS FOR LOW SEROTONIN:

1. 5-HTP. A derivative of tryptophan that also contributes to the creation of serotonin, 5-HTP has been found to be more effective than tryptophan in treating sleep loss related to depression, anxiety and fibromyalgia. 5-HTP appears to increase REM sleep. It also decreases the amount of time required to fall asleep, as well as the number of nighttime awakenings. Take 50 to 400 mg a day, divided into doses throughout the day and before bed. This product should be taken for at least 4 to 6 weeks before reaching optimal benefit.

2. Clear Mood—Serotonin Support Formula (Clear Medicine). Clear Mood supports optimal serotonin levels. It also contains cofactor vitamins to enhance the production of serotonin from 5-HTP. Take 1 to 3 capsules daily, on rising or before bed. I usually suggest before bed to avoid the nausea that sometimes occurs when you take this product on an empty stomach (although this is usually what's required for optimal effectiveness). This product should be taken for at least 4 to 6 weeks for maximum benefit.

3. Inositol. Naturally present in many foods, inositol improves the activity of serotonin in the brain. As a supplement, it is an excellent choice for alleviating anxiety and depression, and supporting nervous system health. I like a product called Cenitol from Metagenics—a powdered form that can be easily added to my morning smoothie. Take 4 to 12 grams a day. When mixed with magnesium, inositol is very effective for calming the nervous system.

HORMONAL IMBALANCE: LOW DOPAMINE

☐ Fatigue, especially in the morning
☐ Poor tolerance for exercise
☐ Restless leg syndrome
☐ Poor memory
☐ Parkinson's disease
☐ Depression
☐ Loss of libido
☐ Feeling a strong need for stimulation or excitement (foods, gambling, partying, sex, etc.)
☐ Addictive eating or binge eating
☐ Cravings for sweets, carbohydrates, junk food or fast food

TOTAL _____ (Warning score: > 4 points)

TREATMENT OPTIONS FOR LOW DOPAMINE:

1. L-tyrosine. Tyrosine is an amino acid, a building block of dopamine, norepinephrine and thyroid hormones in the body, and a supplement available at most health-food stores. It takes 4 weeks to reach full effectiveness, so starting tyrosine at the beginning of a weight-loss program is a good idea, since studies show levels of dopamine decrease after a few weeks of being on a program to reduce weight. Seeing as tyrosine increases the production of both dopamine and thyroid

hormone, it could give you the boost you need to push past your plateau. Take 500 to 1,500 mg a day of L-tyrosine, away from food. Note: Do *not* take this supplement if you have high blood pressure or hyperthyroidism.

2. Clear Energy—Dopamine Support Formula (Clear Medicine). This is my formulation to provide nutritional support for increased brain energy, metabolic support, enhanced mood, appetite control and neurological functioning. Clear Energy has been specially formulated to support dopamine production for improved resistance to stress and increased vitality. I took this product as I was writing this book and found it to be very helpful. Take 2 to 3 capsules on rising and/or in the midafternoon.

HORMONAL IMBALANCE: EXCESS CORTISOL

- ☐ Wrinkling, thinning skin or skin has lost its fullness
- ☐ Feeling wired at night
- ☐ Heart palpitations
- ☐ Loss of muscle tone in arms and legs
- ☐ Cold hands or feet
- ☐ Water retention in face/puffiness
- ☐ Poor memory or concentration
- ☐ Loss of libido
- ☐ Depression, anxiety, irritability or seasonal affective disorder
- ☐ Frequent colds and flus
- ☐ Hives, bronchitis, allergies (food or environmental), asthma or autoimmune disease
- ☐ Fat gain around "love handles" or abdomen
- ☐ A "buffalo hump" of fat on back of neck/upper back
- ☐ Difficulty building or maintaining muscle
- ☐ Cravings for sweets or carbs, hypoglycemia or constant hunger
- ☐ Difficulty falling asleep

☐ Difficulty staying asleep (especially waking between 2 and 4 a.m.)

☐ Less than 7.5 hours of sleep per night

☐ Irritable bowel or frequent gas and bloating

☐ Use of corticosteroids

TOTAL _____ (Warning score: > 8 points)

TREATMENT OPTIONS FOR EXCESS CORTISOL:

1. Relora. Relora can significantly reduce cortisol and raise DHEA within only 2 weeks of use. Take 2 before bed and 1 in the morning to ease the effects of stress and improve your rest.

2. Clear Balance—Stress Modifying Formula (Clear Medicine). I love this formula; it's my favorite to keep cortisol in check, and my patients report that it works incredibly well for stress reduction and sleep. It is a unique blend containing two patent-pending herbal extracts specifically designed to support normal mental functioning during times of stress and anxiety. In addition to Relora, Clear Balance also contains added B vitamins and folic acid for enhanced effectiveness when compared to other Relora formulations. Clear Balance is a potent combination of herbs that have been proven to control irritability, emotional ups and downs, restlessness, tense muscles, poor sleep, fatigue and difficulty concentrating. It is very effective at boosting DHEA levels and reducing cortisol in patients with mild to moderate stress. Take 1 on rising and 2 before bed.

3. Rhodiola. This herbal supplement can enhance learning capacity and memory and may also be useful for treating fatigue, stress and depression. Research suggests rhodiola may enhance mood regulation and fight depression by stimulating the activity of serotonin and dopamine. Take 200 to 400 mg a day in the morning, away from food. Rhodiola is my favorite choice for reducing cortisol, increasing serotonin and dopamine, and

eliminating stress and anxiety, depression, cravings, fatigue, poor concentration and even symptoms of ADHD.

4. Phosphatidylserine (PS). This supplement is ideal for alleviating nighttime worrying. It curbs the inappropriate release of stress hormones and protects the brain from the negative effects of high cortisol. Take 200 to 300 mg before bed.

5. Ashwagandha. Ayurvedic practitioners use this herb to enhance mental and physical performance, improve learning ability, and decrease stress and fatigue. It can be used in stressful situations, especially for insomnia, restlessness or when you are feeling overworked. The typical dosage is 500 to 1,000 mg twice a day for a minimum of 1 to 6 months. Capsules should be standardized to 1.5 percent withanolides per dose. Ashwagandha is my favorite choice for reducing cortisol, increasing thyroid hormones and treating stress with a sluggish metabolism, anxiety, poor concentration and tension.

6. B vitamins. Endurance athletes and stressed or fatigued individuals should take extra B vitamins, especially vitamin B5, which helps the body adapt to stress and supports adrenal gland function. When taken at bedtime, vitamin B6 is also useful in correcting abnormally high cortisol release throughout the night. Vitamin B6 supports the production and function of serotonin in the brain. Take 200 to 500 mg of vitamin B5 and/or 50 to 100 mg of B6 every day, preferably before bed. These are often available in combination.

You have reached the end of Part One, which has taught you all you need to know about carbs, your metabolism, your appetite and how to beat a carb addiction. You are now prepped and ready to begin the CSP 6-week action plan. You are about to embark on a process that has the potential to improve your health at the most fundamental levels.

"Over the past year on the Carb Sensitivity Program, I have dropped 111 pounds! I am now completely off my antidepressants and my pain medication, with the aid of my doctor. I can't believe that I have no more cravings, late-night binges or hunger pangs. My blood pressure is a perfect 120/72, and my resting pulse is 79. I used to have to take an entire cocktail of drugs in order to fall asleep. I am now sleeping naturally from 11 p.m. to 7 a.m. and springing out of bed every morning. I have more energy now than when I was in my twenties. I have no doubt now that I will see 220 pounds on the scale one day soon. If I can do it, anyone can!"

ALAN, 54

STATS	BEFORE	AFTER
Weight	368 lb	259 lb
BMI	49.9	35.1

INITIAL CHIEF COMPLAINTS:

1. Obesity
2. Depression
3. Joint and muscle pain
4. Difficulty sleeping

PART TWO

THE 6-WEEK PRESCRIPTION FOR DETERMINING YOUR CARB SENSITIVITIES

Opportunity does not knock,
it presents itself when you beat down the door.

KYLE CHANDLER

CHAPTER 6

RULES TO LIVE BY:
THE DIETARY RULES COMMON TO
ALL SIX PHASES OF THE CSP

Quality is not an act, it is a habit.

ARISTOTLE

You may have been surprised to learn that dietary fat is not the main culprit that packs on pounds, raises cholesterol and boosts blood pressure—it's *carbohydrates* from all sources, including sugar, grain products, starchy vegetables and sweets. As explained in Part One, this is because carbohydrates lead to the release of insulin in our body. Insulin allows sugar from the bloodstream to enter our cells to be used as fuel. *Insulin is also the one and only hormone that is always instructing the body to store energy from food as fat.* More insulin, therefore, equals more body fat, especially around the abdomen. It can also cause a host of other health problems. If we are carbohydrate sensitive (CS), our body responds by releasing *more insulin*. The interesting variable that forms the foundation of this program is that *we each possess a tolerance for metabolizing carbohydrates that is unique to our physiology.*

During the coming weeks you will discover your body's unique sensitivity to carbohydrates. You will achieve this simply by switching 1 serving of carbohydrates (beans, grains or starchy vegetables), categorized according to their net carbs per serving, in your daily diet each week. Don't worry: You won't have to measure or calculate anything. I have done all the thinking for you and categorized your permitted food selections for each phase of the program.

This process is straightforward, and I will guide you step by step as you progress. Think of it as your "carb rehab" program. The quick overview is this: If you keep losing weight from one week to the next, you should continue the weekly carb-introduction process. If, however, you gain weight, retain water, experience cravings, feel a decrease in energy or experience any other symptom in the Carb Sensitivity Checklist (which follows the permitted food list for each phase in the next chapter), your current tolerance for carbohydrates has been exceeded.

If that happens, the introduction process should be halted and you should enter the Metabolic Repair Program outlined in Part Three. Completing this stage will restore your metabolism and ultimately *improve* your ability to process carbohydrates effectively. The extent of metabolic damage you have now will determine the length of time you need to remain in the Metabolic Repair Program. If damage is minimal, just 4 to 8 weeks could do the trick; however, I have seen patients who need to work on this phase for a year or more. Regardless of the length of time you require, the great news is that you may be able to return to eating carbs without gaining weight. There will even be a weekly cheat meal to make the whole process of metabolic repair a lot more effective, fun and sustainable!

Dietary Rules Common to All Phases of the Program

The ultimate goal of the CSP is to maintain a consistent blood sugar balance, which in turn allows for stable, low insulin levels. A secondary, but no less important, goal is to determine how many carbs your body can handle before your insulin spikes. In order to achieve these goals, the following rules *must* be followed during all phases:

1. **Keep a complete daily diet diary.** You must record *everything* you eat and drink daily. You should also keep a record of your workouts, water intake and sleep habits.
2. **Weigh yourself at the beginning of the program and then at least once a week,** at the same time and under the same circumstances

(for example, in the morning, without clothing, and on the same scale, prior to eating or drinking anything and after emptying your bladder). Record the number in your diet diary. Some individuals like to weigh themselves daily, while others find it can become a fixation. I will leave your weighing frequency up to you but understand that it is one of the ways you will track your reaction to carbs.

3. **Eat the right foods.**

   - You must eat lean protein (P); low-glycemic carbohydrates, which, as we have learned, include fibrous vegetables and fruits (C); and healthy fats (F) at *every* meal and snack. Your choices in each of these categories for each phase are outlined, along with the meal plans, in the next chapter. Following this rule means you will never consume carbohydrates (C) (e.g., fruit) alone. You will always enjoy them with a protein (P) and fat (F) source, such as yogurt or nuts. Please refer to Appendix B for a list of possible protein sources for vegetarians and vegans.

   - Once you have reintroduced starchy carbs, I would like you to continue to limit starchy vegetables or grains at breakfast. Stick to protein for better appetite control and to avoid that midafternoon slump or craving. This means no more toast, cereal or oatmeal for breakfast. Eggs or a protein shake are best, but I have created a large selection of tasty recipes that accommodate each phase.

   - Eat fresh, locally grown organic produce and choose organic or wild sources of meat, fish, eggs and dairy whenever you can. Organic foods are free of added hormones and harmful pesticides and they are also proven to possess higher amounts of vitamins and minerals.

   - Certain foods do a super job of helping you keep insulin in check. Select these "insulin-sensitizing superfoods" as often as you can. You will find an overview of these foods beginning on page 118.

- Drink as much water as possible during the day, between meals. If you consume two glasses of water prior to each meal, you will lose more weight than those who do not, because it aids appetite control.

4. **Eat at the right times.**
   - Eat within 1 hour of rising and limit eating within the 3-hour period before bedtime, unless you absolutely have to. It's best to avoid skipping meals.
   - Eat every 2 to 3 hours, and enjoy your meals at the *same times* every day. It is proven that individuals who do this have better blood sugar balance and lower insulin levels.
   - Always eat within 45 minutes of finishing your workout. This is vital for muscle growth and repair.
   - To ensure optimal performance and strength, never do your weight training on an empty stomach.
   - You may complete your cardio training before eating, if your session is 30 minutes or less.

5. **Avoid these foods 100 percent of the time:**
   - Processed meats and luncheon meats that contain harmful nitrites, sulfites, etc.
   - Trans fatty acids (hydrogenated oils, partially hydrogenated oils, shortenings, margarines) and unhealthy inflammatory fats (vegetable oils, soy oil, peanut oil, cottonseed oil and palm oil). Limit your intake of flax oil, safflower oil and sunflower oil, which can become inflammatory in excess.
   - Peanuts, unless they are organic and free of aflatoxin (which will be stated on the label), a naturally occurring toxin
   - Fructose-sweetened foods or foods containing high-fructose corn syrup (HFCS)
   - Foods and drinks containing aspartame or any other artificial sweeteners

- Farmed salmon
- Foods containing artificial coloring, preservatives, sulfites and nitrites

Once you are following the rules each day and consuming the permitted foods and serving sizes outlined in each phase, you will then use my instructions to guide you through the CSP. Don't worry, complete instructions and a CSP Flowchart to clearly guide you are also repeated at the end of each phase in the next chapter.

A Few of the Most Common CSP Questions Answered
What can I expect to feel when I begin the CSP?
Headaches, fatigue, irritability and general malaise are common for as many as 2 to 5 days at the beginning of the diet, as your body is doing a lot of housecleaning. Allow yourself time to rest if you feel sluggish. Drink lots of water (at least 8 cups daily) and take extra vitamin C to reduce any detox or carb-withdrawal symptoms. Reverse osmosis water is best (check the Resource section for my recommendation); spring water should be your second choice. Distilled water should be avoided because it may leach minerals out of your body. If using bottled water, I prefer the Fiji brand. Even though it is not reverse osmosis, it is alkaline, which aids metabolism and overall health by assisting our natural pH balance. Interestingly, I have prescribed this water to patients with chronic bladder problems or other conditions and it has provided relief.

By the third or fourth day, you should feel your energy increasing and mental focus improving. If you typically drink a lot of coffee, decrease the amounts you consume slowly throughout the first few days to minimize the effects of caffeine withdrawal. Unlike the Hormone Diet detox, you need to avoid caffeine only during Phase One, which lasts for 1 week. But, once reintroduced, should you choose to do so, your daily coffee must remain free of sugar and artificial sweeteners. If you experience increased cravings, sleep disruption or blood sugar imbalance once caffeine is reintroduced into your diet, then I would skip the java. Go for green tea instead.

If you need encouragement and motivation to keep you on track, remember this: *The more severe your detox reactions or carb withdrawal, the more you really needed it!*

Can I exercise while following the CSP?

If you usually exercise, continue with your current routine. Keep in mind that headaches, fatigue or feelings of malaise are common during the first few days. If you experience these symptoms, allow your body to rest, and select less-intense forms of exercise such as yoga, walking or Pilates. And be sure to keep drinking plenty of water.

If you are not exercising at this point, *and you are not ready to commit to continuing to do so,* now is not the time to dive into an intensive workout regimen. Trying to take on too much at once is not advantageous, especially at this stage, when we are determining your carb sensitivities. For now, your workout will focus mostly on walking. In fact, I would like you to take a walk every day, even if only for 15 or 20 minutes.

From this point on, *walking should be part of your life.* Even a short stroll can be a simple and highly beneficial way to avoid cheating and falling off your diet, and lessen the harmful effects of stress and fatty foods on your body. Studies prove that walking after an unhealthy meal can curb the effects of stress by reducing the amounts of fatty acids, sugars and stress hormones that are released into the bloodstream and subsequently stored as fat. Plus, this gentle form of exercise strengthens nearly every aspect of your body. Even a leisurely walk can prevent heart disease and offer excellent stress-reducing effects. Exercise also promotes relaxation and improves the quality of your sleep.

Can I dine out on the CSP?

Yes, you can still dine out. Simply stick to the permitted foods of the phase you are in and always be carb conscious. Salads, most vegetable dishes, stir-fries, seafood and grilled chicken, fish or turkey are all fine, but keep an eye out for hidden sugars and unhealthy oils in sauces, soups and dressings. I often find ordering two or three appetizers can help me to successfully avoid starchy dishes while still consuming enough protein. They also provide a nice variety of tastes and textures. Don't be afraid to ask your server for specific details about what you're ordering. Many restaurants will prepare menu items tailored to your requests (for example, no sauce or dressing). You should absolutely avoid fast-food restaurants, unless you are picking up a salad.

What should I do if I experience constipation during the CSP?

If things are not "moving along" properly at least once (optimally, two to three times) per day, it is tough to feel healthy, let alone slim. Obvious negative issues associated with constipation include feeling bloated, abdominal discomfort, occasional cramping and abdominal distension.

Constipation is not only unpleasant but also can impact other aspects of your health. Simply stated, the longer waste remains in your large intestine, the longer undesirable by-products of digestion and elimination will be permitted to reabsorb into your system. This stagnation can result in headaches, fatigue, increased menstrual pain and cramping, acne and other signs of toxicity. Some evidence suggests chronic constipation can even increase the risk of certain types of cancers. Breast and colon cancer rates, for example, have been found to be higher in women with a history of chronic constipation. I encourage you to take action right away if there is a pattern of constipation in your past, or if you experience constipation in response to reducing grains in your diet.

In my opinion, it is always better to ease constipation without the use of laxatives—even herbal ones such as senna and cascara—if possible. Dependency on laxatives is common with chronic use, and some laxatives can be irritating to the digestive tract lining. Laxatives can also act as a diuretic and cause loose stools. This leads to fluid and electrolyte loss, which in turn places stress on the body's ability to maintain hydration and may result in muscle cramps as potassium and magnesium are depleted. Over time, dehydration and electrolyte imbalance put stress on all internal organs. I formulated Clear Detox—Digestive Health to keep the digestive system moving without any laxatives. It contains 1,000 mg of vitamin C and 200 mg of magnesium, which not only benefit bowel regularity but also have added benefits for your blood sugar and insulin balance. Most people who take this product during their program report their digestion feels great, their sleep is better and, when used in combination with Clear Detox—Hormonal Health, their energy and cravings are improved too.

Keeping your bowels moving regularly is critical at all times. Because you are removing grains, legumes and starchy vegetables—our high-fiber foods—in Phase One, constipation is not uncommon. During this phase, a fiber supplement with 7 to 9 grams of fiber per serving is a necessity. Try one or more of these solutions if you find you need some additional help:

- **Take a probiotic supplement.** The friendly bacteria *Lactobacillus acidophilus* live in our digestive tract. Healthy bacterial balance in our digestive tract is easily affected by poor dietary habits and by the use of medications, such as birth control pills, corticosteroids and antibiotics. Everyone can benefit from the use of probiotics for healthy digestion, regular bowel function and immunity. Healthy bacterial balance is also essential for the breakdown and elimination of estrogen. If a bacterial imbalance is present, estrogen may not be properly broken down and removed from the body, resulting in symptoms such as PMS and other hormonal imbalances. Look for a supplement with 10 to 15 billion cells per capsule, and take it on rising, before breakfast. Clear Flora, a high potency probiotic, is included in the CSP Kit, which is explained in Chapter 8. The complete kit or individual products can be ordered from my Web site www.carbsensitivity.com.

- **Increase your intake of chia seed or flaxseed.** Add 1 or 2 tablespoons daily to your smoothies, salads or water. Whether you purchase them ground or grind your own, flaxseed should be kept in the freezer for maximum freshness.
- **Increase your vitamin C.** Take 3 to 8 grams of vitamin C (spread throughout the day, not all at once). Vitamin C is a natural laxative in higher doses.
- **Take magnesium citrate or glycinate.** This supplement can encourage bowel movements because it's a natural muscle relaxant. Take 200 to 800 mg per day, normally at bedtime. Start with a low dose and increase it gradually. As with vitamin C, do not take your magnesium all at once. However, I usually dose about 300 to 500 mg at bedtime.
- **Consider a fiber supplement.** Fiber not only promotes health but also can reduce the risk of certain chronic diseases such as colon cancer, breast cancer and heart disease. Fiber may help lower LDL cholesterol ("bad" cholesterol), total cholesterol and blood sugar, allowing better treatment and prevention of type 2 diabetes. It also may assist in weight loss. Insoluble fiber helps prevent constipation and promotes regular bowel movements. Foods such as green beans, flaxseed and cauliflower are high in insoluble fiber. A supplement such as Clear Fiber may also be helpful; it contains a mix of both insoluble and soluble fiber and offers 8 grams of fiber per serving, as compared to a couple tablespoons of ground flaxseed or chia seed, which contains only 4 grams.
- **Stay well hydrated.** Always drink 8 cups or more of water each day, between meals. A simple guideline is to drink 2 cups before each meal or snack.

- **Take essential fatty acids to help lubricate the bowels.** If you choose a liquid form, 1 tablespoon per day is usually sufficient. Good brands include Pure Encaps, Essential Balance oil, Nordic Naturals fish oils, Carlson fish oils or NutraSea extra strength fish oils from Signature Supplements. All of these come in liquid form, and many are available in capsules. Liquid forms should be kept in the freezer. If you choose capsules, take 2 to 4 capsules twice a day with food. If you find that fish oil "repeats," put the bottle in the freezer and take it with food, or purchase an enteric-coated formula. Clear Omega high-potency fish oil, in enteric-coated capsules, is also included in the basic CSP Kit.

What can I do about sugar or carb cravings during the CSP?

The five-step prescription for beating carb addiction outlined in Chapter 5 will help solve your carb-craving dilemma over the long haul. But what about *right now?* Many of us experience short-term cravings for sweets, especially late at night, during that midday slump or (for the ladies) just before a menstrual cycle. The causes of these cravings can vary widely, but chief among them are hormonal imbalances, especially low blood sugar (hypoglycemia) and low serotonin levels (common in the winter or with depression or anxiety). These imbalances can be brought on by stress, sleep deprivation, poor eating habits or unbalanced nutrition. If your blood sugar and insulin levels are balanced, you should be free of cravings. In fact, cravings or increased appetite is one of the symptoms I ask you to pay attention to during your CSP process. A recurring pattern of either may indicate your insulin has spiked. And it's not all about the food. Sometimes additional help is needed; lifestyle factors such as stress or sleep deprivation can contribute to pesky sweet cravings, regardless of your best dietary efforts.

You can use one or more of the following simple tips to help keep you on your diet plan, while satisfying your urge to splurge.

TO CURB YOUR CRAVINGS:

- Reach for frozen berries. A ¼ cup serving feels like a frozen treat. It's hard to eat too many and, because they are frozen, you have to eat them more slowly.
- Sip some herbal tea. Those with fruit flavors tend to be more satisfying, and the warm drink will raise your body temperature, which helps appetite and craving control.
- Take glutamine. Open a 500 mg capsule under the tongue to beat your cravings.
- Chew vitamin C tablets. One or two are sweet enough to get you through, while also providing health benefits.
- Try Nusera lozenges from Metagenics. These chocolate-flavored treats contain hydrolyzed milk protein extract, which lowers cortisol and quickly helps to reduce stress, anxiety and tension. (I have two of these before every media interview or lecture.) High stress is a known cause of cravings and weight gain. Enjoy no more than three per day.

TO PREVENT CRAVINGS IN THE FIRST PLACE:

- Make sure you are getting enough protein at each meal. Revisit the allowed proteins and recommended serving sizes in the Foods to Enjoy list for your current phase presented in the next chapter.
- Never miss your afternoon snack. This mini-meal will help balance your blood sugars so you avoid the dreaded "afternoon slump" that often makes us reach for junk food. This snack will also help you achieve greater weight loss.
- Be sure to keep hidden sugars from sneaking into your diet. Be on the lookout for drinks, flavored yogurts, low-fat packaged foods, energy bars, granola bars, sauces, dressings and other processed foods. Most are loaded with extra sugar.

- Increase your fiber intake. Fiber will help you feel fuller longer, and you'll feel more satisfied. Add ground flaxseed or chia seed to your meals, or purchase a nonpsyllium fiber supplement to add to your smoothies.
- Improve your sleep and consider a natural sleep aid, if necessary (see page 80). Sleep deprivation is proven to increase our appetite, particularly our cravings for sweets.

THE CSP TOP TWELVE INSULIN-SENSITIZING SUPERFOODS

Patients ask me all the time if there is a magic supplement they can take to look younger, shed body fat, boost energy or improve their skin. Most are shocked to learn that the answer is food! The right foods, at the right times and in the right quantities, can have a dramatic effect on your appearance and overall health. Following is a list of twelve functional foods that help to improve insulin sensitivity and balance blood sugars, which makes them ideal components of the Carb Sensitivity Program.

Blueberries. Free radicals in the body cause cellular damage, accelerate aging and contribute to the development of diseases such as cancer and Alzheimer's. Antioxidants fight free radical damage, and blueberries are absolutely loaded with them. They contain fiber, which when combined with antioxidants, will keep you feeling full and looking younger. Blueberries are low in naturally occurring sugars, and contain a potent dose of proanthocyanidins beneficial for skin, cognitive function and cardiovascular health. According to a groundbreaking study published in the *Journal of Nutrition* (2010), a daily dose of the bioactive ingredients from blueberries also increases sensitivity to insulin and may reduce the risk of developing diabetes in at-risk individuals. Researchers discovered that obese, nondiabetic and insulin-resistant participants who consumed a blueberry smoothie daily for 6 weeks experienced a 22 percent change in insulin sensitivity, compared to only 4.9 percent in the placebo group. These results put blueberries at the top of my insulin super-food list.

Whey protein isolate. Protein is essential for immunity, maintaining healthy body composition, blood sugar balance, tissue repair and muscle growth. Adding just a bit of whey protein to your meal will also *reduce* your food intake. According to research from the University of Toronto, published in the *Journal of the American College of Nutrition* (2007), whey protein can contribute to the regulation of body weight by providing satiety signals that affect both short- and long-term food intake regulation. Whey protein is considered to be one of the best sources of branched-chain amino acids, especially leucine, which is unique in its ability to initiate muscle protein synthesis. Researchers at McMaster University discovered that study participants who consumed 10 grams of whey protein with 21 grams of fructose following resistance exercise exhibited a greater ability to repair and build muscle compared to a group that consumed an equal amount of carbohydrates only (remember from *The Hormone Diet* that weight training improves your insulin sensitivity, and postworkout your insulin receptors are primed to accept carbohydrates). Whey protein is not only good for you, but also tastes great.

Avocados. Avocados contain glutathione, one of the most potent antioxidants and disease-fighting agents available. High in monounsaturated fats, avocados got an undue bad rap during the recent low-fat era. Yet studies show that people sustain their nutrition program longer and see greater weight loss on a diet that contains about 30 percent healthy monounsaturated fat, such as that found in avocados, rather than a strictly low-fat diet. This is because fats, when eaten in the proper balance with carbohydrates, can help to slow the release of sugars into the bloodstream, which leads to less insulin release. Avocados also contain a unique weight loss–friendly carbohydrate called mannoheptulose, which has been specifically found to lower insulin secretions.

Studies show that avocados are also rich in beta-sitosterol, a natural substance shown to significantly lower blood cholesterol levels. In an article published in the *American Journal of Medicine* (1999), researchers discovered that beta-sitosterol reduced cholesterol in 16 human studies. Another wonderful benefit of beta-sitosterol is that it helps to balance cortisol, even during exercise. It may also help to restore low DHEA and decrease the inflammation typically associated with the stress of intense exercise. Despite all these benefits, fat does have twice the amount of calories as carbs or protein, so limit your avocado consumption to one-quarter at a time, enjoyed as a healthy fat source with a meal.

Chia seed. This ancient gluten-free grain can be added to just about any food. On a per gram basis, chia is touted to be the highest source of omega-3s in nature, with 65 percent of its total fat from omega-3 fatty acids. It is also a substantial source of fiber, as well as magnesium, potassium, folic acid, iron and calcium. Chia stabilizes blood sugar, manages the effects of diabetes, improves insulin sensitivity and aids symptoms related to metabolic syndrome, including imbalances in cholesterol, blood pressure and high blood sugar after meals. It is highly anti-inflammatory and reduces high-sensitivity C-reactive protein, a blood marker of inflammation. This wondrous little grain also contains tryptophan, the amino acid precursor of serotonin and melatonin. Add 1 to 2 tablespoons to your meals, salads or smoothies daily.

Flaxseed. Flaxseed, a must-have in your smoothie-making arsenal, is rich in thiamin, magnesium, copper, phosphorus and manganese. Flaxseed's high fiber content helps lower blood sugar, improve cholesterol levels and aid weight loss. Flaxseed is also full of lignans—phytoestrogenic compounds that have been proven to help protect us against certain kinds of cancers, especially of the breast, prostate and colon. Adding 2 to 3 tablespoons of flaxseed to your smoothies, oatmeal, salads or cereals daily can reduce your cancer risk and also provide a healthy hit of fiber and essential fatty acids. The oils in flaxseed can go rancid quickly, so be sure to purchase ground flaxseed in a vacuum-sealed package and store it in the freezer. Better yet, you can grind your own daily.

Spices. It turns out that your favorite spice mix not only helps your food taste great but also can reduce your waistline. According to the *Journal of Medicinal Food* (2005), a food seasoning spice mixture containing various spices improved glucose and cholesterol metabolism in rats fed a high-fructose diet to increase their insulin levels. Treatment with these spices significantly reduced blood sugar and insulin levels and improved blood-cholesterol balance. Additional research published in the *Research Journal of Pharmaceutical, Biological and Chemical Sciences* (2010) confirmed the antidiabetic effect of various spices. In particular, fenugreek seeds, garlic, onion and turmeric have been documented to possess antidiabetic potential by either lowering blood sugar or reducing insulin. In a limited number of studies, cumin seeds, ginger, mustard, curry leaves and coriander have been reported to help lower blood sugar, which is always great for lowering insulin too. This is very promising if you like a little spice in your life.

Olive oil. Olives and olive oil are rich in antioxidant compounds called polyphenols, which are known to have anti-inflammatory, anticancer and anticoagulant benefits. Olive oil also provides a rich source of plant sterols to curb inflammation, aid hormonal balance and control cholesterol. But the weight-loss benefits of olive oil could be what is most exciting. When we include monounsaturated fats such as olive oil (and avocados) in our daily diet, they encourage the release of our appetite-suppressing hormone leptin. Olive oil, in particular, has been shown to improve our sensitivity to insulin. In a study published in the July 2007 issue of *Diabetes Care*, 11 subjects with insulin resistance and increased abdominal fat used three different diets for 28 days. Each diet had equal calories but different compositions: One was a high saturated-fat diet, the second was high in carbohydrates and the third was rich in monounsaturated fats. At the end of the 28-day period, researchers measured the effects of each diet on body-fat distribution, insulin resistance and levels of adiponectin, a hormone released by our fat cells and known to improve insulin sensitivity, reduce inflammation and offer protection against obesity and metabolic syndrome. Of the three diets, the one rich in olive oil showed the best outcome, preventing not only belly fat accumulation but also insulin resistance and the drop in adiponectin typically seen in people who eat a high carbohydrate diet.

Olive oil helps you not only lose weight but also keep it off. In a 2007 study published in the *Journal of the American College of Nutrition*, weight maintenance was best with an olive oil–rich diet, especially when this fat was consumed at breakfast. Improved fasting insulin, blood sugar balance (after meals), good HDL cholesterol and other signs of insulin balance were noted in the 12 insulin-resistant subjects who participated in the study. If you do not enjoy the taste of olive oil, consider my supplement

Glyci-Med Forte. Patients who take 2 capsules at breakfast daily enjoy better appetite control, fewer cravings and greater loss of belly fat.

Cinnamon. Just a little cinnamon in your smoothies or on top of your oatmeal can go a long way toward balancing your insulin levels. A study published in the journal *Diabetes Care* (2003) showed that cinnamon may cause muscle and liver cells to respond more readily to insulin, thereby improving weight loss. Better response to insulin means better blood sugar balance and, therefore, less insulin in your body. Cinnamon also seems to reduce several risk factors for cardiovascular disease, including high blood sugar, triglycerides, LDL cholesterol and total cholesterol. Just ½ teaspoon a day for 20 days is enough to improve your insulin response and lower blood sugar by up to 20 percent. An additional research group from the Beltsville Human Nutrition Research Center found that cinnamon reduced blood sugar, total cholesterol and LDL cholesterol in subjects with type 2 diabetes after just 40 days of consuming 1 to 6 grams per day.

Eggs. Believe it or not, our grandparents had it right—eggs for breakfast, regardless of how you prepare them, improve appetite control and boost energy levels. In a 2005 study published in the *Journal of the American College of Nutrition,* researchers found that participants who consumed eggs for breakfast had greater feelings of satiety and consumed significantly fewer calories at lunch. In fact, calorie intake following the egg breakfast remained lower for the entire day, as well as for the next 36 hours. In a second study, published in the *International Journal of Obesity* (2008), overweight and obese subjects given two eggs a day for breakfast lost 65 percent more weight than those eating a similar breakfast without eggs. The researchers concluded that eating eggs may control hunger by reducing the postmeal insulin response and control appetite by preventing large fluctuations in both glucose and insulin levels.

Cherries. Cherries are the new wonder food, and not just because they taste great and can satisfy your urge for something sweet. This fruit contains red-pigmented antioxidants, is high in soluble fiber and is low in calories, all of which can help improve insulin sensitivity. Scientists have identified a group of naturally occurring chemicals called anthocyanins, abundant in cherries and other red fruits, that may help to lower blood sugar levels in people with diabetes. In early studies published in the American Chemical Society's *Journal of Agricultural and Food Chemistry*, anthocyanins were found to reduce insulin production by 50 percent. Anthocyanins are also potent antioxidants, which may protect against heart disease and cancer. This research is promising for both the prevention of type 2 diabetes and for helping control glucose levels in those who already have diabetes.

Vinegar. Research has found that your salad dressing may play a role in your glucose levels following your meal. According to a 2005 study in the *European Journal of Clinical Nutrition,* vinegar has been found to blunt blood sugar and insulin increases, and increase the sensation of fullness after a higher-carbohydrate meal. The study, conducted at the Department of Nutrition at Arizona State University, found that each of the groups showed improved blood sugar and insulin profiles following meals that started with a vinegar drink. In subjects with type 2 diabetes who drank vinegar, blood sugar concentrations were cut by about 25 percent compared to those who consumed a placebo. In subjects with prediabetic conditions who drank vinegar, blood sugar concentrations were cut *by nearly half* compared to prediabetics who drank a placebo. And here's the most surprising result: Prediabetic subjects who drank vinegar actually had lower blood sugar levels than subjects with normal insulin sensitivity who also drank vinegar. The acetic acid that gives vinegar its tart taste improves postmeal insulin sensitivity, even in those who are currently insulin resistant. From white vinegar to apple cider vinegar, it's worth it to develop a taste for vinegar's sour bite. Just watch out for balsamic vinegar, which contains more sugar.

Nuts and nut butters. Nuts are not only tasty, but a great source of "good fats" such as monounsaturated and polyunsaturated fats, which reduce insulin resistance and improve cholesterol levels. Nuts are also rich in antioxidant vitamins, minerals, plant protein and dietary fiber. Researchers from the Harvard School of Public Health have found that women who consumed nuts or peanut butter five times a week or more significantly lowered their risk for type 2 diabetes compared to those who rarely or never ate nuts or peanut butter. In fact, the nut lovers *reduced their risk of type 2 diabetes by almost 30 percent* compared to those who rarely or never ate nuts. If you reach for nut butters, be sure to select natural, sugar-free types, and avoid peanut butter.

You may recall my two detox shakes from *The Supercharged Hormone Diet*. (I have repeated the recipes for you on pages 136–138.) One contains whey protein, fiber, cinnamon, ice (optional) and almond butter—3 of the 12 superfoods! The other contains blueberries, whey protein and fiber—2 insulin-sensitizing superfoods! No wonder they work so well.

Should I be concerned with body pH balance?

When your body becomes acidic, minerals such as potassium, sodium, magnesium and calcium may be stolen from your vital organs and bones to combat or buffer the acid. If these mineral losses and metabolic abnormalities continue, there is increased risk for a number of conditions including:

- Obesity, slow metabolism and inability to lose weight
- Chronic inflammation
- High blood pressure
- Weight gain, obesity and diabetes
- Bladder and kidney conditions, including kidney stones
- Weakened immunity
- Premature aging
- Osteoporosis; weak, brittle bones, fractures and bone spurs
- Joint pain, aching muscles and lactic acid buildup
- Low energy and chronic fatigue
- Mood swings
- Slow digestion and elimination
- Yeast/fungal overgrowth

If you have a health problem, you are likely a walking acid trip. No matter what type of therapy you choose to treat your condition, resolution will not come until your pH balance is restored. The pH scale runs from 0 to 14, and measures the acidity or alkalinity of a substance. A lower pH number means a higher level of acidity and generally indicates that less oxygen is present. A higher pH indicates a greater level of alkalinity. A solution is considered neutral, neither acid nor alkaline, when it has a pH of 7. Our body continually strives to maintain its normal pH balance of about 7.0–7.4. We experience health problems when the pH of our body fluids, digestive system and tissues is pushed out of its comfortable neutral zone.

You will enjoy the most dramatic results from the CSP process when your body is slightly alkaline. Acidity decreases your body's ability to absorb the vitamins and minerals from your foods and supplements. It interferes with your ability to detoxify. It disrupts your metabolism and it makes you more prone to fatigue and mood changes.

You can test your body fluids (saliva or urine) using litmus paper strips purchased from your local health-food store. Test your pH first thing in the morning or 1 hour before a meal or 2 hours after eating.

For the saliva test: *Before* brushing your teeth, fill your mouth with saliva and swallow; repeat once; *spit directly on the pH test strip.* This three-step process will ensure a clean saliva sample. Measure your saliva pH in the same manner again later in the day, at least 2 hours after eating.

To do the urine test: Collect a small sample of your first morning urine in a clean glass container, then dip the pH strip in the container.

Quickly, match your strip to the associated color on the package of pH papers to determine your body pH. Ideally your pH strip should turn the same color matched with 7.2–7.4 on the package (usually dark green or bluish depending on the brand of pH papers you purchase).

What's normal?

If the pH of your saliva stays between 7.0 and 7.4 all day, your body is functioning within a healthy range. If your urinary pH fluctuates between 6.0 and 6.5 in the morning and 6.5 and 7.0 in the evening, your body is within a healthy pH range. First morning urine should be slightly more acidic as you eliminate waste accumulated throughout the night. Continue to measure your pH daily if your values are abnormal, otherwise testing once a week will suffice.

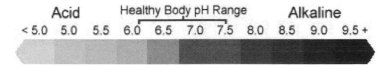

	Acid			Healthy Body pH Range				Alkaline		
< 5.0	5.0	5.5	6.0	6.5	7.0	7.5	8.0	8.5	9.0	9.5 +

The nutritional approach of the CSP, along with the recommended supplements, are often enough to restore optimal pH balance. If you find, however, that your pH does not improve, add fresh lemon juice to your water daily. You may also consider a pH balance supplement, which is available at your local health-food store.

Do I need to pay attention to nutrition labels?

In short, yes. You should read the label of all food selections whenever a label is present. I have outlined my approach for carb-conscious shopping below. But you can skip the label-reading work too if you wish, and enjoy a hormone-friendly shopping experience by referring to Chapter 8 of *The Supercharged Hormone Diet*. There I have identified your best selection in each grocery store—soups, dressings, breads, cereals and more—according to their protein, fat and carbohydrate content, as well as your permitted ingredients. Whenever possible, stick to the brands I have recommended and ensure the item fits the phase of the CSP that you are in. I have done a lot of research and evaluation to find the products that best suit your intake guidelines.

Here are some additional tips for every shopping trip:

- **Read the ingredients.** If the product contains any hormone-hindering ingredients that you are to avoid 100 percent of the time (such as high-fructose corn syrup, hydrogenated oils, artificial sweeteners, etc.), put it back on the shelf.
- **Check the serving size for the nutrition information provided.** Sometimes foods look as though they are a good choice for you, but only because the serving size used to report the nutrition values is completely unrealistic. A serving size of five potato chips, for example, doesn't make much sense based on the amount most of us would really eat in a sitting.
- **Check the carbohydrates.** First, make sure the source of the carbohydrates is permitted for your dietary phase. For

instance, reading the carbohydrate content in a sweet potato soup is pointless unless you are in Phase Five or Six, in which consuming sweet potatoes is permitted. Read the amount listed on the label and measure it against the total amount of carbohydrate you should consume per meal and snack (see the next page). If the product contains a lot more than these amounts, look for something else.

- **Check the amount of protein.** Remember this simple guideline: If the product contains equal amounts of protein and carbohydrate or *more* protein than carbs per serving, it is a good choice for you. For example: Vanilla soy milk has 11 grams of carbs and 6 grams of protein; plain soy milk has 3 grams of carbs and 6 grams of protein. In this case, the plain soy milk is a much better bet. Also, compare the protein to the amount you need to consume in meals or snacks (specified on the next page).
- **Check the fat content.** Compare it to the total amount of fat you should consume in a meal or snack (see the next page). Check the saturated fat content, in particular, and aim for little to none.
- **Check the fiber content.** Products that contain fewer than 2 grams of fiber per serving are not great choices. If you have a number of brands to choose from, select the product that's highest in fiber.
- **Check the sodium content.** Products with fewer than 140 mg of salt are considered to be low-sodium choices. Remember, you should consume only 2,300 mg of sodium per day, which is equal to about 1 teaspoon of salt. When comparing products, pick the one that's lowest in sodium.
- **Check the calorie content.** About 300 to 500 calories per meal is a good guideline. But remember that the source of your calories is the most important factor, not the total calories you consume.

Optimize Your Protein, Carb and Fat Intake at Meals and Snacks

The numbers listed below are the only bits of information I expect you, just like my patients, to memorize, if you want to become truly nutrition savvy. In general, these numbers highlight how much you should eat at meals and snacks. Pay attention mostly to the meal sizes, since snacks are basically just half the amount listed for a meal.

You can be low on carbs at a meal or snack, but avoid being low on fat or protein. This simple habit optimizes your metabolism and improves appetite control. Review the ideal parameters below for selecting your meals and snacks. You will notice that many of the Phase One recipes have a slightly higher protein and fat content to make up for the removal of starchy carbs. Think of each meal as a full glass of water, split into three types of liquid—protein, fat and carbs. You always want to keep the same amount of water in the glass (i.e., the total number of calories) despite removing a portion of the liquid. Following this formula will help you maintain your metabolism. You may change the components in the meal slightly, but we always want to keep the glass "full" to keep our fat-burning furnace revving at all times. And the CSP will help you to determine which type of carbs should be included in your diet.

WOMEN		MEN	
MEALS (3)	SNACKS (2)	MEALS (3)	SNACKS (2–3)
Protein: 25–30 g	10–15 g	Protein: 35–40 g	15–20 g
Carbs: 20–30 g	15–20 g	Carbs: 30–40 g	15–20 g
Fats: 10–14 g	5–7 g	Fats: 14–18 g	7–8 g

If you eat a food that does not come with a nutrition label, you can look up its nutritional values on www.calorieking.com. I love

GET TO KNOW YOUR FATS

Remember, we need to eat healthy fat in order to lose body fat. The key is choosing the right fats and avoiding those that sit high on the list of hormone-hindering foods.

TYPE OF FAT	FOOD SOURCES	RISKS/BENEFITS
Monounsaturated fat	Olive oil, canola oil, peanut oil, avocados	Aids appetite control, lowers harmful LDL cholesterol, reduces inflammation, promotes heart health
Polyunsaturated fat	Vegetable oils such as soybean, corn, safflower and sunflower. Two types: Omega-3s: flaxseed oil, omega-3 eggs, deepwater fish and fish oil, walnuts and walnut oil Omega-6s: raw nuts, seeds, legumes, borage oil, grapeseed oil and primrose oil	Can lower good HDL cholesterol if eaten in excess; can promote inflammation. Balance of omega-6 to omega-3 is very important. Allergies, eczema, inflammatory conditions (e.g., arthritis, colitis), constipation, attention deficit disorder and other learning disabilities have all been linked to a deficiency of this precious fat.
Saturated fat	Red meats (beef, pork and lamb), dairy products. Note: Coconut oil is a saturated fat yet it is good for you.	Raises harmful LDL cholesterol and increases inflammation
Trans fats (may appear on labels as "hydrogenated" or "partially hydrogenated" fats)	Margarines, snack foods, many packaged foods, microwave popcorn and fried foods	Increase bad LDL cholesterol and decrease good HDL cholesterol. There is no safe level of intake for trans fats!

this site because it is user friendly and the information changes according to the serving size you select. For instance, it was here that I learned rapini was such a fabulous source of protein and fiber.

Armed with these rules that you must live by to balance your blood sugar, and subsequently insulin, you are ready to venture into the meal plans for the various CSP phases. Let me reiterate that these guidelines I have just shared are powerful, should you choose to implement them. I hope I have clearly answered most, if not all, of the questions you may have. However, if you have a question or concern that I have not touched on here, please feel free to post your inquiries or comments on our Facebook page at www.facebook.com /carbsensitivity. If you have a question, chances are other people are wondering the same thing too.

CSP SUCCESS STORY: SUZANNE

"I got married in April at the age of 34 and was pregnant by August. Unfortunately, I ended up having a miscarriage and two more after that. I had no problems getting pregnant; I just couldn't hold on to the pregnancies. I went to a fertility clinic and had a successful pregnancy and now have a beautiful baby boy who is 14 months old. However, I did not lose all of my baby weight and tried this year for 6 months straight at the fertility clinic to get pregnant again, with no luck. I started to see Dr. Natasha Turner, and she put me on the Carb Sensitivity Program. I lost 17 pounds in 6 weeks! I followed many of her delicious recipes and guidelines and had no cravings for sweets or carbs at all. After losing the weight and maintaining her program, I was again successful in becoming pregnant. I am now 6 months along and am still following Dr. Turner's program—and I feel great! I truly believe had I not gone on Dr. Turner's program and lost the weight from my first baby, I would not be pregnant today. I recommend it to anyone who is in my situation or looking to improve their health."

SUZANNE, 37

STATS	BEFORE	AFTER
Weight	140 lb	123 lb
BMI	23.3	20.5

INITIAL CHIEF COMPLAINTS:
1. Infertility
2. Thyroid problems
3. Excess weight

CHAPTER 7

THE CARB SENSITIVITY PROGRAM— WEEKLY MEAL PLANS AND PERMITTED FOOD LISTS

Always do your best.
What you plant now, you will harvest later.

OG MANDINO

It's now time to implement what you have learned and begin the journey that will uncover your carb sensitivities and restore your insulin balance. In this chapter, you will find your suggested meal plans. At the end of each 7-day phase, you will also find a handy list of permitted foods, along with recommended serving sizes. Carb-sensitizing recipes to accompany each phase, and my favorite time-saving tips, have been laid out for you in Part Four.

In general, this is how the CSP nutrition plan works:

- *Fat and protein selections remain the same through all six phases, and into your maintenance program.*
- *Carb intake from permitted fruits, nuts and nonstarchy vegetable options will also remain the same in all phases.*
- *Your starchy carbohydrate options will vary from one phase to the next.* For example, the first group of carbs you will introduce into your diet is sourced from a selection of starchy vegetables. Upon entering the next phase, these will be removed as an option and you will then choose from a selection of legumes. You must go through the CSP process exactly as prescribed; each phase has been scientifically designed to test your tolerance to a new group of carbs with progressively higher net-carb contents.

- *The new carb additions and other changes are shaded in each phase's permitted foods list, so you can easily identify the changes from one phase to the next.*
- *At the end of each phase, you will complete the Carb Sensitivity Checklist.* Your answers to this quiz will determine the dietary route you should follow next. You will either progress to the next phase of the plan, or be directed to the Metabolic Repair Program outlined in Part Three, which is designed to improve your level of carb sensitivity.
- *Each phase includes two snacks and three meals daily.* In addition to the snack recipes I have included in Part Four, you can use the following list of approved snack options or the Carb Sensitivity Shake, both of which require very little preparation time. I suggest avoiding the dairy options if they cause you digestive discomfort.
    - 2 servings of Cabot 75% reduced-fat Cheddar cheese or low-fat Jarlsberg cheese with a piece of permitted fruit
    - 1 small organic apple with 1 tablespoon almond butter
    - ½ cup of plain Fage Total 0% yogurt or goat yogurt with a piece of allowed fruit and 4 walnuts or 5 almonds
    - A Simply Bar or Simply Snack, if you want a lower-calorie option (available at most health-food stores or through our online store at www.carbsensitivity.com)
    - ½ cup berries mixed with ½ cup ricotta cheese
    - 12 tamari-roasted almonds with ½ cup blackberries
    - 2 hard-cooked eggs with a handful of veggie sticks such as celery, cucumber and green bell pepper
    - 2 to 3 slices of nitrite- and sulfite-free turkey or chicken with 1 tablespoon of almonds
    - 2 to 3 tablespoons pumpkin seeds
    - 7 walnuts with a piece of permitted fruit or ½ cup berries or 1 serving low-fat Swiss cheese

- 2 large tomato slices, topped with 1½ ounces Nu Tofu nonfat Cheddar cheese alternative and ¼ avocado
- 8 almonds and 1½ ounces firm tofu
- Blend ½ cup Fage Total 0% plain yogurt, ½ scoop whey protein isolate, 3 walnuts or 5 almonds, and ¼ cup raspberries or blackberries until smooth and creamy.
- One Protein Fusion Bar, Quest Protein Bar or homemade protein bar (see page 423)
- Select any smoothie recipe from the recipe section, split into two portions and place in the freezer for at least 1 to 2 hours. When you are ready to eat, simply remove one from the freezer, let thaw slightly, grab a spoon and enjoy! You can save the other half for another time.
- Mix ¼ cup berries with ½ cup cottage cheese and 1 tablespoon slivered almonds.
- The ingredients of the Carb Sensitivity Shakes have been selected because they lower insulin. Here are your four options:

OPTION #1

1	serving whey protein isolate, any flavor (or rice, hemp or vegan protein)
2	tablespoons ground flaxseed or chia seed or 1 serving of a fiber supplement (optional, but highly recommended)
1	tablespoon almond, hazelnut, cashew or pumpkin seed butter
¼	teaspoon cinnamon
½–¾	cup water or unsweetened almond milk

3–4   ice cubes (optional)

      Stevia (optional)

Place all ingredients in a blender and blend on high speed until smooth and creamy. Alternatively, you can toss all the ingredients except the water into a protein shaker cup. When you are ready for a snack, add the water, shake well and drink.

OPTION #2

1   serving whey protein isolate, any flavor (or rice, hemp or vegan protein)

½–¾   cup water or unsweetened almond milk

½   cup blueberries

2   tablespoons ground flaxseed or chia seed or 1 serving of a fiber supplement (optional, but highly recommended)

3–4   ice cubes (optional)

      Stevia (optional)

Place all ingredients in a blender and blend on high speed until smooth and creamy.

OPTION #3

1   serving whey protein isolate, any flavor (or rice, hemp or vegan protein)

1   scoop Clear Recovery

½–¾   cup water

Combine ingredients and drink. This is a great "on the go" option because it does not require a blender.

OPTION #4

½–¾   cup unsweetened almond milk

½   cup pitted fresh or frozen cherries

2   tablespoons ground flaxseed or chia seed or
     1 serving of a fiber supplement (optional, but
     highly recommended)
¾   cup Fage Total 0% plain yogurt or goat yogurt
     *Place all ingredients in a blender and blend on high until
     smooth and creamy.*

THE CSP METABOLIC MASTER BREW

½ to 1 organic lemon, juiced

1-inch piece of fresh gingerroot, peeled and sliced (you can leave
    this out completely or add more, if you wish)

A pinch (or more) of cayenne pepper

8 cups reverse osmosis water

Because this simple concoction offers such wonderful metabolic benefits, I had to give it an encore presentation in the CSP. (It first appeared in *The Supercharged Hormone Diet*, as the Supercharged Hormone Diet Detox Water.) While it may sound like a strange brew, consider this: The spices in this mixture increase metabolism, lower insulin, support digestion and improve liver function. Capsaicin, which is the active ingredient in cayenne, may boost sympathetic nervous system activity in a way that dampens hunger and caloric intake later in the day. This drink can be enjoyed hot or cold. Try to drink as many cups as possible per day of this flavorful formula.

Phase One Meal Plan and Permitted Foods List

Phase One of the Carb Sensitivity Program is designed to break your addiction to carbohydrates, stabilize your blood sugar and set you on the path toward improved insulin balance. It is the strictest of the six phases because all "starchy" carbs, including grains, legumes and starchy vegetables, are removed from the menu plan. In exchange, you will find the protein and fat content of some of the meals are higher, which will keep you feeling full and your fat-burning hormones primed. I promise you will not feel hungry. Note that there are also prescribed times for all your meals and snacks. Coffee and caffeinated tea (except green tea) should be avoided during this phase.

Feel free to mix and match snacks and meals from the meal plans. These suggestions are just for your guidance. The meals and snacks are interchangeable *within each phase*. Note that nutrition content per meal may vary slightly, depending on the brand of the food selected for recipes in all phases of the diet. You may also visit the Book Extras section of the Carb Sensitivity Program at www .carbsensitivity.com, or the Facebook page, for additional recipe options and tips for your success. Instructional videos on the CSP process may be found here as well.

During Phase One, your daily dietary sources of carbs will be derived from unlimited nonstarchy vegetables, 1 to 2 servings of low–GI fruits and 2 servings of nuts or nut butters per day. The complete list of Phase One foods to enjoy and foods to avoid is summarized on pages 147–150. Although the first few days may bring about the standard detox reaction symptoms for some—including headaches, fatigue or irritability—you should experience relief by day 3 to 5. At that time you will find that your cravings will cease, your hunger will subside, your moods will balance and your energy will increase, all as a result of stable blood sugar and lower insulin. As an added bonus, the scale will reflect your brand-new lifestyle— most people lose 2 to 8 pounds during Phase One.

Day 1

Breakfast (7 a.m. to 8 a.m.)
Awesome Avocado and Egg Breakfast (page 360)

Midmorning Snack (10 a.m.)
Carb Sensitivity Shake (page 419), or CSP–approved Snack
Options (pages 135–38)

Lunch (12 p.m. to 1 p.m.)
Blueberry Chicken Salad (page 365)

Midafternoon Snack (3 p.m. to 4 p.m.)
Carb Sensitivity Shake (page 419), or CSP–approved Snack
Options (pages 135–38)

Dinner (6 p.m. to 8 p.m. at the latest)
Selenium-boosting Shrimp and Salsa (page 376)

Bedtime (10 p.m. to 11 p.m. at the latest)

Day 2

Breakfast (7 a.m. to 8 a.m.)
Portobello Mushroom Omelette (page 361)

Midmorning Snack (10 a.m.)
Carb Sensitivity Shake (page 419), or CSP–approved Snack
Options (pages 135–38)

Lunch (12 p.m. to 1 p.m.)
Curry Chicken Soup, served cold or hot (page 377)

Midafternoon Snack (3 p.m. to 4 p.m.)
Carb Sensitivity Shake (page 419), or CSP–approved Snack
Options (pages 135–38)

Dinner (6 p.m. to 8 p.m. at the latest)
Wasabi Whitefish with Almond Crust (page 380)

Bedtime (10 p.m. to 11 p.m. at the latest)

Day 3

Breakfast (7 a.m. to 8 a.m.)
Breakfast Salsa Dish (page 364)

Midmorning Snack (10 a.m.)
Carb Sensitivity Shake (page 419), or CSP–approved Snack
Options (pages 135–38)

Lunch (12 p.m. to 1 p.m.)
Crispy Chicken and Lettuce Wraps (page 379)

Midafternoon Snack (3 p.m. to 4 p.m.)
Carb Sensitivity Shake (page 419), or CSP–approved Snack
Options (pages 135–38)

Dinner (6 p.m. to 8 p.m. at the latest)
Salmon with Spinach and Strawberry Salsa (page 381)

Bedtime (10 p.m. to 11 p.m. at the latest)

Day 4

Breakfast (7 a.m. to 8 a.m.)
Chocolate Banana Smoothie (page 351)

Midmorning Snack (10 a.m.)
Carb Sensitivity Shake (page 419), or CSP–approved Snack
Options (pages 135–38)

Lunch (12 p.m. to 1 p.m.)
Immunity-boosting Ginger Chicken (page 374)

Midafternoon Snack (3 p.m. to 4 p.m.)
Carb Sensitivity Shake (page 419), or CSP–approved Snack
Options (pages 135–38)

Dinner (6 p.m. to 8 p.m. at the latest)
Cauliflower and Kale Soup (page 382) with Turkey Breast

Bedtime (10 p.m. to 11 p.m. at the latest)

Day 5

Breakfast (7 a.m. to 8 a.m.)
Mint Chocolate Smoothie (page 352)

Midmorning Snack (10 a.m.)
Carb Sensitivity Shake (page 419), or CSP–approved Snack
Options (pages 135–38)

Lunch (12 p.m. to 1 p.m.)
Tuna Waldorf Salad (page 383)

Midafternoon Snack (3 p.m. to 4 p.m.)
Carb Sensitivity Shake (page 419), or CSP–approved Snack
Options (pages 135–38)

Dinner (6 p.m. to 8 p.m. at the latest)
Sautéed Shrimp and Green Beans (page 373)

Bedtime (10 p.m. to 11 p.m. at the latest)

Day 6

Breakfast (7 a.m. to 8 a.m.)
Strawberry Shortcake Smoothie (page 352)

Midmorning Snack (10 a.m.)
Carb Sensitivity Shake (page 419), or CSP–approved Snack
Options (pages 135–38)

Lunch (12 p.m. to 1 p.m.)
Baby Bok Choy and Chicken (page 375)

Midafternoon Snack (3 p.m. to 4 p.m.)
Carb Sensitivity Shake (page 419), or CSP–approved Snack
Options (pages 135–38)

Dinner (6 p.m. to 8 p.m. at the latest)
Spicy Pepper Salmon with Pear Salsa (page 384)

Bedtime (10 p.m. to 11 p.m. at the latest)

Day 7

Breakfast (7 a.m. to 8 a.m.)
Pepper and Spinach Omelette (page 363)

Midmorning Snack (10 a.m.)
Carb Sensitivity Shake (page 419), or CSP–approved Snack
Options (pages 135–38)

Lunch (12 p.m. to 1 p.m.)
Immunity-boosting Ginger Chicken (page 374)

Midafternoon Snack (3 p.m. to 4 p.m.)
Carb Sensitivity Shake (page 419), or CSP–approved Snack
Options (pages 135–38)

Dinner (6 p.m. to 8 p.m. at the latest)
Selenium-boosting Shrimp and Salsa (page 376)

Bedtime (10 p.m. to 11 p.m. at the latest)

Phase One: Summary of Foods to Enjoy and Avoid

Permitted carbs: 2 servings of nuts, unlimited nonstarchy vegetables, and 1 to 2 servings of low–GI fruit.

C = CARB, P = PROTEIN AND F = FAT

Foods to Enjoy and Suggested Serving Sizes

C: GRAINS AND STARCHY VEGETABLES

None of these foods are permitted this week.

C: FRUITS

> A maximum of 2 servings of fruit are allowed daily— 1 selection should be berries.

Cherries—12
Apricots—3
Prunes—3
Berries—½ cup
Peaches—1 small
Pears—1 small

Apples—1 small
Plums—1 small
Oranges—1 small
Kiwi—1 small
Grapefruit—1 whole
Watermelon—1 cup
Banana—½ (preferably in protein shakes only for less of an impact on blood sugars)

C: NONSTARCHY VEGETABLES

(1 to 2 cups per meal)
All green/nonstarchy vegetables: spinach, peppers, tomatoes, eggplant, zucchini, cauliflower, onion, leek, artichokes, broccoli, rapini, green beans, asparagus, etc.

C/P: LEGUMES

No legumes are permitted this week.

F/C/P: NUTS & SEEDS

(2 servings a day)
Walnuts—8
Cashews—6
Pistachios—15
Macadamia nuts—4

> Consider your nut selections primarily as the fat source in your snacks and meals, rather than as a protein source.

Almonds—10 to 12
Pecans—6 to 7
Seeds—2 to 3 tablespoons
Nut butters, preferably almond butter or pumpkin seed butter with no salt or sugar added— 1 tablespoon

P: PROTEINS

Chicken, turkey (including ground meats and sausage products)
Shellfish, fish
Liquid egg whites— ½ cup = 24 grams protein

> 3 servings the size and width of your palm, and 2 half-servings for snacks each day. For women: 4 ounces or 25–30 grams per meal. For men: 6 ounces or 35–40 grams per meal. Organic or free-range selections are best.

Eggs—Women: 2 whole eggs or 4 egg whites and 1 yolk. Men: 3 whole eggs or 6 egg whites and 1 yolk
Tofu or tempeh
Lamb
Bison and venison
Cottage cheese, ricotta cheese—½ cup for a snack, ¾ cup for a meal

P: PROTEINS *(continued)*

Organic pressed cottage cheese—
  ½ cup for a meal
Cabot 75% reduced-fat Cheddar
  (regular or habañero flavor) or
  low-fat Jarlsberg—2 ounces =
  meal; 1 ounce = snack
Fage Total 0% plain yogurt—
  1 cup = meal; ½ cup = snack
Fage Total Classic plain yogurt—
  1 cup = meal; ½ cup = snack
Lean red meat (preferably organic/
  grass fed)—
  1 serving per
  week

Protein Powder
Supplements
(must be free of
sugar and artificial
sweeteners)
100% whey
  protein isolate
  powder
Rice, pea or hemp
  protein powder

> **Protein bars** should contain 14–20 grams of protein and a maximum of 24 grams of net carbs, and must be free of sugar, harmful oils and artificial sweeteners. Maximum 1 per day as a meal replacement. Recommended brands include Protein Fusion Bar, UltraMeal Bar, Jay Robb Protein Bar, The Simply Bar and Quest Bar.

F/C/P: DAIRY AND SUBSTITUTES

Plain soy milk
  (unsweetened)—½ cup
Almond milk—¾ cup
Goat's milk, goat cheese, sheep
  cheese—1 tablespoon
Goat yogurt—½ cup

F: OILS

(3 to 4 servings a day)
Olive oil (must have daily)—
  1 tablespoon
Avocado—⅛ to ¼
Mayonnaise (canola or olive-oil
  based)—1 teaspoon
Olives—5 to 6
Butter—1 teaspoon
Flaxseed (ground)—1 to
  3 tablespoons
Omega-3 egg yolks—2 for women;
  3 for men
Organic coconut butter/oil—
  1 tablespoon

SPICES AND CONDIMENTS

All spices, unless otherwise
  indicated, are allowed. Examples
  include: carob, cinnamon, cumin,
  dill, garlic, ginger, oregano,
  parsley, rosemary, tarragon,
  thyme, turmeric, etc.
Mustards free of sugar
Mayonnaise and salad dressings
  (canola or olive-oil based) are
  allowed, but consider these as a
  fat source

DRINKS

Sodium-free soda water; Perrier
All herbal teas
Reverse osmosis water is preferred—
  at least 4 cups a day
Green tea

Foods to Avoid

C: GRAINS AND STARCHY VEGETABLES

White bread

White pasta, couscous

Bagels

Muffins

Pastries and pies

Cookies

Anything labeled as an "energy" bar

Spelt products

Crackers

Granola bars

Sesame snacks

Rye bread and crackers

Kamut products

Quinoa

Amaranth

Buckwheat

Whole-wheat products

Whole-grain cereals

Ezekiel bread, pastas, tortillas, English muffins

Stone Mills glycemically tested bread

Brown rice, white rice and all rice products including pasta, crackers, rice puffs

Millet

Oats and oatmeal

Starchy vegetables including sweet potatoes, squash, corn, polenta, potatoes, beets, carrots, etc.

C: FRUITS

Melons (cantaloupe, honeydew, etc.)

Dates

Raisins

Pineapple

Papaya

Mango

Grapes

Dried fruits

Fruit juices

C: VEGETABLES

Green peas, corn, white potatoes, parsnips, beets, carrots, squash, turnip, sweet potatoes; basically any starchy vegetable that grows below the ground

C/P: LEGUMES

All legumes must be avoided, including black beans, lentils, chickpeas, kidney beans, navy beans, refried beans, etc.

F/C/P: NUTS

Peanuts

Exception: permitted protein bar selections that contain peanuts

P: PROTEINS

Luncheon meats containing nitrites and sulphites, regular-fat cold cuts, sausage, bacon

> Limit red meats (beef and pork) to once per week.

All full-fat cheeses made from cow's milk

Marbled meats

Deep-fried foods

Whey protein concentrates and any protein powder containing sugar or artificial sweeteners

Protein bars containing sugar, artificial sweeteners, an imbalanced ratio of protein and carbs (i.e., significantly more carbs than protein). Most bars freely available on shelves are not CSP friendly.

F/C/P: DAIRY AND SUBSTITUTES
Rice milk

F: OILS
Always avoid:
Hydrogenated oils and trans fatty
    acids
Palm oil
Soy oil
Corn oil
Cottonseed oil
Vegetable oil, shortening and all
    margarines

Limit your intake of:
Safflower and sunflower oil
Flaxseed oil

SPICES AND CONDIMENTS
Chocolate syrups
Relish and all types of pickles that
    contain sugar
Honey, maple syrup, jam, apple butter
Chutney
Soy sauce
Barbecue sauce, ketchup and other
    condiments containing sugar

DRINKS
All drinks that contain sugar or
    artificial sweeteners
Juices
Specialty coffees
Sparkling water or juices with sugar
    added
Alcohol
Caffeine (except green tea)

Phase One Carb Sensitivity Checklist

Review the following checklist of possible carb sensitivity reactions
at the end of Phase One to determine your next step.

☐ Failure to lose 1 to 2 pounds

☐ Increased cravings

☐ Fatigue or sleepiness after meals

☐ Brain fogginess or difficulty concentrating

☐ Water retention or puffiness

☐ Increased appetite or obsession with food

☐ Increased weight gain (especially around the middle)

☐ Intestinal bloating or excess gas

☐ Increased blood pressure

☐ Depression or related mood changes

☐ Burning feet or sensation of hot feet at night

☐ Low blood sugar (hypoglycemia)

If you experienced one or more of these symptoms on most days during the past week, you should enter the Metabolic Repair Program outlined in Part Three. Your Metabolic Repair Diet is outlined on pages 260–64. It is very similar to Phase One; however, no fruits are permitted and your protein and fat intake is increased. You should enjoy a cheat meal once weekly, the details of which are explained in on pages 203–5. After 4 weeks you may retry Phase One.

If you purchased the basic CSP supplements, continue to use these products until they are finished before moving on to one or more of the products I have recommended in Chapter 10 as the Metabolic Repair Supplement Plan to repair your metabolism and improve carbohydrate tolerance (see page 264–84).

CSP FLOWCHART FOR PHASE ONE

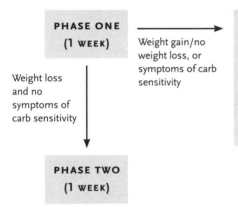

PHASE ONE
(1 WEEK) ⟶ Weight gain/no weight loss, or symptoms of carb sensitivity

Weight loss and no symptoms of carb sensitivity

PHASE TWO
(1 WEEK)

Metabolic Repair Program:
Your Metabolic Repair Diet is for those who did not progress beyond Phase One (see Chapter 10, pages 260–64) and add weekly cheat meal. Begin the Metabolic Repair Supplements and Workout (pages 264–342). Stick with this for 4 weeks then retry Phase One.

For additional assistance, visit www.carbsensitivity.com to view my instructional video on how to progress from one phase to the next.

Phase Two Meal Plan and Permitted Foods List

In Phase One, the foods that could trigger excess insulin release and spur inflammation or cravings were removed completely from your diet. This not only primes your body for weight loss but also reduces water retention and tames an excessive appetite. In Phase Two, you will continue to include 2 servings of nuts or nut butters, unlimited nonstarchy vegetables and 1 to 2 servings of the recommend fruit options. You will, however, add in 1 serving of low-glycemic starchy vegetables. All other rules of the CSP, as outlined in Chapter 6, remain the same. The complete list of Phase Two foods to enjoy and avoid is summarized on pages 159–62.

Day 1

Breakfast (7 a.m. to 8 a.m.)
Skinny Banana Split Smoothie (page 353)

Midmorning Snack (10 a.m.)
Carb Sensitivity Shake (page 419), or CSP–approved Snack Options (pages 135–38)

Lunch (12 p.m. to 1 p.m.)
Sautéed Shrimp and Green Beans (page 373)

Midafternoon Snack (3 p.m. to 4 p.m.)
Carb Sensitivity Shake (page 419), or CSP–approved Snack Options (pages 135–38)

Dinner (6 p.m. to 8 p.m. at the latest)
Scrumptious Edamame Salad (page 385)

Bedtime (10 p.m. to 11 p.m. at the latest)

Day 2

Breakfast (7 a.m. to 8 a.m.)
Orange Vanilla Shake (page 353)

Midmorning Snack (10 a.m.)
Carb Sensitivity Shake (page 419), or CSP–approved Snack
Options (pages 135–38)

Lunch (12 p.m. to 1 p.m.)
Cucumber and Cottage Cheese Salad (page 373)

Midafternoon Snack (3 p.m. to 4 p.m.)
Carb Sensitivity Shake (page 419), or CSP–approved Snack
Options (pages 135–38)

Dinner (6 p.m. to 8 p.m. at the latest)
Carrot and Ginger Soup (page 387) with Baked Chicken

Bedtime (10 p.m. to 11 p.m. at the latest)

Day 3

Breakfast (7 a.m. to 8 a.m.)
Breakfast Cooler Smoothie (page 354)

Midmorning Snack (10 a.m.)
Carb Sensitivity Shake (page 419), or CSP–approved Snack
Options (pages 135–38)

Lunch (12 p.m. to 1 p.m.)
Grilled Mediterranean Salad (page 369)

Midafternoon Snack (3 p.m. to 4 p.m.)
Carb Sensitivity Shake (page 419), or CSP–approved Snack
Options (pages 135–38)

Dinner (6 p.m. to 8 p.m. at the latest)
Summer Squash and Sesame Chicken (page 388)

Bedtime (10 p.m. to 11 p.m. at the latest)

Day 4

Breakfast (7 a.m. to 8 a.m.)
Wild Berry Breakfast (page 354)

Midmorning Snack (10 a.m.)
Carb Sensitivity Shake (page 419), or CSP–approved Snack
Options (pages 135–38)

Lunch (12 p.m. to 1 p.m.)
Perfect Peppercorn Fish (page 378)

Midafternoon Snack (3 p.m. to 4 p.m.)
Carb Sensitivity Shake (page 419), or CSP–approved Snack
Options (pages 135–38)

Dinner (6 p.m. to 8 p.m. at the latest)
Warm Beet and Goat Cheese Salad (page 389)

Bedtime (10 p.m. to 11 p.m. at the latest)

Day 5

Breakfast (7 a.m. to 8 a.m.)
Jelly Sandwich Smoothie (page 357)

Midmorning Snack (10 a.m.)
Carb Sensitivity Shake (page 419), or CSP–approved Snack
Options (pages 135–38)

Lunch (12 p.m. to 1 p.m.)
Crispy Chicken and Lettuce Wraps (page 379)

Midafternoon Snack (3 p.m. to 4 p.m.)
Carb Sensitivity Shake (page 419), or CSP–approved Snack
Options (pages 135–38)

Dinner (6 p.m. to 8 p.m. at the latest)
Curried Pumpkin and Green Beans (page 390)

Bedtime (10 p.m. to 11 p.m. at the latest)

Day 6

Breakfast (7 a.m. to 8 a.m.)
Breakfast Cooler Smoothie (page 354)

Midmorning Snack (10 a.m.)
Carb Sensitivity Shake (page 419), or CSP–approved Snack
Options (pages 135–38)

Lunch (12 p.m. to 1 p.m.)
Wasabi Whitefish with Almond Crust (page 380)

Midafternoon Snack (3 p.m. to 4 p.m.)
Carb Sensitivity Shake (page 419), or CSP–approved Snack
Options (pages 135–38)

Dinner (6 p.m. to 8 p.m. at the latest)
Summerlicious Squash with Yogurt Chicken (page 391)

Bedtime (10 p.m. to 11 p.m. at the latest)

Day 7

Breakfast (7 a.m. to 8 a.m.)
Root Beer Float Smoothie (page 356)

Midmorning Snack (10 a.m.)
Carb Sensitivity Shake (page 419), or CSP–approved Snack
Options (pages 135–38)

Lunch (12 p.m. to 1 p.m.)
Baby Bok Choy and Chicken (page 375)

Midafternoon Snack (3 p.m. to 4 p.m.)
Carb Sensitivity Shake (page 419), or CSP–approved Snack
Options (pages 135–38)

Dinner (6 p.m. to 8 p.m. at the latest)
Chilled Dill and Beet Salad (page 386)

Bedtime (10 p.m. to 11 p.m. at the latest)

Phase Two: Summary of Foods to Enjoy and Avoid

Permitted carbs: 1 serving of starchy vegetables, 2 servings of nuts, unlimited nonstarchy vegetables and 1 to 2 servings of low–GI fruit

C = CARB, P = PROTEIN AND F = FAT

Foods to Enjoy and Suggested Serving Sizes

C: GRAINS AND STARCHY VEGETABLES
(1 serving a day)
Carrots (cooked)—½ cup
Soybeans/edamame (shelled)—½ cup
Summer squash—1 cup
Baby carrots (raw)—½ cup
Beets (sliced)—½ cup
Celery root/celeriac—1 cup
Spaghetti squash—1 cup
Peas—½ cup
Turnip—½ cup
Pumpkin—½ cup

C: FRUITS
Cherries—12

A maximum of 2 servings of fruit are allowed daily—1 selection should be berries.

Apricots—3
Prunes—3
Berries—½ cup
Peaches—1 small
Pears—1 small
Apples—1 small
Plums—1 small
Oranges—1 small
Kiwi—1 small
Grapefruit—1 whole
Watermelon—1 cup
Banana—½ (preferably in protein shakes only)

C: NONSTARCHY VEGETABLES
(1 to 2 cups per meal)
All green/nonstarchy vegetables: spinach, peppers, tomatoes, eggplant, zucchini, cauliflower, onion, leek, artichokes, broccoli, rapini, green beans, asparagus, etc.

C/P: LEGUMES
No legumes are permitted this week.

F/C/P: NUTS & SEEDS
(2 servings a day)
Walnuts—8
Cashews—6
Pistachios—15
Macadamia nuts—4
Almonds—10 to 12
Pecans—6 to 7
Seeds—2 to 3 tablespoons
Nut butters, preferably almond butter or pumpkin seed butter with no salt or sugar added—1 tablespoon

> Consider your nut selections primarily as the fat source in your snacks and meals, rather than as a protein source.

P: PROTEINS
Chicken or turkey (including ground meats and sausage products)
Shellfish, fish
Liquid egg whites—½ cup = 24 grams protein

> 3 servings the size and width of your palm, and 2 half-servings for snacks each day. Women: 4 ounces or 25–30 grams per meal. Men: 6 ounces or 35–40 grams per meal. Organic or free-range selections are best.

PROTEINS *(continued)*

Eggs—Women: 2 whole eggs or 4 egg
   whites and 1 yolk. Men: 3 whole
   eggs or 6 egg whites and 1 yolk

Tofu or tempeh

Lamb

Bison and venison

Cottage cheese, ricotta cheese—½ cup
   for a snack, ¾ cup for a meal

Organic pressed cottage cheese—
   ½ cup for a meal

Cabot 75% reduced-fat Cheddar
   (regular or habañero flavor) or
   low-fat Jarlsberg—2 ounces =
   meal; 1 ounce = snack

Fage Total 0% plain yogurt—
   1 cup = meal; ½ cup = snack

Fage Total Classic
   plain yogurt—
   1 cup = meal;
   ½ cup = snack

Lean red meat
   (preferably
   organic/grass
   fed)—1 serving
   per week

> **Protein bars** should
> contain 14–20 grams of
> protein and a maximum
> of 24 grams of net-carbs,
> and must be free of
> sugar, harmful oils and
> artificial sweeteners.
> Maximum 1 per day as a
> meal replacement.
> Recommended brands
> include Protein Fusion
> Bar, UltraMeal Bar, Jay
> Robb Protein Bar, The
> Simply Bar and Quest Bar.

Protein Powder
Supplements
**(must be free of
sugar and artificial
sweeteners)**

100% whey protein isolate powder

Rice, pea or hemp protein powder

F/C/P: DAIRY AND SUBSTITUTES

Plain soy milk (unsweetened)—½ cup

Almond milk—¾ cup

Goat's milk, goat cheese, sheep
   cheese—1 tablespoon

Goat yogurt—½ cup

F: OILS

(3 to 4 servings a day)

Olive oil (must have daily)—
   1 tablespoon

Avocado—⅛ to ¼

Mayonnaise (canola or olive-oil
   based)—1 teaspoon

Olives—5 to 6

Butter—1 teaspoon

Flaxseed (ground)—1 to 3 tablespoons

Omega-3 egg yolks—2 for women;
   3 for men

Organic coconut butter/oil—
   1 tablespoon

SPICES AND CONDIMENTS

All spices, unless otherwise indicated,
   are allowed. Examples include:
   carob, cinnamon, cumin, dill,
   garlic, ginger, oregano, parsley,
   rosemary, tarragon, thyme,
   turmeric, etc.

Mustards free of sugar

Mayonnaise and salad dressings—
   canola or olive-oil based are
   allowed, but consider these as a
   fat source

DRINKS

Sodium-free soda water; Perrier

All herbal teas

Reverse osmosis water is preferred—
   at least 4 cups a day

Green tea

Coffee or regular tea—1 cup a day is
   permitted from this phase on.
   Skip the java if you feel it triggers
   sugar or carb cravings. Your best
   options are organic coffees and
   teas, and these should be
   consumed before noon.

Foods to Avoid

C: GRAINS
White bread

White pasta, couscous

Bagels

Muffins

Pastries and pies

Cookies

Anything labeled as an "energy" bar

Spelt products

Crackers

Granola bars

Sesame snacks

Rye bread and crackers

Amaranth

Buckwheat

Whole-wheat products

Whole-grain cereals

Ezekiel bread, pastas, tortillas,
English muffins

Kamut products

Quinoa

Brown rice, white rice and all rice
products including pasta,
crackers, rice puffs

Millet

Oats and oatmeal

C: FRUITS
Melons (cantaloupe, honeydew, etc.)

Dates

Raisins

Pineapple

Papaya

Mango

Grapes

Dried fruits

Fruit juices

C: VEGETABLES
Corn, white potatoes, parsnips

C/P: LEGUMES
All legumes must be avoided,
including black beans, lentils,
chickpeas, kidney beans, navy
beans, refried beans, etc.

F/C/P: NUTS
Peanuts

Exception: permitted protein bar
selections that contain peanuts

P: PROTEINS
Luncheon meats
containing nitrites
and sulphites,
regular-fat cold
cuts, sausage, bacon

> Limit red meats (beef and pork) to once per week.

All full-fat cheeses made from cow's
milk

Marbled meats

Deep-fried foods

Whey protein concentrates and any
protein powder containing sugar
or artificial sweeteners

Protein bars containing sugar,
artificial sweeteners, an imbalanced ratio of protein and carbs
(i.e., significantly more carbs than
protein). Most bars freely
available on shelves are not CSP
friendly.

F/C/P: DAIRY AND SUBSTITUTES
Rice milk

F: OILS

Always avoid:

Hydrogenated oils and trans fatty acids

Palm oil

Soy oil

Corn oil

Cottonseed oil

Vegetable oil, shortening and all margarines

Limit your intake of:

Safflower and sunflower oil

Flaxseed oil

SPICES AND CONDIMENTS

Chocolate syrups

Relish and all types of pickles that contain sugar

Honey, maple syrup, jam, apple butter

Chutney

Soy sauce

Barbecue sauce, ketchup and other condiments containing sugar

DRINKS

All drinks that contain sugar or artificial sweeteners

Juices

Specialty coffees

Sparkling water or juices with sugar added

Alcohol

Phase Two Carb Sensitivity Checklist

Review the following checklist of possible carb sensitivity reactions at the end of Phase Two to determine your next step.

- ☐ Failure to lose 1 to 2 pounds
- ☐ Increased cravings
- ☐ Fatigue or sleepiness after meals
- ☐ Brain fogginess or difficulty concentrating
- ☐ Water retention or puffiness
- ☐ Increased appetite or obsession with food
- ☐ Increased weight gain (especially around the middle)
- ☐ Intestinal bloating or excess gas
- ☐ Increased blood pressure
- ☐ Depression or related mood changes
- ☐ Burning feet or sensation of hot feet at night
- ☐ Low blood sugar (hypoglycemia)

If you remained free of these symptoms on most days this week, you are ready to move on to Phase Three. If, however, you experienced

one or more of these symptoms on most days during the past week, you should enter the Metabolic Repair Program outlined in Part Three. Your Metabolic Repair Diet should include Phase One permitted foods (listed on pages 147–50), and you should enjoy a cheat meal once a week, the details of which are explained for you on pages 203–5. After 4 weeks of the Metabolic Repair Program, you may retry Phase Two.

If you purchased the basic CSP supplements, continue to use these products until they are finished before moving on to the Metabolic Repair Supplements in Chapter 10 to repair your metabolism and improve carbohydrate tolerance (see pages 264–84).

CSP FLOWCHART FOR PHASE TWO

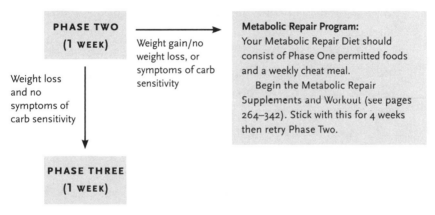

PHASE TWO
(1 WEEK) ⟶ Weight gain/no weight loss, or symptoms of carb sensitivity

Weight loss and no symptoms of carb sensitivity

PHASE THREE
(1 WEEK)

Metabolic Repair Program:
Your Metabolic Repair Diet should consist of Phase One permitted foods and a weekly cheat meal.
Begin the Metabolic Repair Supplements and Workout (see pages 264–342). Stick with this for 4 weeks then retry Phase Two.

For additional assistance, visit www.carbsensitivity.com to view my instructional video on how to progress from one phase to the next.

Phase Three Meal Plan and Permitted Foods List

If you breezed through Phase One and had a smooth ride through Phase Two, your carb tolerance is looking pretty good so far. During Phase Three, your test selection of carbohydrates extends into the realm of legumes, which have a higher net-carb count than the starchy vegetables you tried in the previous phase. (If you know from past experiences that you cannot tolerate legumes, you can skip this phase completely and move on to Phase Four now.) The complete list of Phase Three foods to enjoy and foods to avoid is summarized on pages 172–75. Remember: the rules common to all phases of the CSP, as outlined in Chapter 6, still apply.

While you should still be on the lookout for any symptoms of carbohydrate intolerance, these should not be confused with your body's natural adaptation to a high-fiber bean dish, which can initially include flatulence or stomach discomfort. Unlike the symptoms of an intolerance to carbohydrates, these reactions typically pass as your body gets used to the food. Beans contain a sugar called oligosaccharide, and our body lacks the enzyme required to break down this sugar. When the sugar arrives in your lower intestinal tract intact, it ferments, creating a buildup of gas, which is then expelled. You can allay this problem by preparing your own beans rather than using canned. Allow the beans to soak thoroughly and change the soaking water a few times. If you do use canned beans, rinsing them thoroughly can also help remove the indigestible complex sugars.

Day 1

Breakfast (7 a.m. to 8 a.m.)
Coco-Vanilla Smoothie (page 356)

Midmorning Snack (10 a.m.)
Carb Sensitivity Shake (page 419), or CSP–approved Snack
Options (pages 135–38)

Lunch (12 p.m. to 1 p.m.)
Salmon with Spinach and Strawberry Salsa (page 381)

Midafternoon Snack (3 p.m. to 4 p.m.)
Carb Sensitivity Shake (page 419), or CSP–approved Snack
Options (pages 135–38)

Dinner (6 p.m. to 8 p.m. at the latest)
Curried Red Lentils with Shrimp or Tofu (page 392)

Bedtime (10 p.m. to 11 p.m. at the latest)

Day 2

Breakfast (7 a.m. to 8 a.m.)
Cinnamon Roll Smoothie (page 355)

Midmorning Snack (10 a.m.)
Carb Sensitivity Shake (page 419), or CSP–approved Snack
Options (pages 135–38)

Lunch (12 p.m. to 1 p.m.)
Garlic Chicken and Asparagus (page 370)

Midafternoon Snack (3 p.m. to 4 p.m.)
Carb Sensitivity Shake (page 419), or CSP–approved Snack
Options (pages 135–38)

Dinner (6 p.m. to 8 p.m. at the latest)
Lovely Lemongrass Tofu (page 393)

Bedtime (10 p.m. to 11 p.m. at the latest)

Day 3

Breakfast (7 a.m. to 8 a.m.)
Piña Colada Smoothie (page 357)

Midmorning Snack (10 a.m.)
Carb Sensitivity Shake (page 419), or CSP–approved Snack
Options (pages 135–38)

Lunch (12 p.m. to 1 p.m.)
Apricot-glazed Chicken and Kale (page 372)

Midafternoon Snack (3 p.m. to 4 p.m.)
Carb Sensitivity Shake (page 419), or CSP–approved Snack
Options (pages 135–38)

Dinner (6 p.m. to 8 p.m. at the latest)
Halibut and Rapini in Portobello Mushroom Sauce (page 394)

Bedtime (10 p.m. to 11 p.m. at the latest)

Day 4

Breakfast (7 a.m. to 8 a.m.)
Alkalizing Breakfast Smoothie (page 358)

Midmorning Snack (10 a.m.)
Carb Sensitivity Shake (page 419), or CSP–approved Snack
Options (pages 135–38)

Lunch (12 p.m. to 1 p.m.)
Ahi Tuna Steak and Salad (page 367)

Midafternoon Snack (3 p.m. to 4 p.m.)
Carb Sensitivity Shake (page 419), or CSP–approved Snack
Options (pages 135–38)

Dinner (6 p.m. to 8 p.m. at the latest)
Beautiful Bean and Protein Salad (page 396)

Bedtime (10 p.m. to 11 p.m. at the latest)

Day 5

Breakfast (7 a.m. to 8 a.m.)
Orange Vanilla Shake (page 353)

Midmorning Snack (10 a.m.)
Carb Sensitivity Shake (page 419), or CSP–approved Snack
Options (pages 135–38)

Lunch (12 p.m. to 1 p.m.)
Garlic Chicken and Asparagus (page 370)

Midafternoon Snack (3 p.m. to 4 p.m.)
Carb Sensitivity Shake (page 419), or CSP–approved Snack
Options (pages 135–38)

Dinner (6 p.m. to 8 p.m. at the latest)
Summer Tomato Lentils (page 395)

Bedtime (10 p.m. to 11 p.m. at the latest)

Day 6

Breakfast (7 a.m. to 8 a.m.)
Apricot Yogurt Smoothie (page 350)

Midmorning Snack (10 a.m.)
Carb Sensitivity Shake (page 419), or CSP–approved Snack
Options (pages 135–38)

Lunch (12 p.m. to 1 p.m.)
Miso Salad (page 368)

Midafternoon Snack (3 p.m. to 4 p.m.)
Carb Sensitivity Shake (page 419), or CSP–approved Snack
Options (pages 135–38)

Dinner (6 p.m. to 8 p.m. at the latest)
Spicy Lentil Burgers (page 399)

Bedtime (10 p.m. to 11 p.m. at the latest)

Day 7

Breakfast (7 a.m. to 8 a.m.)
Awesome Avocado and Egg Breakfast (page 360)

Midmorning Snack (10 a.m.)
Carb Sensitivity Shake (page 419), or CSP–approved Snack
Options (pages 135–38)

Lunch (12 p.m. to 1 p.m.)
Blueberry Chicken Salad (page 365)

Midafternoon Snack (3 p.m. to 4 p.m.)
Carb Sensitivity Shake (page 419), or CSP–approved Snack
Options (pages 135–38)

Dinner (6 p.m. to 8 p.m. at the latest)
Curried Red Lentils with Shrimp or Tofu (page 392)

Bedtime (10 p.m. to 11 p.m. at the latest)

Phase Three: Summary of Foods to Enjoy and Avoid

Permitted carbs: 1 serving of legumes, 2 servings of nuts, unlimited
nonstarchy vegetables and 1 to 2 servings of low–GI fruit

C = CARB, P = PROTEIN AND F = FAT

Foods to Enjoy and Suggested Serving Sizes

C: GRAINS AND STARCHY VEGETABLES

None of these foods are permitted this week. This means the starchy vegetables permitted last week must be excluded again, as you attempt to assess your sensitivity to a new group of carbs (legumes).

C: FRUITS

> A maximum of 2 servings of fruit are allowed daily— 1 selection should be berries.

Cherries—12
Apricots—3
Prunes—3
Berries—½ cup
Peaches—1 small
Pears—1 small
Apples—1 small
Plums—1 small
Oranges—1 small
Kiwi—1 small
Grapefruit—1 whole
Watermelon—1 cup
Banana—½ (preferably in protein shakes only)

C: NONSTARCHY VEGETABLES
(1 to 2 cups per meal)

All green/nonstarchy vegetables: spinach, peppers, tomatoes, eggplant, zucchini, cauliflower, onion, leek, artichokes, broccoli, rapini, green beans, asparagus, etc.

C/P: LEGUMES
(1 serving only—a serving is ½ cup)

Calico beans
Broad beans (fava beans)
Cannellini beans
Lentils
Split peas
Mung beans
Black beans
Butter beans
Kidney beans
Navy beans
Note: Once you have reintroduced legumes, they should be considered primarily as a carbohydrate source rather than as a protein.

F/C/P: NUTS & SEEDS
(2 servings a day)

Walnuts—8
Cashews—6
Pistachios—15
Macadamia nuts—4
Almonds—10 to 12
Pecans—6 to 7
Seeds—2 to 3 tablespoons
Nut butters, preferably almond butter or pumpkin seed butter with no salt or sugar added— 1 tablespoon

> Consider your nut selections primarily as the fat source in your snacks and meals, rather than as a protein source.

P: PROTEINS

3 servings the size and width of your palm, and 2 half-servings for snacks each day. Women: 4 ounces or 25–30 grams per meal. Men: 6 ounces or 35–40 grams per meal. Organic or free-range selections are best.

Protein bars should contain 14–20 grams of protein and a maximum of 24 grams of net-carbs, and must be free of sugar, harmful oils and artificial sweeteners. Maximum 1 per day as a meal replacement. Recommended brands include Protein Fusion Bar, UltraMeal Bar, Jay Robb Protein Bar, The Simply Bar and Quest Bar.

Chicken, turkey (including ground meats and sausage products)
Shellfish, fish
Liquid egg whites—½ cup = 24 grams protein
Eggs—Women: 2 whole eggs or 4 egg whites and 1 yolk. Men: 3 whole eggs or 6 egg whites and 1 yolk
Tofu or tempeh
Lamb
Bison and venison
Cottage cheese, ricotta cheese—½ cup for a snack, ¾ cup for a meal
Organic pressed cottage cheese— ½ cup for a meal
Cabot 75% reduced-fat Cheddar (regular or habañero flavor) or low-fat Jarlsberg— 2 ounces = meal; 1 ounce = snack
Fage Total 0% plain yogurt— 1 cup = meal; ½ cup = snack
Fage Total Classic plain yogurt— 1 cup = meal; ½ cup = snack
Lean red meat (preferably organic/grass fed)—1 serving per week

Protein Powder Supplements (must be free of sugar and artificial sweeteners)
100% whey protein isolate powder
Rice, pea or hemp protein powder

F/C/P: DAIRY AND SUBSTITUTES
Plain soy milk (unsweetened)—½ cup
Almond milk—¾ cup
Goat's milk, goat cheese, sheep cheese—1 tablespoon
Goat yogurt—½ cup

F: OILS
(3 to 4 servings a day)
Olive oil (must have daily)— 1 tablespoon
Avocado—⅛ to ¼
Mayonnaise (canola or olive-oil based)—1 teaspoon
Olives—5 to 6
Butter—1 teaspoon
Flaxseed (ground)— 1 to 3 tablespoons
Omega-3 egg yolks—2 for women; 3 for men
Organic coconut butter/oil— 1 tablespoon

SPICES AND CONDIMENTS
All spices, unless otherwise indicated, are allowed. Examples include: carob, cinnamon, cumin, dill, garlic, ginger, oregano, parsley, rosemary, tarragon, thyme, turmeric, etc.
Mustards free of sugar
Mayonnaise and salad dressings (canola or olive-oil based) are allowed, but consider these as a fat source

DRINKS

Sodium-free soda water; Perrier

All herbal teas

Reverse osmosis water is preferred—
at least 8 cups per day

Green tea

Coffee or regular tea—1 cup a day,
preferably organic and consumed
before noon

Foods to Avoid

**C: GRAINS AND STARCHY
VEGETABLES**

White bread

White pasta, couscous

Bagels

Muffins

Pastries and pies

Cookies

Anything labeled as an "energy" bar

Spelt products

Crackers

Granola bars

Sesame snacks

Rye bread and crackers

Amaranth

Buckwheat

Whole-wheat products

Whole-grain cereals

Ezekiel bread, pastas, tortillas,
English muffins

Kamut products

Quinoa

Brown rice, white rice and all rice
products including pasta,
crackers, rice puffs

Millet

Oats and oatmeal

C: FRUITS

Melons (cantaloupe, honeydew, etc.)

Dates

Raisins

Pineapple

Papaya

Mango

Grapes

Dried fruits

Fruit juices

C: VEGETABLES

Green peas, corn, white potatoes,
parsnips, beets, carrots, squash,
turnip, sweet potatoes; basically
any starchy vegetable that grows
below the ground must be
avoided during this week.

C/P: LEGUMES

Lima beans, chickpeas and white
beans (these are high in net-carbs
and have been included in the next
phase of test foods)

F/C/P: NUTS

Peanuts

Exception: permitted protein bar
selections that contain peanuts

P: PROTEINS

Luncheon meats
containing
nitrites and
sulphites,
regular-fat cold cuts, sausage,
bacon

All full-fat cheeses made from
cow's milk

Marbled meats

> Limit red meats
> (beef and pork) to
> once per week.

Deep-fried foods

Whey protein concentrates and any protein powder containing sugar or artificial sweeteners

Protein bars containing sugar, artificial sweeteners, an imbalanced ratio of protein and carbs (i.e., significantly more carbs than protein). Most bars freely available on shelves are not CSP friendly.

F/C/P: DAIRY AND SUBSTITUTES
Rice milk

F: OILS
Always avoid:

Hydrogenated oils and trans fatty acids

Palm oil

Soy oil

Corn oil

Cottonseed oil

Vegetable oil, shortening and all margarines

Limit your intake of:

Safflower and sunflower oil

Flaxseed oil

SPICES AND CONDIMENTS
Chocolate syrups

Relish and all types of pickles that contain sugar

Honey, maple syrup, jam, apple butter

Chutney

Soy sauce

Barbecue sauce, ketchup and other condiments containing sugar

DRINKS
All drinks that contain sugar or artificial sweeteners

Juices

Specialty coffees

Sparkling water or juices with sugar added

Alcohol

Phase Three Carb Sensitivity Checklist
Review the following checklist of possible carb sensitivity reactions at the end of Phase Three to determine your next step.

- ☐ Failure to lose 1 to 2 pounds
- ☐ Increased cravings
- ☐ Fatigue or sleepiness after meals
- ☐ Brain fogginess or difficulty concentrating
- ☐ Water retention or puffiness
- ☐ Increased appetite or obsession with food
- ☐ Increased weight gain (especially around the middle)
- ☐ Intestinal bloating or excess gas
- ☐ Increased blood pressure
- ☐ Depression or related mood changes

☐ Burning feet or sensation of hot feet at night
☐ Low blood sugar (hypoglycemia)

If you remained free of these symptoms on most days during the past week, you may carry on to Phase Four. If, however, you experienced one or more of these symptoms on most days, you should enter the Metabolic Repair Program outlined in Part Three. Your Metabolic Repair Diet will include Phase Two and earlier permitted foods (listed on pages 147–50 and 159–62), and you should enjoy a cheat meal once weekly. The specifics of your cheat meal are explained for you on pages 203–5. After 4 weeks of the Metabolic Repair Program, you may retry Phase Three.

If you purchased the basic CSP supplements, continue to use these products until they are finished before moving on to the Metabolic Repair Supplements I have recommended in Chapter 10 to repair your metabolism and improve carbohydrate tolerance (see pages 264–84).

CSP FLOWCHART FOR PHASE THREE

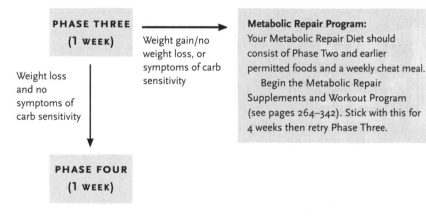

For additional assistance, visit www.carbsensitivity.com to view my instructional video on how to progress from one phase to the next.

Phase Four Meal Plan and Permitted Foods List

During Phase Four, we test the first selection of low-glycemic grains. This week includes some of my favorites: Ezekiel products, quinoa and rye. The complete list of Phase Four foods to enjoy and foods to avoid is summarized on pages 185–88. For many, this phase is a true litmus test because it involves crossing the threshold from starchy vegetables and legumes into the world of grains and higher net-carb foods. The risk of uncovering a carb sensitivity certainly increases in this phase and the next.

I should point out that this is the first phase that contains possible sources of *gluten*, a protein found in certain grains that is a common allergen. You may want to pay special attention to how you feel after you eat these foods, specifically the Ezekiel and rye products. This is especially important if you tend to suffer from inflammatory conditions such as allergies, autoimmune disease, arthritis, asthma, eczema, acne, obesity, headaches, joint stiffness, depression or sinus disorders.

While my recommended meal plans place your starchy carbohydrate meal at the end of the day (for improved sleep and a serotonin boost), feel free to move it to your lunch if this better suits your needs or schedule.

Day 1

Breakfast (7 a.m. to 8 a.m.)
Breakfast Salsa Dish (page 364)

Midmorning Snack (10 a.m.)
Carb Sensitivity Shake (page 419), or CSP–approved Snack
Options (pages 135–38)

Lunch (12 p.m. to 1 p.m.)
Cucumber and Cottage Cheese Salad (page 373)

Midafternoon Snack (3 p.m. to 4 p.m.)
Carb Sensitivity Shake (page 419), or CSP–approved Snack
Options (pages 135–38)

Dinner (6 p.m. to 8 p.m. at the latest)
Cherry Tomato Salmon in Wine Broth (page 404)

Bedtime (10 p.m. to 11 p.m. at the latest)

Day 2

Breakfast (7 a.m. to 8 a.m.)
Piña Colada Smoothie (page 357)

Midmorning Snack (10 a.m.)
Carb Sensitivity Shake (page 419), or CSP–approved Snack
Options (pages 135–38)

Lunch (12 p.m. to 1 p.m.)
Apricot-glazed Chicken and Kale (page 372)

Midafternoon Snack (3 p.m. to 4 p.m.)
Carb Sensitivity Shake (page 419), or CSP–approved Snack
Options (pages 135–38)

Dinner (6 p.m. to 8 p.m. at the latest)
Quick Cinnamon Quinoa (page 403)

Bedtime (10 p.m. to 11 p.m. at the latest)

Day 3

Breakfast (7 a.m. to 8 a.m.)
Berrylicious Iron-booster Smoothie (page 351)

Midmorning Snack (10 a.m.)
Carb Sensitivity Shake (page 419), or CSP–approved Snack
Options (pages 135–38)

Lunch (12 p.m. to 1 p.m.)
Feta Cheese Meatballs with Grilled Vegetables (page 371)

Midafternoon Snack (3 p.m. to 4 p.m.)
Carb Sensitivity Shake (page 419), or CSP–approved Snack
Options (pages 135–38)

Dinner (6 p.m. to 8 p.m. at the latest)
Apple, Arugula and Chicken Salad (page 405)

Bedtime (10 p.m. to 11 p.m. at the latest)

Day 4

Breakfast (7 a.m. to 8 a.m.)
Chocolate Banana Smoothie (page 351)

Midmorning Snack (10 a.m.)
Carb Sensitivity Shake (page 419), or CSP–approved Snack
Options (pages 135–38)

Lunch (12 p.m. to 1 p.m.)
Grilled Mediterranean Salad (page 369)

Midafternoon Snack (3 p.m. to 4 p.m.)
Carb Sensitivity Shake (page 419), or CSP–approved Snack
Options (pages 135–38)

Dinner (6 p.m. to 8 p.m. at the latest)
Ezekiel Crumb-coated Chicken (page 406)

Bedtime (10 p.m. to 11 p.m. at the latest)

Day 5

Breakfast (7 a.m. to 8 a.m.)
Mint Chocolate Smoothie (page 352)

Midmorning Snack (10 a.m.)
Carb Sensitivity Shake (page 419), or CSP–approved Snack
Options (pages 135–38)

Lunch (12 p.m. to 1 p.m.)
Mexican Summer Salad (page 366)

Midafternoon Snack (3 p.m. to 4 p.m.)
Carb Sensitivity Shake (page 419), or CSP–approved Snack
Options (pages 135–38)

Dinner (6 p.m. to 8 p.m. at the latest)
Chicken with Bulgur and Mushrooms (page 407)

Bedtime (10 p.m. to 11 p.m. at the latest)

Day 6

Breakfast (7 a.m. to 8 a.m.)
Skinny Banana Split Smoothie (page 353)

Midmorning Snack (10 a.m.)
Carb Sensitivity Shake (page 419), or CSP–approved Snack
Options (pages 135–38)

Lunch (12 p.m. to 1 p.m.)
Cucumber and Cottage Cheese Salad (page 373)

Midafternoon Snack (3 p.m. to 4 p.m.)
Carb Sensitivity Shake (page 419), or CSP–approved Snack
Options (pages 135–38)

Dinner (6 p.m. to 8 p.m. at the latest)
Grilled Chicken Skewer Wraps (page 408)

Bedtime (10 p.m. to 11 p.m. at the latest)

Day 7

Breakfast (7 a.m. to 8 a.m.)
Strawberry Shortcake Smoothie (page 352)

Midmorning Snack (10 a.m.)
Carb Sensitivity Shake (page 419), or CSP–approved Snack
Options (pages 135–38)

Lunch (12 p.m. to 1 p.m.)
Immunity-boosting Ginger Chicken (page 374)

Midafternoon Snack (3 p.m. to 4 p.m.)
Carb Sensitivity Shake (page 419), or CSP–approved Snack
Options (pages 135–38)

Dinner (6 p.m. to 8 p.m. at the latest)
Turkey Bacon Scallops (page 402) with
Fresh Mint Chickpea Salad (page 397)

Bedtime (10 p.m. to 11 p.m. at the latest)

Phase Four: Summary of Foods to Enjoy and Avoid

Permitted carbs: 1 serving of low net-carb grains, 2 servings of
nuts, unlimited nonstarchy vegetables and
1 to 2 servings of low–GI fruit

C = CARB, P = PROTEIN AND F = FAT

Foods to Enjoy and Suggested Serving Sizes

**C: GRAINS, SELECT LEGUMES AND
STARCHY VEGETABLES**

(1 serving a day)

All-Bran Extra Fiber—½ cup
Kashi GoLean—½ cup
Fiber One—½ cup
Bran Buds—⅓ cup
Ezekiel bread—1 slice
Ezekiel wrap—1 wrap
Ezekiel English muffin—1 muffin
Wasa crispbread (only Crisp 'n Light
    Mild Rye, Fiber, Multi-Grain
    flavors)—3 crackers
Ryvita crispbread (Tomato & Basil, and
    Garlic & Rosemary)—3 crackers
Ryvita crispbread (Sunflower Seeds &
    Oats, Multigrain, Sesame, Dark
    Rye, and Original)—4 crackers
Bulgur—½ cup
Buckwheat groats/kasha—½ cup
Rye bread—1 slice
Quinoa—½ cup
Winter squashes (acorn and
    butternut)—1 cup
Lima beans—½ cup
Chickpeas/garbanzo beans—½ cup
White beans—½ cup

C: FRUITS

Cherries—12
Apricots—3
Prunes—3
Berries—½ cup

Peaches—1 small
Pears—1 small
Apples—1 small
Plums—1 small
Oranges—1 small
Kiwi—1 small
Grapefruit—1 whole
Watermelon—1 cup
Banana—½ (preferably in protein
    shakes only)

> A maximum of 2 servings
> of fruit are allowed
> daily—1 selection should
> be berries

C: NON-STARCHY VEGETABLES

(1 to 2 cups per meal)

All green/nonstarchy vegetables:
    spinach, peppers, tomatoes,
    eggplant, zucchini, cauliflower,
    onion, leek, artichokes, broccoli,
    rapini, green beans, asparagus, etc.

C/P: LEGUMES

Chickpeas, white beans or lima beans
    are permitted. I have listed them
    as a starchy carb source because
    of their high net-carb content.

F/C/P: NUTS & SEEDS (2 servings
a day)

Walnuts—8
Cashews—6
Pistachios—15
Macadamia nuts—4
Almonds—10 to 12
Pecans—6 to 7

NUTS & SEEDS (continued)

Nut butters, preferably almond butter or pumpkin seed butter with no salt or sugar added—

1 tablespoon

> Consider your nut selections primarily as the fat source in your snacks and meals, rather than as a protein source.

P: PROTEINS

Chicken, turkey (including ground meats and sausage products)

Shellfish, fish

Liquid egg whites—½ cup = 24 grams protein

> 3 servings the size and width of your palm, and 2 half-servings for snacks each day. Women: 4 ounces or 25–30 grams per meal. Men: 6 ounces or 35–40 grams per meal. Organic or free-range selections are best.

Eggs—Women: 2 whole eggs or 4 egg whites and 1 yolk. Men: 3 whole eggs or 6 egg whites and 1 yolk

Tofu or tempeh

Lamb

Bison and venison

Cottage cheese, ricotta cheese—½ cup for a snack, ¾ cup for a meal

Organic pressed cottage cheese— ½ cup for a meal

Cabot 75% reduced-fat Cheddar (regular or habañero flavor) or low-fat Jarlsberg—2 ounces = meal; 1 ounce = snack

Fage Total 0% plain yogurt— 1 cup = meal; ½ cup = snack

Fage Total Classic plain yogurt— 1 cup = meal; ½ cup = snack

Lean red meat (preferably organic/ grass fed)—1 serving per week

Protein Powder Supplements (must be free of sugar and artificial sweeteners)

100% whey protein isolate powder

Rice, pea or hemp protein powder

F/C/P: DAIRY AND SUBSTITUTES

Plain soy milk (unsweetened)—½ cup

Almond milk—¾ cup

Goat's milk, goat cheese, sheep cheese—1 tablespoon

Goat yogurt—½ cup

F: OILS (3 to 4 servings a day)

Olive oil (must have daily)— 1 tablespoon

Avocado—⅛ to ¼

Mayonnaise (canola or olive-oil based)—1 teaspoon

Olives—5 to 6

Butter—1 teaspoon

Flaxseed (ground)— 1 to 3 tablespoons

Omega-3 egg yolks—2 for women; 3 for men

Organic coconut butter/oil— 1 tablespoon

SPICES AND CONDIMENTS

All spices, unless otherwise indicated, are allowed. Examples include: carob, cinnamon, cumin, dill, garlic, ginger, oregano, parsley,

> **Protein bars** should contain 14–20 grams of protein and a maximum of 24 grams of net-carbs, and must be free of sugar, harmful oils and artificial sweeteners. Maximum 1 per day as a meal replacement. Recommended brands include Protein Fusion Bar, UltraMeal Bar, Jay Robb Protein Bar, The Simply Bar and Quest Bar.

rosemary, tarragon, thyme,
turmeric, etc.
Mustards free of sugar
Mayonnaise and salad dressings—
canola or olive-oil based are
allowed, but consider these as a
fat source

DRINKS
Sodium-free soda water; Perrier
All herbal teas
Reverse osmosis water is preferred—
at least 8 cups a day
Green tea
Coffee or regular tea—1 cup a day,
preferably organic and consumed
before noon

Foods to Avoid

**C: GRAINS AND STARCHY
VEGETABLES**
White bread
White pasta, couscous
Bagels
Muffins
Pastries and pies
Cookies
Anything labeled as an "energy" bar
Spelt products
Crackers
Granola bars
Sesame snacks
Kamut products
Amaranth
Whole-wheat products
Whole-grain cereals
Brown rice, white rice
and all rice products including
pasta, crackers, rice puffs
Millet
Oats and oatmeal
Starchy vegetables including squash,
sweet potatoes, corn, potatoes,
beets, carrots, etc.
Buckwheat

C: FRUITS
Melons (cantaloupe, honeydew, etc.)
Dates
Raisins

Pineapple
Papaya
Mango
Grapes
Dried fruits
Fruit juices

C: VEGETABLES
Green peas, corn, white potatoes,
parsnips, beets, carrots, squash,
turnip, sweet potatoes; basically
any starchy vegetable that grows
below the ground.

C/P: LEGUMES
All legumes, with the exception of lima
beans, chickpeas or white beans
must be avoided, including black
beans, lentils, kidney beans, navy
beans, refried beans, etc., as we
are testing your tolerance for
higher net carbs during this week.

F/C/P: NUTS
Peanuts
Exception: permitted protein bar
selections that contain peanuts

P: PROTEINS
Luncheon meats
containing

Limit red meats (beef and
pork) to once per week.

P: PROTEINS *(continued)*

nitrites and sulphites, regular-fat cold cuts, sausage, bacon

All full-fat cheeses made from cow's milk

Marbled meats

Deep-fried foods

Whey protein concentrates and any protein powder containing sugar or artificial sweeteners

Protein bars containing sugar, artificial sweeteners, an imbalanced ratio of protein and carbs (i.e., significantly more carbs than protein). Most bars freely available on shelves are not CSP friendly.

F/C/P: DAIRY AND SUBSTITUTES

Rice milk

F: OILS

Always avoid:

Hydrogenated oils and trans fatty acids

Palm oil

Soy oil

Corn oil

Cottonseed oil

Vegetable oil, shortening and all margarines

Limit your intake of:

Safflower and sunflower oil

Flaxseed oil

SPICES AND CONDIMENTS

Chocolate syrups

Relish and all types of pickles that contain sugar

Honey, maple syrup, jam, apple butter

Chutney

Soy sauce

Barbecue sauce, ketchup and other condiments containing sugar

DRINKS

All drinks that contain sugar or artificial sweeteners

Juices

Specialty coffees

Sparkling water or juices with sugar added

Alcohol

Phase Four Carb Sensitivity Checklist

Review the following checklist of possible carb sensitivity reactions at the end of Phase Four to determine your next step.

- ☐ Failure to lose 1 to 2 pounds
- ☐ Increased cravings
- ☐ Fatigue or sleepiness after meals
- ☐ Brain fogginess or difficulty concentrating
- ☐ Water retention or puffiness
- ☐ Increased appetite or obsession with food
- ☐ Increased weight gain (especially around the middle)
- ☐ Intestinal bloating or excess gas
- ☐ Increased blood pressure

☐ Depression or related mood changes
☐ Burning feet or sensation of hot feet at night
☐ Low blood sugar (hypoglycemia)

If you remained free of these symptoms on most days, progress to Phase Five. If, however, you experienced one or more of these symptoms on most days during the past week, you should enter the Metabolic Repair Program outlined in Part Three. Your Metabolic Repair Diet will include Phase Three and earlier permitted foods (see pages 172–75), and you should enjoy a cheat meal once weekly. The specifics of your cheat meal are explained for you on pages 203–5. Keep in mind that selections of carbs from earlier phases (for instance, the starchy vegetables in Phase Two) may be included as an option for your single daily serving of starchy carbs. After 4 weeks, you may retry Phase Four.

If you purchased the basic CSP supplements, continue to use these products until they are finished before moving on to the Metabolic Repair Supplements I have recommended in Chapter 10 to repair your metabolism and improve carbohydrate tolerance (see pages 264–84).

CSP FLOWCHART FOR PHASE FOUR

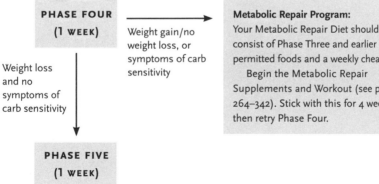

PHASE FOUR
(1 WEEK) → Weight gain/no weight loss, or symptoms of carb sensitivity

Metabolic Repair Program: Your Metabolic Repair Diet should consist of Phase Three and earlier permitted foods and a weekly cheat meal. Begin the Metabolic Repair Supplements and Workout (see pages 264–342). Stick with this for 4 weeks then retry Phase Four.

Weight loss and no symptoms of carb sensitivity

PHASE FIVE
(1 WEEK)

For additional assistance, visit www.carbsensitivity.com to view my instructional video on how to progress from one phase to the next.

Phase Five Meal Plan and Permitted Foods List

By now you will likely have dropped anywhere from 5 to 20 pounds and are beginning to look and feel like a whole *new you*. It's been at least 4 weeks since you have had some of the foods that have contributed to a possible carbohydrate addiction and compromised insulin levels.

During this final phase of test carbs, you will try low-glycemic, high-fiber, less-processed grains such as whole-wheat pasta, kamut products and brown rice. I hope these foods will continue to be your ongoing replacements for the high-glycemic, low-fiber, over-processed options such as white rice and refined pasta, which may have been a staple (or a weakness!) in your diet prior to starting the CSP. Enjoy this testing phase—permitted foods and those to be avoided are outlined on pages 198–201. Once you make it through, you will finally be free of carb sensitivities, and your metabolism will be amazingly healthy.

Day 1

Breakfast (7 a.m. to 8 a.m.)
Orange Vanilla Shake (page 353)

Midmorning Snack (10 a.m.)
Carb Sensitivity Shake (page 419), or CSP–approved Snack
Options (pages 135–38)

Lunch (12 p.m. to 1 p.m.)
Sautéed Shrimp and Green Beans (page 373)

Midafternoon Snack (3 p.m. to 4 p.m.)
Carb Sensitivity Shake (page 419), or CSP–approved Snack
Options (pages 135–38)

Dinner (6 p.m. to 8 p.m. at the latest)
Cinnamon Sweet Potato Pancakes (page 414)

Bedtime (10 p.m. to 11 p.m. at the latest)

Day 2

Breakfast (7 a.m. to 8 a.m.)
Breakfast Cooler Smoothie (page 354)

Midmorning Snack (10 a.m.)
Carb Sensitivity Shake (page 419), or CSP–approved Snack
Options (pages 135–38)

Lunch (12 p.m. to 1 p.m.)
Blueberry Chicken Salad (page 365)

Midafternoon Snack (3 p.m. to 4 p.m.)
Carb Sensitivity Shake (page 419), or CSP–approved Snack
Options (pages 135–38)

Dinner (6 p.m. to 8 p.m. at the latest)
Rosemary Salmon Steaks (page 415)

Bedtime (10 p.m. to 11 p.m. at the latest)

Day 3

Breakfast (7 a.m. to 8 a.m.)
Root Beer Float Smoothie (page 356)

Midmorning Snack (10 a.m.)
Carb Sensitivity Shake (page 419), or CSP–approved Snack
Options (pages 135–38)

Lunch (12 p.m. to 1 p.m.)
Crispy Chicken and Lettuce Wraps (page 379)

Midafternoon Snack (3 p.m. to 4 p.m.)
Carb Sensitivity Shake (page 419), or CSP–approved Snack
Options (pages 135–38)

Dinner (6 p.m. to 8 p.m. at the latest)
Spicy Turkey Muffins (page 416)

Bedtime (10 p.m. to 11 p.m. at the latest)

Day 4

Breakfast (7 a.m. to 8 a.m.)
Breakfast Salsa Dish (page 364)

Midmorning Snack (10 a.m.)
Carb Sensitivity Shake (page 419), or CSP–approved Snack
Options (pages 135–38)

Lunch (12 p.m. to 1 p.m.)
Feta Cheese Meatballs with Grilled Vegetables (page 371)

Midafternoon Snack (3 p.m. to 4 p.m.)
Carb Sensitivity Shake (page 419), or CSP–approved Snack
Options (pages 135–38)

Dinner (6 p.m. to 8 p.m. at the latest)
Sweet tooth–satisfying Salmon (page 417)

Bedtime (10 p.m. to 11 p.m. at the latest)

Day 5

Breakfast (7 a.m. to 8 a.m.)
Alkalizing Breakfast Smoothie (page 358)

Midmorning Snack (10 a.m.)
Carb Sensitivity Shake (page 419), or CSP–approved Snack
Options (pages 135–38)

Lunch (12 p.m. to 1 p.m.)
Curry Chicken Soup, served cold or hot (page 377)

Midafternoon Snack (3 p.m. to 4 p.m.)
Carb Sensitivity Shake (page 419), or CSP–approved Snack
Options (pages 135–38)

Dinner (6 p.m. to 8 p.m. at the latest)
Red Potato and Asparagus Casserole (page 418)

Bedtime (10 p.m. to 11 p.m. at the latest)

Day 6

Breakfast (7 a.m. to 8 a.m.)
Cheesecake Smoothie (page 358)

Midmorning Snack (10 a.m.)
Carb Sensitivity Shake (page 419), or CSP–approved Snack
Options (pages 135–38)

Lunch (12 p.m. to 1 p.m.)
Perfect Peppercorn Fish (page 378)

Midafternoon Snack (3 p.m. to 4 p.m.)
Carb Sensitivity Shake (page 419), or CSP–approved Snack
Options (pages 135–38)

Dinner (6 p.m. to 8 p.m. at the latest)
Barley and Spinach-stuffed Bell Peppers (page 411)

Bedtime (10 p.m. to 11 p.m. at the latest)

Day 7

Breakfast (7 a.m. to 8 a.m.)
Portobello Mushroom Omelette (page 361)

Midmorning Snack (10 a.m.)
Carb Sensitivity Shake (page 419), or CSP–approved Snack
Options (pages 135–38)

Lunch (12 p.m. to 1 p.m.)
Grilled Mediterranean Salad (page 369)

Midafternoon Snack (3 p.m. to 4 p.m.)
Carb Sensitivity Shake (page 419), or CSP–approved Snack
Options (pages 135–38)

Dinner (6 p.m. to 8 p.m. at the latest)
Sweet Apple Cinnamon Delight (page 412)

Bedtime (10 p.m. to 11 p.m. at the latest)

Phase Five: Summary of Foods to Enjoy and Avoid

Permitted carbs: 1 serving of higher net-carb grains, 2 servings
of nuts, unlimited nonstarchy vegetables and
1 to 2 servings of low–GI fruit

C = CARB, P = PROTEIN AND F = FAT

Foods to Enjoy and Suggested Serving Sizes

C: GRAINS AND STARCHY VEGETABLES
(1 serving a day)
Oat bran—½ cup
Potatoes (boiled)—1 medium
Oatmeal (measured dry)—⅓ cup
Steel-cut oats—¼ cup
Kamut pasta—½ cup
Plantains (cooked)—½ cup
Sweet potato (peeled)—½ cup
Brown rice—½ cup
Basmati rice—¼ cup
Whole-wheat pasta—½ cup
Pearl barley—½ cup

C: FRUITS

A maximum of 2 servings of fruit are allowed daily—1 selection should be berries.

Cherries—12
Apricots—3
Prunes—3
Berries—½ cup
Peaches—1 small
Pears—1 small
Apples—1 small
Plums—1 small
Oranges—1 small
Kiwi—1 small
Grapefruit—1 whole
Watermelon—1 cup
Banana—½ (preferably in protein
  shakes only)

C: NONSTARCHY VEGETABLES
(1 to 2 cups per meal)
All green/nonstarchy vegetables:
  spinach, peppers, tomatoes,
  eggplant, zucchini, cauliflower,
  onion, leek, artichokes, broccoli,
  rapini, green beans, asparagus, etc.

C/P: LEGUMES
No legumes are permitted this week.

F/C/P: NUTS & SEEDS
(2 servings a day)
Walnuts—8
Cashews—6
Pistachios—15
Macadamia nuts—4
Almonds—10 to 12
Pecans—6 to 7
Seeds—2 to 3
  tablespoons
Nut butters, preferably almond
  butter or pumpkin seed butter
  with no salt or sugar added—
  1 tablespoon

Consider your nut selections primarily as the fat source in your snacks and meals, rather than as a protein source.

P: PROTEINS
Chicken, turkey (including ground
  meats and sausage products)
Shellfish, fish
Liquid egg whites—½ cup =
  24 grams protein

> 3 servings the size and width of your palm, and 2 half-servings for snacks each day. Women: 4 ounces or 25–30 grams per meal. Men: 6 ounces or 35–40 grams per meal. Organic or free-range selections are best.

Eggs—Women: 2 whole eggs or 4 egg whites and 1 yolk. Men: 3 whole eggs or 6 egg whites and 1 yolk
Tofu or tempeh— 8 ounces
Lamb
Bison and venison
Cottage cheese, ricotta cheese— ½ cup for a snack, ¾ cup for a meal
Organic pressed cottage cheese— ½ cup for a meal
Cabot 75% reduced-fat Cheddar (regular or habañero flavor) or low-fat Jarlsberg—2 ounces = meal; 1 ounce = snack
Fage Total 0% plain yogurt— 1 cup = meal; ½ cup = snack
Fage Total Classic plain yogurt— 1 cup = meal; ½ cup = snack
Lean red meat (preferably organic/ grass fed)—1 serving per week

Protein Powder Supplements (must be free of sugar and artificial sweeteners)
100% whey protein isolate powder
Rice, pea or hemp protein powder

> **Protein bars** should contain 14–20 grams of protein and a maximum of 24 grams of net-carbs, and must be free of sugar, harmful oils and artificial sweeteners. Maximum 1 per day as a meal replacement. Recommended brands include Protein Fusion Bar, UltraMeal Bar, Jay Robb Protein Bar, The Simply Bar and Quest Bar.

F/C/P: DAIRY AND SUBSTITUTES

Plain soy milk (unsweetened)—½ cup
Almond milk—¾ cup
Goat's milk, goat cheese, sheep cheese—1 tablespoon
Goat yogurt—½ cup

F: OILS

(3 to 4 servings a day)
Olive oil (must have daily)— 1 tablespoon
Avocado—⅛ to ¼
Mayonnaise (canola or olive-oil based)—1 teaspoon
Olives—5 to 6
Butter—1 teaspoon
Flaxseed (ground)— 1 to 3 tablespoons
Omega-3 egg yolks—2 for women; 3 for men
Organic coconut butter/oil— 1 tablespoon

SPICES AND CONDIMENTS

All spices, unless otherwise indicated, are allowed. Examples include: carob, cinnamon, cumin, dill, garlic, ginger, oregano, parsley, rosemary, tarragon, thyme, turmeric, etc.
Mustards free of sugar
Mayonnaise and salad dressing— canola or olive-oil based are allowed, but consider these as a fat source

DRINKS

Sodium-free soda water; Perrier
All herbal teas
Reverse osmosis water is preferred— at least 8 cups a day
Green tea

DRINKS *(continued)*

Coffee or regular tea—1 cup a day,
 preferably organic and consumed
 before noon

Foods to Avoid

C: GRAINS AND STARCHY VEGETABLES

White bread

White pasta, couscous

Bagels

Muffins

Pastries and pies

Cookies

Anything labeled as an "energy" bar

Spelt products

Crackers

Granola bars

Sesame snacks

Amaranth

Buckwheat

Whole-grain cereals

Ezekiel bread, pastas, tortillas,
 English muffins

Millet

Quinoa

Starchy vegetables including squash,
 corn, beets, carrots, etc.

C: FRUITS

Melons (cantaloupe, honeydew, etc.)

Dates

Raisins

Pineapple

Papaya

Mango

Grapes

Dried fruits

Fruit juices

C: VEGETABLES

Green peas, corn, parsnips, beets,
 carrots, squash, turnip; basically
 any starchy vegetable that grows
 below the ground, except potatoes
 and sweet potatoes

C/P: LEGUMES

All legumes must be avoided
 including black beans, lentils,
 chickpeas, kidney beans, navy
 beans, refried beans, etc.

F/C/P: NUTS

Peanuts

Exception: permitted protein bar
 selections that contain peanuts

P: PROTEINS

Luncheon meats
 containing
 nitrites and
 sulphites, regular-fat cold cuts,
 sausage, bacon

Limit red meats (beef and pork) to once per week.

All full-fat cheeses made from cow's
 milk

Marbled meats

Deep-fried foods

Whey protein concentrates and any
 protein powder containing sugar
 or artificial sweeteners

Protein bars containing sugar,
 artificial sweeteners, an imbalanced ratio of protein and carbs

(i.e., significantly more carbs than protein). Most bars freely available on shelves are not CSP friendly.

F/C/P: DAIRY AND SUBSTITUTES
Rice milk

F: OILS
Always avoid:
Hydrogenated oils and trans fatty acids
Palm oil
Soy oil
Corn oil
Cottonseed oil
Vegetable oil, shortening and all margarines

Limit your intake of:
Safflower and sunflower oil
Flaxseed oil

SPICES AND CONDIMENTS
Chocolate syrups
Relish and all types of pickles that contain sugar
Honey, maple syrup, jam, apple butter
Chutney
Soy sauce
Barbecue sauce, ketchup and other condiments containing sugar

DRINKS
All drinks that contain sugar or artificial sweeteners
Juices
Specialty coffees
Sparkling water or juices with sugar added
Alcohol

Phase Five Carb Sensitivity Checklist
Review the following checklist of possible carb sensitivity reactions at the end of Phase Five to determine your next step.

☐ Failure to lose 1 to 2 pounds
☐ Increased cravings
☐ Fatigue or sleepiness after meals
☐ Brain fogginess or difficulty concentrating
☐ Water retention or puffiness
☐ Increased appetite or obsession with food
☐ Increased weight gain (especially around the middle)
☐ Intestinal bloating or excess gas
☐ Increased blood pressure
☐ Depression or related mood changes
☐ Burning feet or sensation of hot feet at night
☐ Low blood sugar (hypoglycemia)

If you remained free of these symptoms on most days, you can progress to the final maintenance phase of the CSP. If, however, you experienced one or more of these symptoms on most days during the past week, you should enter the Metabolic Repair Program outlined in Part Three. Your Metabolic Repair Diet will include Phase Four and earlier permitted foods (see pages 185–88), plus a cheat meal once weekly, the details of which are highlighted on pages 203–5. Keep in mind that selections of carbs from all earlier phases (for instance, the legumes in Phase Three and the starchy vegetables in Phase Two) may also be included as an option for your daily serving of starchy carbs. After 4 weeks you may retry Phase Five.

If you purchased the basic CSP supplements, continue to use these products until they are finished before moving on to the Metabolic Repair Supplements I have recommended in Chapter 10 to repair your metabolism and improve carbohydrate tolerance (see pages 264–84).

CSP FLOWCHART FOR PHASE FIVE

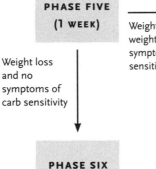

PHASE FIVE
(1 WEEK)

Weight gain/no weight loss, or symptoms of carb sensitivity

Weight loss and no symptoms of carb sensitivity

Metabolic Repair Program:
Your Metabolic Repair Diet should consist of Phase Four and earlier permitted foods and a weekly cheat meal.
Begin the Metabolic Repair Supplements and Workout (see pages 264–342). Stick with this for 4 weeks then retry Phase Five.

PHASE SIX

For additional assistance, visit www.carbsensitivity.com to view my instructional video on how to progress from one phase to the next.

Phase Six and Beyond Meal Plan and Permitted Foods List

Congratulations! You have entered the maintenance stage of the Carb Sensitivity Program! Your daily serving of starchy carb selections may be chosen from all earlier phases, which includes the starchy vegetables in Phase Two, the legumes from Phase Three, the low net-carb grains from Phase Four and the grains highest in net carbs from Phase Five. Pages 213–15 show the complete lists of permitted foods for Phase Six and beyond. Getting to this point indicates that you have a very low sensitivity to carbohydrates, that your insulin response is balanced and that your metabolism is healthy. To keep it that way, be sure to incorporate a strength-training program (such as the one in Chapter 11), include a cheat meal once a week and stick to the list of permitted foods in this phase 80 to 90 percent of the time.

Why the Cheat Meal?

While it may seem counterintuitive, I emphasize including a weekly "cheat" meal, which can include some of your high-carb favorites. Why? Continuous, extreme caloric restriction is not an effective long-term fat-loss solution; it is simply not sustainable. The short-term victories achieved with this type of eating are *always* followed by rebound weight gain. Whether we like it or not, our hormones will kick in to return the body to status quo.

From a psychological perspective, this cheat meal can certainly help keep you motivated, but it also offers physiological benefits. This meal serves to increase your thyroid hormone and to lower levels of reverse T3, a hormone that can block the action of the active thyroid hormone that influences metabolism, and which naturally increases with dieting. It will also generally boost your metabolism—this is the absolute truth! Remember, the human body is an adaptation machine. When we reduce calories overall, our body adapts by lowering our metabolism as a survival mechanism. And let's face it: A zero-tolerance diet policy rarely lasts. Having a cheat meal keeps our metabolism guessing, thereby *increasing* our long-term success. This meal also prevents hunger, quells cravings and refuels our muscle stores of energy, particularly glycogen, which helps to maintain strength and endurance for the workouts that are essential for our metabolic repair. And let's not forget that a hit of carbs can give a little boost to your serotonin levels and lower your stress hormones such as cortisol.

QUICK GUIDELINES FOR YOUR WEEKLY CHEAT MEAL:

- Have your cheat meal as your last meal of the day rather than your first. Otherwise, you will be more prone to continue cheating all day long.
- Keep your fat intake low and your carb intake high, but don't exceed 100 grams of carbs or go over 1 hour of eating time.
- Take the time and care to really enjoy your cheat meal. Plan it ahead of time, and have it at the dinner table or at a restaurant.
- Once you leave the table, stop eating. Don't be tempted to continue through the evening.
- Good examples of a cheat meal are:
  - Pancakes with a small amount of syrup and fruit
  - High-sugar, low-fat yogurt selections
  - A small bowl of pasta with tomato sauce
  - Sushi or sashimi with white sticky rice, or teriyaki stir-fry with rice
  - Cereal with milk
  - All cheat meals may include dessert such as cake; pie; cookies; pudding; low-fat ice cream or low-fat frozen yogurt (I highly recommend Ben & Jerry's Chocolate Fudge Brownie Low Fat Frozen Yogurt!); high-sugar, low-fat yogurts (those that are more like pudding than yogurt); etc. One glass of wine, one beer or a mixed drink may also be included, if desired.

- Bad examples of cheat meals (the high-fat *and* high-carb varieties) are:
  - Pizza, especially deep dish
  - Pasta with cream sauce
  - Cheesecake or any other high-fat dessert selection
  - High-fat dips (such as artichoke or creamy spinach) with chips or pita bread

A bit of water retention after a cheat meal is normal, but if your weight is still up a few days later, it means that you may have overdone it *or* you included selections that don't particularly agree with your body chemistry. In that case, I recommend avoiding things such as sugar, dairy or gluten and opt for other higher-carb alternatives.

If you have more than *40 pounds* to lose, aim to have a cheat meal every *second* week versus every week in order to expedite your weight-loss efforts.

Day 1

Breakfast (7 a.m. to 8 a.m.)
Chocolate Hazelnut Coffee Smoothie (page 350)

Midmorning Snack (10 a.m.)
Carb Sensitivity Shake (page 419), or CSP–approved Snack
Options (pages 135–38)

Lunch (12 p.m. to 1 p.m.)
Mexican Summer Salad (page 366)

Midafternoon Snack (3 p.m. to 4 p.m.)
Carb Sensitivity Shake (page 419), or CSP–approved Snack
Options (pages 135–38)

Dinner (6 p.m. to 8 p.m. at the latest)
Bison Chili and Beans (page 398)

Bedtime (10 p.m. to 11 p.m. at the latest)

Day 2

Breakfast (7 a.m. to 8 a.m.)
Berrylicious Iron-booster Smoothie (page 351)

Midmorning Snack (10 a.m.)
Carb Sensitivity Shake (page 419), or CSP–approved Snack
Options (pages 135–38)

Lunch (12 p.m. to 1 p.m.)
Cauliflower and Kale Soup (page 382)

Midafternoon Snack (3 p.m. to 4 p.m.)
Carb Sensitivity Shake (page 419), or CSP–approved Snack
Options (pages 135–38)

Dinner (6 p.m. to 8 p.m. at the latest)
Turkey Bacon Scallops (page 402)

Bedtime (10 p.m. to 11 p.m. at the latest)

Day 3

Breakfast (7 a.m. to 8 a.m.)
Cinnamon Roll Smoothie (page 355)

Midmorning Snack (10 a.m.)
Carb Sensitivity Shake (page 419), or CSP–approved Snack
Options (pages 135–38)

Lunch (12 p.m. to 1 p.m.)
Miso Salad (page 368) with Shrimp

Midafternoon Snack (3 p.m. to 4 p.m.)
Carb Sensitivity Shake (page 419), or CSP–approved Snack
Options (pages 135–38)

Dinner (6 p.m. to 8 p.m. at the latest)
Quinoa Salad with Orange, Walnuts and Mint (page 401)

Bedtime (10 p.m. to 11 p.m. at the latest)

Day 4

Breakfast (7 a.m. to 8 a.m.)
Piña Colada Smoothie (page 357)

Midmorning Snack (10 a.m.)
Carb Sensitivity Shake (page 419), or CSP–approved Snack
Options (pages 135–38)

Lunch (12 p.m. to 1 p.m.)
Apricot-glazed Chicken and Kale (page 372)

Midafternoon Snack (3 p.m. to 4 p.m.)
Carb Sensitivity Shake (page 419), or CSP–approved Snack
Options (pages 135–38)

Dinner (6 p.m. to 8 p.m. at the latest)
Lovely Lemongrass Tofu (page 393)

Bedtime (10 p.m. to 11 p.m. at the latest)

Day 5

Breakfast (7 a.m. to 8 a.m.)
Sweet Apple Pie Smoothie (page 359)

Midmorning Snack (10 a.m.)
Carb Sensitivity Shake (page 419), or CSP–approved Snack
Options (pages 135–38)

Lunch (12 p.m. to 1 p.m.)
Garlic Chicken and Asparagus (page 370)

Midafternoon Snack (3 p.m. to 4 p.m.)
Carb Sensitivity Shake (page 419), or CSP–approved Snack
Options (pages 135–38)

Dinner (6 p.m. to 8 p.m. at the latest)
Curried Pumpkin and Green Beans (page 390)

Bedtime (10 p.m. to 11 p.m. at the latest)

Day 6

Breakfast (7 a.m. to 8 a.m.)
Portobello Mushroom Omelette (page 361)

Midmorning Snack (10 a.m.)
Carb Sensitivity Shake (page 419), or CSP–approved Snack
Options (pages 135–38)

Lunch (12 p.m. to 1 p.m.)
Ahi Tuna Steak and Salad (page 367)

Midafternoon Snack (3 p.m. to 4 p.m.)
Carb Sensitivity Shake (page 419), or CSP–approved Snack
Options (pages 135–38)

Dinner (6 p.m. to 8 p.m. at the latest)
Grilled Chicken Skewer Wraps (page 408)

Bedtime (10 p.m. to 11 p.m. at the latest)

Day 7

Breakfast (7 a.m. to 8 a.m.)
Breakfast Cooler Smoothie (page 354)

Midmorning Snack (10 a.m.)
Carb Sensitivity Shake (page 419), or CSP–approved Snack
Options (pages 135–38)

Lunch (12 p.m. to 1 p.m.)
Salmon and Dill Omelette (page 362)

Midafternoon Snack (3 p.m. to 4 p.m.)
Carb Sensitivity Shake (page 419), or CSP–approved Snack
Options (pages 135–38)

Dinner (6 p.m. to 8 p.m. at the latest)
Honey Chicken and Sweet Potatoes (page 413)

Bedtime (10 p.m. to 11 p.m. at the latest)

Phase Six and Beyond:
Summary of Foods to Enjoy and Avoid

Permitted carbs: 1 serving of grains, select legumes or vegetables; an optional serving of legumes; 2 servings of nuts; unlimited nonstarchy vegetables; and 1 to 2 servings of low–GI fruit

C = CARB, P = PROTEIN AND F = FAT

Foods to Enjoy and Suggested Serving Sizes

C: GRAINS AND STARCHY VEGETABLES

(1 serving a day)

Carrots (cooked)—½ cup
Soybeans/edamame (shelled)—½ cup
Summer squash—1 cup
Baby carrots (raw)—½ cup
Beets (sliced) ½ cup
Celery root/celeriac— 1 cup
Spaghetti squash—1 cup
Peas—½ cup
Turnip—½ cup
Pumpkin—½ cup
All-Bran Extra Fiber—½ cup
Kashi GoLean—½ cup
Fiber One—½ cup
All-Bran Buds—⅓ cup
Ezekiel bread—1 slice
Ezekiel wrap—1 wrap
Ezekiel English muffin—1 muffin
Wasa crispbread (only Crisp'n Light
    Mild Rye, Fiber, Multi Grain
    flavors)—3 crackers
Ryvita crispbread (Tomato & Basil,
    Garlic & Rosemary)—3 crackers
Ryvita crispbread (Sunflower Seeds
    & Oats, Multigrain, Sesame, Dark
    Rye, Original)—4 crackers
Bulgur—½ cup
Buckwheat groats/kasha—½ cup
Rye bread—1 slice

Quinoa—½ cup
Winter squashes (acorn and
    butternut—1 cup
Oat bran—½ cup
Potatoes (boiled)—1 medium
Oatmeal (measured dry)—⅓ cup
Steel-cut oats—¼ cup
Kamut pasta—½ cup
Plantains (cooked)—½ cup
Sweet potato (peeled)—½ cup
Brown rice—½ cup
Basmati rice—¼ cup
Whole-wheat pasta—½ cup
Pearl barley—½ cup

C: FRUITS

Cherries—12
Apricots—3
Prunes—3
Berries—½ cup
Peaches—1 small
Pears—1 small
Apples—1 small
Plums—1 small
Oranges—1 small
Kiwi—1 small
Grapefruit—1 whole
Watermelon—1 cup
Banana—½ (preferably in protein
    shakes only)

> A maximum of 2 servings of fruit are allowed daily— 1 selection should be berries.

C: NONSTARCHY VEGETABLES

(1 to 2 cups per meal)

All green/nonstarchy vegetables:
spinach, peppers, tomatoes,
eggplant, zucchini, cauliflower,
onion, leek, artichokes, broccoli,
rapini, green beans, asparagus, etc.

C/P: LEGUMES

(optional 1 serving a day)

Calico beans—½ cup
Broad beans/fava beans—½ cup
Cannellini beans—½ cup
Lentils—½ cup
Split peas—½ cup
Mung beans—½ cup
Black beans—½ cup
Butter beans—½ cup
Kidney beans—½ cup
Navy beans—½ cup

Note: Consider these legumes as a
starchy carb selection if you discover
that enjoying 1 daily serving of
starchy carbs (listed on page 213)
along with 1 serving of legumes
triggers symptoms of carb sensitivity.

F/C/P: NUTS AND SEEDS

(2 servings a day)

Walnuts—8
Cashews—6
Pistachios—15
Macadamia nuts—4
Almonds—10 to 12
Pecans—6 to 7

Seeds—2 to 3
tablespoons
Nut butters,
preferably
almond butter
or pumpkin

> Consider your nut
> selections primarily as
> the fat source in your
> snacks and meals, rather
> than as a protein source.

seed butter with no salt
or sugar added—
1 tablespoon

P: PROTEINS

Chicken, turkey
(including
ground meats
and sausage
products)
Shellfish, fish
Liquid egg whites—
½ cup = 24
grams protein
Eggs—Women:
2 whole eggs or
4 egg whites and
1 yolk. Men: 3
whole eggs or 6 egg whites
and 1 yolk

> 3 servings the size
> and width of your
> palm, and 2
> half-servings for
> snacks each day.
> Women: 4 ounces
> or 25–30 grams
> per meal.
> Men: 6 ounces or
> 35–40 grams per
> meal. Organic
> or free-range
> selections are best.

Tofu or tempeh
Lamb
Bison and venison
Cottage cheese, ricotta cheese—
½ cup for a snack, ¾ cup for
a meal
Organic pressed cottage cheese—
½ cup for a meal
Cabot 75% reduced-fat
Cheddar (regular or habañero
flavor) or low-fat Jarlsberg—
2 ounces = meal;
1 ounce = snack
Fage Total 0% plain yogurt—
1 cup = meal;
½ cup = snack
Fage Total Classic plain yogurt—
1 cup = meal;
½ cup = snack
Lean red meat (preferably organic/
grass fed)—1 serving per week

Protein Powder Supplements
(must be free of sugar and artificial
sweeteners)

100% whey protein isolate powder

Rice, pea or hemp protein powder

F/C/P: DAIRY AND SUBSTITUTES
Plain soy milk (unsweetened)— ½ cup

Almond milk— ¾ cup

Goat's milk, goat cheese, sheep cheese— 1 tablespoon

Goat yogurt— ½ cup

F: OILS (3 to 4 servings a day)
Olive oil (must have daily)— 1 tablespoon

Avocado—⅛ to ¼

Mayonnaise (canola or olive-oil based)—1 teaspoon

Olives—5 to 6

Butter—1 teaspoon

Flaxseed (ground)—1 to 3 tablespoons

Omega-3 egg yolks—2 for women; 3 for men

Organic coconut butter/oil— 1 tablespoon

SPICES AND CONDIMENTS
All spices, unless otherwise indicated, are allowed. Examples include: carob, cinnamon, cumin, dill, garlic, ginger, oregano, parsley, rosemary, tarragon, thyme, turmeric, etc.

Mustards free of sugar

Mayonnaise and salad dressings— canola or olive-oil based are allowed, but consider these as a fat source

DRINKS
Sodium-free soda water; Perrier

All herbal teas

Reverse osmosis water is preferred— at least 8 cups a day

Green tea

Coffee or regular tea—1 cup a day, preferably organic and consumed before noon

Foods to Avoid

C: GRAINS (except for your cheat meal once a week)

White bread

White pasta, couscous

Bagels

Muffins

Pastries and pies

Cookies

Anything labeled as an "energy" bar

Spelt products

Crackers

Granola bars

Sesame snacks

C: FRUITS (except for your cheat meal once a week)

Melons (cantaloupe, honeydew, etc.)

Dates

Raisins

Pineapple

Papaya

Mango

FRUITS *(continued)*
Grapes
Dried fruits
Fruit juices

C: VEGETABLES (except for your cheat meal once a week)
Corn, white potatoes, parsnips

C/P: LEGUMES
Remember to consider chickpeas, lima beans and white beans as a starchy carb source.

F/C/P: NUTS (except for your cheat meal once a week)
Peanuts
Exception: permitted protein bar selections that contain peanuts

P: PROTEINS (except for your cheat meal once a week)

Limit red meats (beef and pork) to once per week.

Luncheon meats containing nitrites and sulphites, regular-fat cold cuts, sausage, bacon
All full-fat cheeses made from cow's milk
Marbled meats
Deep-fried foods
Whey protein concentrates and any protein powder containing sugar or artificial sweeteners
Protein bars containing sugar, artificial sweeteners, an imbalanced ratio of protein and carbs (i.e., significantly more carbs than protein). Most bars freely available on shelves are not CSP friendly.

F/C/P: DAIRY AND SUBSTITUTES
(except for your cheat meal once a week)
Rice milk

F: OILS
Always avoid:
Hydrogenated oils and trans fatty acids
Palm oil
Soy oil
Corn oil
Cottonseed oil
Vegetable oil, shortening and all margarines

Limit your intake of:
Safflower and sunflower oil
Flaxseed oil

SPICES AND CONDIMENTS
(except for your cheat meal once a week)
Chocolate syrups
Relish and all types of pickles that contain sugar
Honey, maple syrup, jam, apple butter
Chutney
Soy sauce
Barbecue sauce, ketchup and other condiments containing sugar

DRINKS (except for your cheat meal once a week)
All drinks that contain sugar or artificial sweeteners

Continue to avoid all foods and drinks that contain artificial sweeteners 100 percent of the time.

Juices
Specialty coffees
Sparkling water or juices with sugar added
Alcohol

"I went in to my doctor for a regular checkup and some routine blood work. He called me back and told me my platelets were dropping. I was not sure what that meant, but I knew it was not a good thing. He was sending me to a specialist, but it would take about 6 months to get the appointment. I decided to do something myself while I waited for the specialist. I contacted a friend of mine, Dr. Natasha Turner. She suggested the Carb Sensitivity Program. In the first week I lost 7 pounds, and within 1 month I lost a total of 15. The weight kept on dropping. I was down 20 pounds after 2 months, and, after 3 months, down 25. I stopped needing my stomach pills 4 days into the detox and have not had one since. My family doctor has now taken me off my high blood pressure pills, which I had been taking for over 10 years. My platelets have gone up for the first time in almost 10 years. I now have lots of energy and feel 100 percent—all with no added exercise, just the proper diet given to me by Dr. Turner. She has taken 10 years off my looks and has added 10 years to my life. I feel fantastic. I did not think it would be this easy to lose weight and get my health back."

ANDREW, 45

STATS	BEFORE	AFTER
Weight	197 lb	170 lb
BMI	27.5	23.7

INITIAL CHIEF COMPLAINTS:

1. Weight gain
2. High blood pressure
3. Low platelets

CHAPTER 8

SUPPORTIVE SUPPLEMENTS
FOR THE SIX CSP PHASES

Change is such hard work.

BILLY CRYSTAL

While you are on the CSP weekly plan, you should include the supplements I have outlined in this section. Even though they are not a mandatory part of your program, they will enhance both how you feel and your results considerably. I certainly don't want you taking heaps of supplements (until you "rattle when you walk," as a good friend once said must be the case with me), but there is no doubt in my mind that the right nutrients will be of great help. Remember, these are *optional*, but they are strongly recommended.

The supplements discussed in the pages that follow will serve to:

- Detox the liver and digestive system, which aids metabolism and reduces inflammation
- Improve the metabolism and the elimination of harmful excess hormones from the body, including estrogen and cortisol
- Prevent cravings and constipation
- Provide additional antioxidant and anti-inflammatory protection
- Boost your energy and increase your metabolic rate
- Assist with appetite control
- Improve your sleep

While I have recommended specific brands, don't feel that you have to purchase these exact products. Products with similar ingredients should be fine, provided they are from a reputable company. You can certainly ask the staff at your local health-food store for advice. If you don't have a health-food store near you, try searching the Internet for companies that deliver their products to your door. You can also visit www.carbsensitivity.com to place an order for the CSP Kit, which contains the first four supplements I have listed below as recommended for use during the basic CSP phases. Note that a vitamin D3 supplement is not included in the kit, as I find most patients tend to have this on hand.

Basic Supplement Recommendations for All Six CSP Phases

1. **A high-quality probiotic supplement**: Healthy bacterial balance in the digestive system is vital for overall health, particularly for the breakdown and elimination of estrogen. Probiotics assist with bowel cleansing, preventing constipation, reducing allergy symptoms, boosting immunity and promoting skin health. While yogurt naturally contains probiotics, supplements are more effective as a concentrated source. Most probiotic supplements should be refrigerated. During the CSP weekly process, as well as the Metabolic Repair Program (should you be directed there), I recommend a probiotic with at least 10 to 15 billion cells per capsule, such as Clear Flora. A good maintenance dose is 1 to 2 billion of both *lactobacilli* and *bifidobacteria* cells once a day, best taken away from food. Some people experience bloating when they first begin taking probiotic supplements. If you are bothered by this effect, simply reduce the dosage and slowly increase it as your body adapts. Recommended brands include:
   - **Clear Flora**—2 capsules on rising
   - **MultiBiotic 4000** (Douglas Labs)—2 capsules on rising and/or before bed
   - **Bio-K+**—1 jar (away from food) or 1 capsule per day (with food)

- **Live Probio+ 03mega** (Genuine Health)—1 to 2 capsules on rising
- **Smooth Food 2** or **All Flora** (New Chapter)—2 capsules per day
- **ProbioMax Daily** (Xymogen)—1 capsule on rising (an excellent option if you don't want a supplement requiring refrigeration)

2. **An herbal cleansing formula for the liver and/or bowels that contains milk thistle, dandelion, turmeric, artichoke and/or beet leaf:** These herbs improve the flow of bile, aid liver function, reduce inflammation, improve estrogen and cortisol metabolism, and reduce fatty liver, a factor known to accelerate insulin imbalance and aging. In addition to these herbs, you should also include B vitamins and magnesium. These nutrients aid your metabolism, blood sugar balance, insulin balance, estrogen detoxification and energy. Recommended brands include:
   - **Clear Detox—Hormonal Health** (Clear Medicine)—1 pack per day on rising. This product not only contains nutrients to support liver detoxification but also ingredients to support the breakdown and elimination of harmful excess estrogen. Clear Detox—Hormonal Health also includes a B complex and magnesium pill, along with calcium-d-glucarate, a fantastic anticancer and weight loss–enhancing supplement. I initially formulated this product with all the ingredients necessary to help free the body from estrogen dominance, but the majority of people who used it reported increased energy and decreased cravings—two wonderful side effects!
   - **L-Trepein** (Thorne Research)—2 capsules with breakfast and dinner
   - **Choline-Inositol** (Metagenics)—2 capsules with breakfast and dinner
   - **Liver–G.I. Detox** (Pure Encapsulations)—1 to 2 capsules with breakfast and dinner

If you choose one of the three liver formulas previously listed instead of Clear Detox—Hormonal Health, you may wish to purchase a B complex and a 100 to 250 mg magnesium citrate or glycinate supplement from your health-food store and take 1 capsule of each at breakfast.

3. **One serving a day of a bowel-cleansing formula containing a mix of soluble and insoluble fiber:** Choices include oat, apple, beet or flax fibers, glutamine, the herb triphala and preferably herbs to coat and heal the digestive tract wall, such as deglycyrrhizinated licorice (DGL), aloe and/or marshmallow. This type of product will promote healthier, more frequent bowel movements while you detox your liver and digestive system during the CSP. It will also help maintain the integrity of your digestive tract wall, thereby reducing inflammation and leaky gut syndrome, two causes of metabolic imbalance and toxic weight gain.

   Soluble fiber is fermented in your large intestine by your intestinal microflora and will help create an intestinal environment that allows beneficial bacteria to thrive. When taken with appropriate amounts of water, soluble fiber also bulks up the stool to support larger, softer stools and healthy bowel movements. As the bulk moves through your intestine, it helps to collect and eliminate other waste and toxins from your intestinal walls.

   Triphala is a standardized blend of three fruit extracts—*Terminalia chebula, Terminalia belerica* and *Emblica officinalis*—in equal proportions. It is an Ayurvedic herbal blend commonly used for supporting intestinal detoxification, occasional constipation and overall colon health. Recommended brands include:
   - **Clear Detox—Digestive Health**—1 pack per day before dinner or bedtime, with a full glass of water. In addition to fiber, probiotics, herbs and other nutrients for digestive support, this pack contains 1,000 mg of vitamin C and

200 mg of magnesium, which can benefit insulin and blood sugar balance.

- **G.I. Fortify** (Pure Encapsulations)—1 serving per day, usually mixed with water and taken before bed
- **FiberSMART** (Renew Life)—1 serving per day, usually mixed with water and taken before bed

4. **Omega-3 fish oils:** Our dietary fatty acid intake determines the healthy composition of all our cells. When we eat fatty acids such as those in fish oils—eicosapentaenoic acid (EPA) and docosahexaenoic acid (DHA)—our cell membranes become more receptive to insulin. The more insulin receptors we have on the surface of our cells, the lower our insulin levels. Healthy cell membranes allow us to enjoy greater wellness benefits and weight loss, as we prime our body for better insulin sensitivity.

Saturated fats such as those found in animal products have the opposite effects on our cells. You definitely need to choose your fats wisely for wellness! In addition to avoiding a high intake of saturated fat, you can prevent the harmful effects of saturated fats by including a DHA supplement in your diet. In one study, when rats fed saturated fats were also provided with DHA fish oils, symptoms of insulin resistance were vastly improved or prevented entirely. Dr. Yvonne Denkins, a nutrition researcher at the Pennington Biomedical Research Institute at Louisiana State University, also found that 3 months of daily supplementation with DHA produced a significant improvement in insulin sensitivity in overweight study participants.

According to a study in the February 2007 edition of the *British Journal of Nutrition,* the EPA component of fish oils is also important for improving insulin resistance and aiding fat loss. These findings were suspected to be the result of the anti-inflammatory and adiponectin-enhancing (fat-burning) benefits of EPA.

- They possess documented insulin-sensitizing effects.
- They protect our liver from the harmful effects of a high-fat diet and improve the insulin sensitivity of liver cells.
- They stimulate the secretion of leptin, one of the hormones that decrease our appetite and promote fat burning.
- They boost adiponectin, a fat-burning and insulin-sensitizing hormone.
- They help us lose fat by activating the fat-burning pathways in our liver and muscle.
- They encourage the storage of carbs as glycogen (in our liver and muscles) rather than fat.
- They are natural anti-inflammatory agents. Remember: Inflammation causes weight gain and can prevent fat loss by interfering with the fat-burning pathways in our liver and muscle tissue.

The insulin-sensitizing ability of DHA, the anti-inflammatory benefits of EPA and the adiponectin-boosting benefits of both make choosing a supplement containing significant amounts of each a good idea. Recommended brands:

- **Clear Omega—Extra Strength Fish Oils** (Clear Medicine)— These are extra strength, enteric-coated capsules that each contain 300 mg EPA and 200 mg DHA. Take 2 to 3 capsules twice daily.
- **o3mega extra strength** (Genuine Health)—2 to 3 capsules twice daily
- **proDHA Capsules** or **ProEFA** (Nordic Naturals)—2 to 3 capsules twice daily
- **Super DHA Capsules** or **MedOMEGA Liquid Fish Oil** (Carlson)—2 to 3 capsules twice daily or 1 teaspoon

- **Nutra Sea High Potency Capsules** or **Liquid Fish Oil**
  (Ascenta)—2 to 3 capsules twice daily or 1 teaspoon

5. **Vitamin D3:** Vitamin D has been proven to lower insulin, improve serotonin levels, enhance the immune system, control appetite and even improve fat-loss efforts. A study completed by a team at Massey University, published in the March 2010 edition of the *British Journal of Nutrition,* showed women who were given a daily dose of 4,000 IU of vitamin D3 showed improvements in their insulin resistance after 6 months of supplementation. You may wish to have your blood level of vitamin D3 tested by your doctor at some point; the participants whose vitamin D levels reached 119 nmol/l had the most improvements. This is not surprising to me. In Appendix A, you'll see that I've indicated an optimal blood value of 50 ng/mL (125 nmol/l) for ideal insulin balance and carb sensitivity.

   The study noted above is not the first to connect vitamin D and diabetes. A February 2011 article in the journal *Diabetes Metabolism* summarized clinical and in vitro observations and found that higher blood levels of vitamin D lowered diabetes risk and improved insulin sensitivity. Vitamin D was also found to prevent increases in blood sugar and insulin resistance and to reduce systolic blood pressure in type 2 diabetic patients.

   If all of this is not enough to convince you to dose daily with vitamin D, a study conducted at the University of Minnesota found that higher vitamin D levels in the body at the start of a low-calorie diet improved weight-loss success. Researchers determined that as vitamin D increased in the blood, subjects ended up losing almost a half pound more on their calorie-restricted diet. Moreover, higher baseline vitamin D levels predicted greater loss of abdominal fat. Take 2,000 to 5,000 IU daily for optimal results during your CSP.

6. **Whey protein isolate:** Whey is fantastic for fat loss, building muscle and boosting our fat-burning hormones. It is also rich in the antioxidant glutathione, aids immunity and supports the removal of harmful heavy metals and, of course, it's one of my favorite insulin-sensitivity superfoods. The metabolic benefits of whey protein isolate are vast and may prevail even when we consume a high-fat diet, according to a study in the February 2011 edition of the *Journal of Nutrition*.

   According to a study published in the September 2010 *British Journal of Nutrition*, whey protein isolate renders a powerful effect on body composition, lipids, insulin and glucose in overweight and obese individuals. Researchers found that subjects using a whey isolate (versus a mixed or casein protein powder, which unlike whey isolate, is not as highly absorbable, and is less allergenic or lactose free) experienced a significant decrease in total cholesterol and LDL cholesterol over 12 weeks. Fasting insulin levels were also significantly decreased in the whey group compared to their counterparts. Another study in the *American Journal of Clinical Nutrition* (April 2010) found that when whey protein is ingested before a meal it reduces the overall food intake as well as pre- and postmeal satiety. This is a *big* reason why I recommend whey protein in your midmorning and midafternoon snacks. This "secret ingredient" will reduce your appetite at lunch and dinner. Moreover, it also lowers postmeal glucose and insulin response.

   Your whey protein smoothie is not only quick, easy and tasty but also an important part of your plan to improve your carb sensitivities. Available in powder form, whey protein isolate is simple to mix into smoothies and is easily absorbed by the body. Just be sure to choose a product free of artificial sweeteners and sugar. Recommended brands include:
   - **Dream Protein**—1 to 2 servings daily. A favorite of our

patients and readers, this product is the best-tasting protein supplement they say they have ever tried.

- **Proteins +** (Genuine Health)—1 to 2 servings daily. This is 100 percent whey protein isolate that is free of sugar and artificial sweeteners.

SKIP THE SALT AND PILE ON POTASSIUM

Reducing your salt intake is one of several ways you can keep your blood pressure within a healthy range and manage your risk of stroke, heart disease and kidney disease. It's also an easy means of freeing yourself from water-related weight gain. Here are some simple salt guidelines:

- The majority of the salt in our diet comes from processed foods, so this recommendation certainly won't be a shock: Choose and prepare foods with little salt. Products containing no more than 200 mg (maximum 300 mg) of sodium per serving are your best options.
- You should consume less than 2,300 mg of sodium per day—the equivalent of approximately 1 teaspoon of salt.
- If you have high blood pressure, or if you are middle aged or older, you should consume no more than 1,500 mg of sodium per day. In this instance, opt for low-sodium foods, which contain 140 mg of salt or less per serving.
- At the same time, pack your diet with potassium-rich foods such as:

  Fresh fruits: bananas (I recommend bananas in your smoothies only to avoid consuming too many carbohydrates without a balance of protein), strawberries, watermelon, cantaloupe (like bananas, this high-glycemic melon is best consumed in small amounts and only in postworkout smoothies), oranges, pears, apricots

Fresh vegetables: beets, greens, spinach, peas, tomatoes, mushrooms, avocado, cucumber

Dried vegetables: beans, peas

Fresh meats: turkey, fish, beef

Potassium is an essential mineral for maintaining the pH balance of our bodily fluids. It can also help to offset the effects of excess sodium in our diet. It plays a vital role in regulating blood pressure, maintaining bone mass and ensuring the healthy function of your nervous system, muscles, heart, kidneys and adrenal glands. The long-term outcome of potassium deficiency is serious and may include high blood pressure, stroke and heart irregularities. On a day-to-day basis, low levels of potassium also leave us feeling less than our best. A whole host of health problems can result, including:

- Trouble losing weight
- Water retention
- A general feeling of weakness
- Constant fatigue
- Difficulty concentrating
- Concerns with muscle coordination, spasms or cramping

7. **A fiber supplement to toss into your smoothies:** Many carbs, especially grains, are a good source of fiber, which can help with regular bowel movements. So temporarily removing carbs as you attempt to determine your tolerance can be tricky if it tends to lead to a nasty case of constipation. Aside from its ability to "keep things moving," fiber can have a dramatic impact on your blood sugar and insulin levels. A study featured in the December 2010 edition of *Applied Physiology, Nutrition and Metabolism* found that supplementation with soluble fiber improved insulin resistance and various markers of metabolic syndrome in overweight men. Over a period of 12 weeks, the test group using

the daily fiber supplement had reductions in glucose and insulin and improvements in cholesterol levels.

A hypoallergenic source of fiber, in supplement form, can quickly become a must-have in your regimen. In the past, I have recommended ground flaxseed or chia seed in smoothies, but these sources provide a surprisingly small dose of just 4 grams of fiber for every tablespoon. I now suggest using these sources at mealtimes—sprinkling them on salad or into yogurt—and using a supplement that provides a more beneficial 7 to 8 grams in your smoothie instead. This simple shift in your fiber-dosing habits will allow you to reach my recommended daily intake of 35 grams of fiber much more easily.

Recommended brands include:

- **Clear Fiber** (Clear Medicine)
- **Gentle Fibers** (Jarrow)
- **Fiber-Tastic!** (Renew Life)
- **Organic Clear Fiber** (Renew Life)

You may purchase all the supplements you need for the first 4 to 6 weeks of the CSP through www.carbsensitivity.com. The CSP Kit contains Clear Detox—Hormonal Health; Clear Detox—Digestive Health; Clear Flora; and Clear Omega—Extra Strength Fish Oil capsules. Clear Recovery—Strength and Exercise formula, the great-tasting whey protein powder Dream Protein (available in chocolate or vanilla), a fiber supplement, and a high-potency vitamin D3 supplement in pill or drop form can also be added, if you do not have these products on hand.

Should you be directed to the Metabolic Repair Program prior to finishing the 4-week supply of products, just finish these supplements before moving on to the supplement prescription for Metabolic Repair. You will notice, however, that many similar supplements are also recommended as part of that plan.

These prescribed products will help you to cruise through the CSP feeling energized, balanced and free of cravings. And the CSP exercise plan in the next part will only help to enhance their effects. For a printable version of your daily dosing guidelines, visit www.carbsensitvity.com.

Daily Supplement Prescription for the 6-Week CSP

TIME OF DAY	SUPPLEMENT	BENEFIT

Upon rising (before food)	1 Clear Flora
	Alternative:
	  See page 219
		Probiotic supplements reduce inflammation, aid estrogen detoxification and improve digestion and immunity.
		  According to the latest research, the bacteria in our gut are also directly related to healthy insulin balance.

Breakfast	1 pack Clear Detox–Hormonal Health Alternative: See page 220	This mixture of herbs and nutrients eliminates toxic estrogen, aids fat loss, increases energy, controls cravings and detoxes the liver.
	2 Clear Omega Alternative: See page 223	Omega-3 oils reduce inflammation and improve insulin sensitivity. They also aid fat loss, especially when combined with exercise, and decrease cravings.
	2,000 to 4,000 IU vitamin D3	Vitamin D3 aids insulin balance, serotonin activity in the brain (important for mood and craving control) and immunity.
Postworkout or as a midafternoon snack, combined with whey protein isolate	Clear Recovery Alternative: • Select a sugar-free postworkout drink rich in antioxidants	Clear Recovery contains a mixture of amino acids and antioxidants that aid energy, exercise recovery, insulin balance and cellular repair.

(continued)

Daily Supplement Prescription for the 6-Week CSP (cont.)

TIME OF DAY	SUPPLEMENT	BENEFIT
Dinner	2 Clear Omega Alternative: See page 223	Omega-3 oils reduce inflammation and improve insulin sensitivity. They aid fat loss, especially when combined with exercise, and reduce cravings.
Before bed	1 Pack Clear Detox—Digestive Health Alternative: See page 220	Detoxes the digestive system, aids sleep, helps balance blood sugar and control cravings.

CSP SUCCESS STORY: FLAVIA

"After many years of struggling with polycystic ovarian syndrome (PCOS), I read *The Hormone Diet*, and later I booked a consultation with Dr. Natasha Turner. She started me on the Carb Sensitivity Program shortly thereafter. I lost weight, got my PCOS under control and am expecting my first child in September! And I feel fantastic."

FLAVIA, 31

STATS	BEFORE	AFTER
Weight	150 lb	134 lb
Body Fat	30%	25%
BMI	26.6	23.8

INITIAL CHIEF COMPLAINTS:

1. Weight
2. Irregular menstrual cycle
3. PCOS

PART THREE

THE METABOLIC REPAIR PROGRAM: A DEFINITIVE SYSTEM TO IMPROVE CARBOHYDRATE SENSITIVITY

What you do today can improve all your tomorrows.

RALPH MARSTON

CHAPTER 9

SO YOU HAVE A DAMAGED
METABOLISM . . .

Even if you fall on your face, you're still moving forward.

VICTOR KIAM

If you have jumped to this chapter, it's because you experienced signs of carb sensitivity and an insulin spike at one of the six phases of the CSP. You may be asking yourself, so now what? How did I end up here? Experiencing one or more of the symptoms presented in the Carb Sensitivity Checklist (in Chapter 7) at the end of any given phase, whether weight gain, water retention, increased cravings, fatigue after eating or an inability to lose weight, indicates you have some degree of insulin resistance—not a good thing for anyone wanting to trim down, let alone age gracefully and disease free.

If you want to understand *the how and why* of your carb sensitivity, read this chapter. If you'd rather cut straight to the *"what do I need to do to fix it"* stage, you can fast-forward to Chapter 10.

If you have chosen to stay here and learn more, I encourage you to sit back and get comfortable. We are going to delve into the inner workings of the body for a little Physiology 101.

Metabolic Damage = Increased Carb Sensitivity and Decreased Insulin Sensitivity

If you have arrived at this point after Phase One, your sensitivity to carbohydrates is high, and your body's response to insulin is very poor. It's so low, in fact, we might postulate that you have full-blown insulin resistance. You may even be prediabetic or type 2 diabetic. If you have arrived at this chapter for metabolic repair after Phase Two or Phase Three, you likely have a moderate sensitivity to carbohydrates and a moderate level of insulin resistance. Landing here after Phase Four or Five likely indicates a mild sensitivity to carbohydrates and only a mild degree of insulin resistance.

Regardless of when you arrived, I guarantee you can improve your current metabolic state and further enhance your tolerance for consuming more carbohydrates. Remember, insulin resistance and carb sensitivity are conditions that are *preventable* and even *reversible* with the right dietary and lifestyle habits. The right nutrition, supplements, exercise, stress management and sleep habits will do wonders to repair your insulin response, which ultimately means less insulin release and less sensitivity to carbohydrates. The only question is, how long will it take?

The answer depends on the degree of damage, your genetic makeup, the length of time you have had the imbalance and, clearly, how well you can stick with the program your body needs to restore its metabolic engines. I have had some patients restore balance within just 4 weeks. Others, particularly those who are prediabetic or have type 2 diabetes, saw improvements in their blood sugar balance immediately, but more dramatic changes in body composition followed months later, once their underlying metabolic imbalances had time for greater repair and restoration.

What Is a Damaged Metabolism?

If you currently have signs of metabolic disruption, it means that there are specific imbalances in your body at the cellular level. As we learned back in Part One, *all* cases of carb sensitivity lead to increased insulin resistance. *All* incidences of metabolic damage indicate inflammation is present, and *most* cases also show estrogen dominance. In summary, the conditions associated with metabolic damage are:

1. Inflammation
2. Insulin resistance
3. Leptin resistance
4. Estrogen dominance

Wow, that's a whole lot of medical talk to take in! Based on my research, my sense is that *most of us* have one, two or all of these imbalances. My Metabolic Repair Program benefits *all* imbalances, so distinguishing which one is at play is actually not that important. I do, however, believe that understanding these conditions will provide you with insight into your carbohydrate sensitivity and what it means for your overall health. Don't worry, I will walk you through it. By the end of this chapter, you will understand the imbalances that your Metabolic Repair Program will address.

Inflammation

Within a well-balanced immune system, inflammation ebbs and flows as needed. A certain degree of inflammation is a basic mechanism of a healthy immune system and bodily repair, just as the proper balance of cholesterol is vital to our cellular health. But much in the same way that surplus cholesterol can block an artery, excessive or persistent inflammation leads to tissue destruction and disease.

Chronic activation of our inflammatory response takes a heavy toll on the body and has recently become recognized as the root cause of most diseases associated with aging. Besides the typical inflammatory illnesses we know of, such as arthritis, the list of conditions spurred by inflammation includes cancer, heart disease, obesity, osteoporosis, Alzheimer's disease, autoimmune disease, diabetes, stroke and even wrinkling of our skin.

Researchers are aggressively searching for ways to tackle inflammation as an underlying cause of disease. Findings at the Joslin Diabetes Center in Boston, for example, have already led to a clinical trial of an anti-inflammatory agent for treating type 2 diabetes. Six years ago, Dr. Steven Shoelson, a professor at Harvard Medical School, reported that very high doses of aspirin, a known anti-inflammatory, proved effective in improving insulin-glucose tolerance, boosting insulin sensitivity and lowering blood-lipid levels in rodents.

Carb Sensitivity Means You Are a Hotbed of Inflammation

Excess carbs increase inflammation, and inflammation fuels your body's sensitivity to carbohydrates. Another of those vicious circles! You may not recognize the signs or symptoms of inflammation, but I can guarantee it is an issue you need to address in order to age without serious complications. Inflammation is a health concern for everyone, but particularly for those who also suffer from digestive disorders, allergies, autoimmune disease, arthritis, heart disease, asthma, eczema, acne, obesity, abdominal fat, headaches, joint stiffness, depression and sinus disorders. Two blood tests can identify your current levels of inflammation: high-sensitivity C-reactive protein (hs-CRP) and homocysteine. These are the simplest and best diagnostic tools currently available to assess inflammation, and can easily be ordered by your doctor, though I describe many others in Appendix A.

Our mental health also is linked to inflammation. Depression in obese men is significantly associated with increased levels of CRP, as shown by a 2003 German study published in the journal *Brain, Behavior and Immunity*. This research supports the strong link between our emotions, our hormones and inflammation. In another study conducted in 2004 and published in *Archives of Internal Medicine*, a similar link was found between depression and higher levels of inflammation (as denoted by CRP) in both men and women, though the link was stronger in men. In fact, the men with the most recent bouts of depression showed the highest CRP values.

But here's another interesting piece of the inflammation puzzle. Menopause appears to be linked to an increase in inflammation, especially due to waning estrogen levels at this stage of life. The declining level of testosterone distinctive of andropause in men is also linked to inflammation.

Reducing inflammation is an absolutely vital step in allowing the body to properly respond to insulin. The peroxisome proliferator-activated receptors (PPARs), the masters of the fat-burning pathways in our liver and muscle cells, influence the tight interaction between our insulin sensitivity, inflammation and weight. A PPAR imbalance contributes to inflammation, obesity and insulin resistance. Because of this interaction, I have included anti-inflammatory and insulin-sensitizing supplements and lifestyle habits in your Metabolic Repair Supplements in the next chapter.

THE SIGNS AND SYMPTOMS OF INFLAMMATION

- High cholesterol, uric acid or blood pressure
- Aches and pains, arthritis, bursitis, tendonitis or joint stiffness
- Water retention in hands or feet
- Gas, bloating, constipation or diarrhea
- Fibromyalgia
- Headaches or migraines
- Allergies (food or environmental), hives or asthma
- Autoimmune disease
- Belly fat or generalized weight gain
- Eczema, skin rashes or acne

Insulin Resistance

As discussed in earlier chapters, when insulin is present in excess over a long period, our cells grow accustomed to having so much of it around. As a result, our cellular response to insulin becomes blunted. The pancreas is then called upon to step up its insulin production in an attempt to maintain a normal blood sugar level. This decrease in insulin sensitivity is called insulin resistance.

Insulin resistance primarily develops in the skeletal muscle cells but can also occur in fat cells, the liver and other tissues. Once our cells become resistant to insulin, losing weight becomes harder than ever, and our sensitivity to carbohydrates is heightened. Moreover, physiological changes start to occur.

The fact that you have been directed to this chapter indicates you are somewhat resistant to insulin, and while you may have anticipated this after the "pinch" test on page 47 in Chapter 3, a much more in-depth investigation is necessary to determine insulin resistance in clinical settings. A full workup includes blood tests, blood pressure readings and, in some cases, additional exams such as an abdominal ultrasound to assess the liver. Should you wish to talk to your health-care provider about this type of investigation, I have outlined the tests involved in a complete investigation of insulin resistance and metabolic disruption in Appendix A.

Leptin Resistance

As discussed in Chapter 2, leptin plays a key role in metabolism and the regulation of fatty tissue. It's released by your fat cells in amounts commensurate with overall body-fat stores. In other words, the more body fat you have, the higher your leptin levels will be. When we are responding to leptin properly, it acts as a signal to the brain, allowing us to determine when we are full or when we should continue eating.

While balanced leptin offers many health-promoting, antiaging benefits, too much of this hormone is not a good thing. Excessive saturated fat intake and obesity can lead to soaring leptin levels and ultimately to leptin resistance (and insulin resistance; when we have one of these conditions, we likely have the other). Under this condition, the brain no longer responds to leptin's appetite-suppressing signals. In the absence of leptin's controlling mechanism, appetite can surge, even when plenty of leptin is present!

Leptin resistance is linked directly to obesity, insulin resistance and inflammation, which means it must be addressed right at the onset of an effective treatment plan to allow for optimal weight-loss results. Unfortunately, the discovery of high leptin levels in obese individuals has dampened the hope of using this hormone as a treatment for obesity, but researchers are still investigating this option.

Estrogen Dominance

Women and men both naturally have estrogen in the body. Estrogen balance is essential for achieving and maintaining fat loss. In men and premenopausal women, too much estrogen, a condition called estrogen dominance, causes toxic fat gain, water retention, bloating and a host of other health and wellness issues. While premenopausal women with excess estrogen tend to have the pear-shaped body type with more weight at the hips, both men and menopausal women with this surplus exhibit an apple shape, with more fat accumulation in the abdominal area. Researchers have now identified excess estrogen to be just as great a risk factor for obesity—in both sexes—as poor eating habits and lack of exercise.

Estrogen dominance can be a serious issue for men. As testosterone and progesterone naturally decline with age or stress, estrogen conversely rises. This hormonal shift impacts not only the physique but also prostate health. Statistics show that shockingly high numbers of men who live to the age of 65 and older will develop prostate cancer, likely due to estrogen exposure.

There are only two ways to accumulate excess estrogen in the body: We either produce too much of it on our own (via the fat cells in both sexes and the ovaries in women) or acquire it from our environment or diet. Unfortunately, accumulating excess estrogen is not hard. We are constantly exposed to estrogen-like compounds in foods that contain toxic pesticides, herbicides and growth hormones. Many of these toxins are known to cause weight gain, which serves to fuel the production of more estrogen from our own fat cells. I have included estrogen dominance as a condition linked to metabolic damage because more weight gain leads to insulin resistance, which—you guessed it—increases the risk of estrogen dominance.

Pharmaceutical hormones, such as those used in hormone-replacement therapy (HRT) or the birth control pill, also increase estrogen, whether we take them actively or absorb them when they make their way into our drinking water. We are living in a virtual sea of harmful estrogens, and researchers are only beginning to identify the impact of this exposure on health in humans and other species.

HOW WE BECOME ESTROGEN DOMINANT

In addition to obesity and metabolic disruption, the following factors also contribute to excess estrogen:

1. **Impaired liver function.** Since the liver breaks down estrogen, alcohol consumption, drug use, a fatty liver, liver disease and any other factor that impairs healthy liver function can spur an estrogen buildup.

2. **Poor digestion.** Insufficient dietary fiber, bacterial imbalance in the gut and other problems that compromise digestion interfere with the proper elimination of estrogen from the body via the digestive tract.

3. **Alcohol consumption.** Research shows that as few as one alcoholic drink can spark an increase in estrogen production.

4. **A high-fat diet.** High-fat diets stimulate the production of the harmful form of estrogen.

5. **Nutrient deficiencies.** The body requires sufficient intake of zinc, magnesium, vitamin B6 and other essential nutrients not only to support the breakdown and elimination of

estrogen but also to aid the function of enzymes responsible for the conversion of testosterone to estrogen. Interestingly, these nutrients tend to become depleted with regular use of the birth control pill, which is a concentrated source of estrogen.

6. **Lack of exercise.** This is one more reason that exercise is so essential for reducing the risk of cancer and other diseases.

7. **Sleep deprivation.** Maintaining habits that prevent sufficient, quality sleep causes a reduction in the hormone melatonin, which helps protect against estrogen dominance.

If you are a premenopausal woman with estrogen dominance, you likely have PMS, too much body fat around the hips and difficulty losing weight. Perhaps you have a history of gallstones, varicose veins, uterine fibroids, cervical dysplasia, endometriosis or ovarian cysts. For all you men out there, low libido, poor motivation, depression, loss of muscle mass and increased belly fat are big red flags. You may even notice breast development. These symptoms are very similar to those that result from low testosterone, since estrogen dominance is most often accompanied by suboptimal testosterone.

In both sexes, estrogen dominance is thought to be responsible for many types of cancers. This particular hormone imbalance is currently estimated to be one of the *leading* causes of breast, uterine and prostate cancer. For those of you taking my detox packs Clear Detox—Hormonal Health and Clear Detox—Digestive Health, the good news is that you have already kick-started the process of removing toxic estrogen from your body, since this is exactly what I formulated these products for.

Now that you know the underlying imbalances related to metabolic damage, let's discuss how you got this way.

Why Is Your Metabolism Damaged?

Have you discovered the types and amounts of carbs your body can handle? If you are over 50, my guess is that your tolerance is much lower than most readers in their 30s. Aging causes some metabolic damage, but other factors brought about your intolerance for carbs.

Certain habits in your life have either increased your production of insulin or reduced your cellular sensitivity to insulin. Both lead to high insulin levels and increased carb sensitivity. The graphic on the next page shows a few of the factors. On the upside, even severe instances of metabolic syndrome can be reversed with better habits.

An insulin backup in the bloodstream can be alleviated in two ways. First, we can restore the function of the insulin receptors on your liver, muscle or fat cells so they respond more easily. Exercise and insulin-sensitizing supplements are highly effective for this purpose. Second, we can lessen the insulin load in the first place by reducing the amount of insulin flooding the bloodstream. In other words, identifying your carb sensitivities, adopting better nutritional habits and, most importantly, limiting simple, high-glycemic carbohydrates all lead to an overall reduction in the stimulation of insulin release.

Let's elaborate on the factors that cause metabolic damage. This will help you better understand the principles behind your prescription for metabolic repair in the coming chapters. These factors include:

- Diet debacles (poor nutrition habits)
- Bad digestion blues (poor digestive health and altered gut microflora)
- Environmental toxins and drugs
- Chronic stress
- Nutrient deficiencies
- Sedentary lifestyle/lack of muscle
- Sleep disruption/deprivation
- Yo-yo dieting
- Fatty liver disease
- Aging

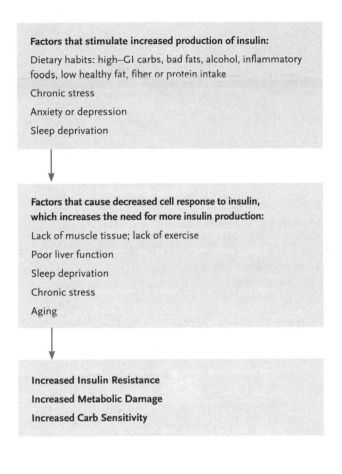

Factors that stimulate increased production of insulin:

Dietary habits: high–GI carbs, bad fats, alcohol, inflammatory foods, low healthy fat, fiber or protein intake

Chronic stress

Anxiety or depression

Sleep deprivation

Factors that cause decreased cell response to insulin, which increases the need for more insulin production:

Lack of muscle tissue; lack of exercise

Poor liver function

Sleep deprivation

Chronic stress

Aging

Increased Insulin Resistance

Increased Metabolic Damage

Increased Carb Sensitivity

Okay, so we definitely can't avoid aging. But we *can* certainly improve how your mind and body responds to it. Every other factor listed on page 242 is 100 percent modifiable and preventable. Amazing!

Dietary Debacles That Cause Excess Insulin

The culprits that trigger insulin release are pretty easily identifiable. What we eat, how much we eat and when we eat can all help or hinder our insulin balance. To have arrived at this point, chances are you have a history of one or more of the eating habits or overindulgences shown on the next few pages.

NASTY NUTRITION HABIT THAT CAUSES HORMONAL IMBALANCES	ASSOCIATED HORMONE IMBALANCE, IMMEDIATE RESULTS AND LONG-TERM RISKS
What We Eat	
Sugars and white processed flours—including glucose, honey, maple syrup, brown rice syrup, molasses, brown sugar, white sugar, sucrose, corn syrup, anything labeled as an "energy" drink or bar, bagels, pastas, white rice, crackers, muffins, pastries, cookies, candies, sweets, granola bars, sesame snacks, sugary juices or specialty coffee drinks, especially those that contain high-fructose corn syrup, such as sodas or energy drinks, as well as any drink containing sucralose, aspartame, saccharin or any other artificial sweetener	All of these foods spike insulin, spur inflammation and increase the risk of leptin resistance.
Chocolate syrups or sauces, ketchup, relish, sweet pickles, honey, jams, apple butter, chutneys, barbecue sauce, store-bought marinades, and other condiments containing sugar (you may have to read the labels for hidden sugars in savory sauces)	Dr. Paresh Dandona, a professor of medicine at the State University of New York at Buffalo who specializes in the topic of metabolism and inflammatory stress, found that overconsumption of any macronutrient—protein, carbohydrate or fat—contributes to inflammation. His team of researchers also identified the immediate effects of specific foods on inflammation. Orange juice, for instance, was shown to have anti-inflammatory properties, red wine was found to be neutral, and cream promoted inflammation. The team also discovered that overweight test subjects experienced significant changes in free radical stress indicators and inflammation just 1 week after starting a more nutritious diet.

NASTY NUTRITION HABIT THAT CAUSES HORMONAL IMBALANCES	ASSOCIATED HORMONE IMBALANCE, IMMEDIATE RESULTS AND LONG-TERM RISKS
What We Eat _(continued)_	
All products containing high-fructose corn syrup (HFCS)	HFCS increases blood sugar and insulin, which ultimately leads to an overactive appetite, overeating, insulin resistance and obesity.
Artificial sweeteners including sucralose, aspartame, saccharin, etc.	Although they may not cause an increase in your blood sugar, foods and drinks containing artificial sweeteners do trigger insulin release. This leads to excess appetite, overeating, insulin resistance and weight gain.
Excess alcohol	Excess alcohol intake leads to insulin resistance and estrogen dominance, and may contribute to symptoms of low testosterone such as loss of muscle and increased belly fat.
Excess caffeine	Moderate caffeine intake (1 cup of organic coffee a day) may help blood sugar and insulin balance. More than 4 cups per day may, however, increase the risk of blood sugar imbalance, high cholesterol, cravings and belly fat. More caffeine appears to stimulate a rise in blood sugar, which eventually spurs more insulin release.
Low-fiber intake	This nasty habit leads to increased blood sugar, insulin and estrogen in the body and increases the risk of insulin resistance, diabetes, heart disease, colon cancer, breast cancer, prostate cancer and obesity.

NASTY NUTRITION HABIT THAT CAUSES HORMONAL IMBALANCES	ASSOCIATED HORMONE IMBALANCE	IMMEDIATE RESULTS AND LONG-TERM RISKS
When and How We Eat		
Overeating (supersizing)	• Increased blood sugar and insulin • Decreased leptin, or increased leptin in the case of leptin resistance • Increased cortisol	Excess appetite, overeating, insulin resistance and weight gain
Late-night eating	• Increased blood sugar and insulin • Decreased melatonin • Decreased growth hormone	Poor sleep quality; excess appetite, overeating, and excess cortisol the following day; weight gain
Failing to balance protein, carbohydrates and fats	• Increased blood sugar and insulin • Increased cortisol • Decreased leptin, or increased leptin in the case of leptin resistance • Increased estrogen in men; increased testosterone in women	Insulin resistance, estrogen dominance, abdominal weight gain, heart disease, diabetes, increased risk of cancer

If you're panicking right now, don't! You will have a cheat meal once a week moving forward, which will allow you to enjoy a sugary treat or a nice bowl of pasta. But until we get your metabolism revving, you will have to curb your urge to indulge in these carb-laden options on all other days of the week. When it comes to hydrogenated oils, inflammatory oils, high-fructose corn syrup and artificial sweeteners, however, I recommend you avoid them 100 percent of the time, even during your weekly cheat meal.

Bad Digestion Blues

Think for a minute about how our eating habits have evolved with our busy lifestyle. We shovel in a fast bite at our desk, in the car or standing over the kitchen counter so we can quickly move on with work or carpooling duties. We eat late at night in front of the television, or we skip meals altogether. Now think about our food choices. Packaged, processed convenience foods loaded with hidden salt, fat and sugar. Sheesh!

Believe it or not, a whopping 60 percent of our immune system is clustered around our digestive tract. That's why anything that compromises digestion—including food allergies, beneficial gut flora (intestinal bacteria)/harmful bacterial imbalance, deficiency of enzymes or acids, yeast overgrowth, parasites and stress—negatively impacts not only the process of digestion itself but also our entire immune system. Painful conditions such as gas, bloating, heartburn, reflux, constipation, diarrhea, irritable bowel syndrome, Crohn's disease and ulcerative colitis are *all* related to inflammation in the digestive system.

Moreover, when our bowels aren't moving properly, waste builds up in our body, creating toxicity and hampering our overall health. A buildup of estrogen by-products is particularly worrisome, since estrogen is metabolized in the liver and excreted into the digestive system in the bile. Bacteria in the large bowel aid the breakdown of estrogen even more. Liver function, bile secretion, bacterial balance and sufficient bowel movements are essential to ridding the body of toxins, especially excess estrogen, which can increase cancer risks.

IS YOUR DIGESTIVE SYSTEM WORKING HARD OR HARDLY WORKING?
Let's face it: Few of us like to spend much time thinking about the contents of our toilet. But together with general feelings in and around your gut, the frequency and quality of your "poop" can give you the real scoop on your digestive health. Use this simple questionnaire to determine whether your digestion could use some help.

QUESTION	YES	NO
Do you have fewer than one bowel movement a day?		
Do you ever have stools that are black in color?		
Have you ever noticed blood in your stool?		
Have you ever noticed mucus in your stool?		
Are your stools very narrow?		
Do you have a tendency toward loose stools or diarrhea?		
Do your stools sink to the bottom of the bowl?		
Do you experience excessive gas?		
Do you experience abdominal bloating?		
Do you have frequent heartburn, indigestion or reflux?		
Do you have recurring nausea?		
Do you have abdominal pain or cramping?		
Do you notice bits of food in your stools (besides corn)?		

If you answered yes to even *one* of these questions, your digestive system needs work.

Optimal bowel function means one bowel movement after every meal, ideally three times a day but a minimum of once daily. If you are experiencing fewer, you're constipated. Quality matters, as well. The perfect bowel movement should be well formed and should float. It should be free of food particles and mucus, and not overly narrow. Mucus in or covering the stool, or narrow stools, suggests inflammation of the bowel. Strong-smelling gas may suggest a deficiency of the enzymes necessary to properly digest protein or an imbalance of healthy gut flora (e.g., parasitic infection). If you wake in the morning with a nice flat stomach but look 5 months pregnant by day's end, your digestion also needs help. Abdominal tenderness is yet another indication that your bowels could be inflamed and that you need to consider your food choices, bacterial balance, enzymes and the state of your digestive tract wall.

Some digestive problems are caused or exacerbated by adverse reactions to particular foods. Such reactions can impair the release of enzymes, the movement of your intestines and the walls of your GI tract. An extreme example is celiac disease, an allergic reaction to gluten that interferes with nutrient absorption. In other cases, the barrier of the intestinal wall can become permeable, allowing foreign substances to pass into the bloodstream. When this disruption occurs, inflammation, immune compromise or allergies may follow and lead to hormonal imbalance.

What Does Your Digestion Have to Do with Your Metabolism?

In a word, everything! It makes sense that what you see *on* your belly essentially begins with what's in your mouth, but it can also be impacted by what's *in* your belly. The health of your digestive system and beneficial gut flora (otherwise known as probiotics) influences the number of calories that are absorbed from your food and stored in your body. The carbohydrates you eat are broken down into sugar through the process of digestion, which begins in the mouth and ends in your small intestine. From there, what's going on in your gut has a huge impact on your metabolic function and your ability to break down toxins, synthesize nutrients, process indigestible food, regulate the immune system and produce the hormones needed to appropriately direct the storage of fat.

Research from the Mayo Clinic (April 2008) has linked favorable intestinal bacteria with the ability to get slim and stay that way. This research suggests that the metabolic activities of the gut flora facilitate the extraction of calories from the foods eaten and help to store these calories in fat tissue for later use. Furthermore, the researchers found that bacterial gut flora of obese mice and humans includes more types of calorie-storing bacteria than that of their lean counterparts. These findings suggest that gut flora may play a key role in regulating weight. The human body, which consists of about 100 trillion cells, carries about 10 times that many micro-organisms in the intestines and GI tract. And anything that affects nutrition absorption in turn impacts the expenditure of calories.

Additional research from the Université Catholique de Louvain in Belgium supports the notion that an increased prevalence of obesity and type 2 diabetes can be attributed not only to changes in dietary habits or reduced activity levels but also to the role, health and type of gut flora present in the body. These researchers found that mice with compromised intestinal bacteria increased their fat mass by about 60 percent and developed insulin resistance within just 2 weeks!

Finally, healthy gut flora promotes healthy immune function and thereby decreases inflammation. A 2010 study published in the *British Journal of Nutrition* found that probiotic bacteria improve insulin sensitivity by doing exactly that, reducing systemic inflam-mation. For this reason and others, the daily use of probiotics is an integral component in the Carb Sensitivity Program during all six phases, as well as in the Metabolic Repair Program.

Toxicity, Medications and Your Metabolism

Now that you know about the link between gut flora and weight gain, you're probably on the probiotics bandwagon, looking to get back in balance. But you may be unwittingly compromising your success because of toxins in your environment and/or the overuse of prescription medications. Under normal circumstances, friendly bacteria found in our digestive system live with us in symbiotic har-mony. Factors such as poor diet, and medications such as birth con-trol pills, antibiotics and corticosteroids, can upset this healthy balance and lead to a host of difficulties, including increased body-fat storage and reduced insulin sensitivity.

While they are designed to help our health, many medications are a source of toxins and hormonal disruption. The biggest culprits are antidepressants, birth control pills, synthetic HRT and corticosteroids. Yes, these medications have a role to play in certain circumstances, but I encourage you to consider trying a natural alternative first. And I strongly recommend that you fully understand the side effects and long-term risks of any and all medications you choose to use. A study published in *Diabetes Care* (December 2010) examined antidepressant medication use as a risk factor for type 2 diabetes and weight gain. Researchers found that more frequent dosages of antidepressants were associated with *double the risk* of diabetes in participants. The study concluded that ongoing use of antidepressant medication was associated with an increase in the risk of type 2 diabetes. When these types of drugs are in your system, total hormonal balance becomes much more difficult to achieve. Antidepressant medications interfere with the liver's detoxification pathways. These pathways are involved with the breakdown and elimination of harmful toxins, and when they are not functioning at their best, more toxins accumulate, which upsets the metabolism. I explain to patients that this process is like mixing alcohol with antidepressant medications—the effects of alcohol are more pronounced while taking one of these medications because of the interference with the detox pathways in the liver. The liver simply does not metabolize and break down the alcohol as quickly. As a result, you will feel the effects of alcohol faster and more intensely while taking antidepressants.

As storage houses in our body, our fat cells also accumulate many types of toxins that need to be neutralized when they are released during a fat-loss program. Your liver must continually metabolize, detoxify and excrete hormone by-products via the bile into the digestive tract for removal from the body at an optimal rate. Think of fat as a hoarder living in your basement—it keeps the good stuff for later use, but it also holds on to the bad stuff, which can be released into the bloodstream. When that happens, it's up to your internal cleaning crew—the liver—to release and dispose of it.

Here is a list of the main metabolic disrupting agents that may be lurking in your medicine cabinet. Please be sure to *consult your health practitioner* before considering making any changes to your medications.

MEDICATION	ALTERNATIVE NAME OR DESCRIPTION
Corticosteroids	Prednisone, hydrocortisone
Antidepressants	SSRIs, MAO inhibitors
Diuretics	Lasix, hydrochlorothiazide
Synthetic progesterone	Provera, Medroxyprogesterone acetate
Antiseizure medications	Tegetol, gabapentin
Antipsychotic medications	Olanzapine, risperidone, quetiapine

BUBBLES AND BODY FAT: METABOLICALLY DAMAGING CHEMICALS IN YOUR BATHROOM

Think of all the products we put on our skin, and imagine how the daily absorption of the chemicals in those products can add up over a lifetime. This long-term exposure is a definite hormonal and health concern. Use the list below to help you to avoid harmful chemicals in your cosmetics and skin care (a more complete list of harmful ingredients can be found at www.saffronrouge.com/learn /ingredients/truth). Some ingredients commonly found in readily available products are not only hormone disruptors but are listed by the US Environmental Protection Agency and the State of California as carcinogen risks. They include:

1. Acrylamide
2. Ethylene oxide
3. Formaldehyde
4. Phthalates

Your cleansing products should be free of sodium lauryl sulphate, a harsh detergent present in shampoos and cleansers. The products you use on your body or face should be free of methyl parabens, propyl parabens, formaldehyde, imidazolidinyl urea, methylisothiazolinone, propylene glycol, paraffin, isopropyl alcohol and sodium lauryl sulphate. You should know that most perfumed products contain many of these harmful chemicals, but the ingredients are not identified on the label. Look for products that contain only natural oils and fragrances. Here are my favorite brands for natural, hormone-healthy skin care:

- Korres. The company makes amazing body butters, lip balms and body lotions.
- Naturopathica. I love their Environmental Defense Mask.
- Juice Beauty. Past readers know I am a fan of their Green Apple Peel as a fabulous, nonabrasive exfoliant. My new faves are the Stem Cellular Repair products for the face and eye area, which really work for combating wrinkles, and Reflecting Lip glosses. They look great and the little tubes are the perfect size to slip inside your jeans pocket.
- Skinceuticals. I love their hyaluronic acid serum and vitamin C serum.
- John Masters. I adore their facial serums that contain green tea and vitamin C , their blood orange and vanilla body milk and all of their shampoos and conditioners.
- As a natural alternative to perfume, use body oils that are scented with natural essential oils.

Check out www.saffronrouge.com for a more complete array of safe skin-care and cosmetic options. Or use the online store at www.juicebeauty.com, which offers a greater array of products than many stores.

Chronic Stress

Our biological stress response has not yet evolved to deal with the plentiful assortment of long-term stressors in everyday modern life. Study after study shows that stress causes abdominal fat, even in people who are otherwise thin. Researchers at Yale University, for example, found slender women with high cortisol had more ab fat than those with lower levels of cortisol. Results published in the journal *Psychosomatic Medicine* in 2000 showed an established link between cortisol and increased storage of abdominal fat. I could cite literally hundreds of studies that prove depression, anxiety, sleep disruption and simply feeling dissatisfied or overwhelmed with life can wreak havoc on the waistline by increasing both appetite and belly fat—two definite signs of insulin and metabolic imbalance.

During temporarily stressful episodes, adrenaline kicks in and taps into fat stores to provide energy to fuel our natural fight-or-flight response. Under prolonged periods of intense stress, however, cortisol seeks out muscle proteins for fuel instead. Over time, this attack on muscle protein leads to the destruction of metabolically active muscle tissue—tissue we need to build in order to boost metabolism and burn energy more efficiently. At the same time, the fuel released from the breakdown of muscle fiber tends to be deposited around the abdomen if it's not burned off right away. As if our metabolism was not already in sufficient jeopardy, cortisol also inhibits the function of thyroid hormone, the master of our metabolic rate.

Over time, this exposure to cortisol decreases cellular response to insulin and leads to increased insulin levels. A long-term study published in the journal *Diabetes Care* (April 2007) followed a group of women for 15 years. The women who reported feeling frequently and intensely angry, tense or stressed also showed increased risk for developing metabolic syndrome. This study was the first to show how depressive symptoms, stressful life events and feelings of anger and tension can be associated with high cortisol and the development of metabolic disease.

Nutrient Deficiencies

There is overwhelming clinical evidence to show that vitamin deficiencies are associated with disease processes and the overall condition of our health. Deficiencies of vitamins, minerals, antioxidants and other essential micronutrients compromise the function of the immune system and contribute to degenerative conditions such as arthritis, cancer, cardiovascular disease, accelerated aging or diabetes.

The nutrients within your cells are involved with metabolism, healthy immunity, reproduction, detoxification, cellular regeneration and growth, as well as many other body processes. It's no wonder that a deficiency can cause problems! For example, an inadequate amount of zinc can lead to lower testosterone levels and cause free radical damage, while lower vitamin D intake has been linked to a risk of obesity, insulin resistance, autoimmune disease and cancer (primarily colorectal cancer, breast cancer and prostate cancer). The most common deficiencies I see in my practice today—which we will discuss in greater detail in the next chapter—include magnesium, zinc, vitamin D, vitamin E, vitamin C, vitamin B12, omega-3 fatty acids (ALA, EPA and DHA) and iodine (potassium iodide).

Lack or Loss of Muscle

With the help of your thyroid hormones, muscle tissue dictates your metabolic rate. Fat is far less metabolically active than muscle, which means the more fat you have, the fewer calories you need to maintain your weight. As a result, it is much easier to gain unwanted weight when you have insufficient muscle, simply because you are less likely to use all the calories you take in each day and more likely to store the excess calories as fat. This is also why some men, who naturally have a higher ratio of muscle to fat, tend to burn up what they eat at a faster rate. An overweight man may, however, have a slower metabolism compared to a slim woman with more muscle tissue.

The metabolic equation is very simple: The more muscle tissue you have, the more calories you will burn. Even the process of breaking down and repairing your muscles postworkout increases your metabolism. Miriam Nelson, a Tufts University researcher, showed that a group of women who followed a weight-loss diet *and* did weight-training exercises lost 44 percent more fat than those who only followed the diet. While aerobic activity can help burn calories during the activity, muscle building via strength training allows you to continue burning more calories at all times, even while you sleep. Muscle cells are also important targets for the action of insulin, since most of our insulin receptors are present within muscle tissue.

As we age and naturally lose muscle, the risk of carb sensitivity, reduced insulin sensitivity and insulin resistance increases. Remember from Chapter 3 that insulin resistance also fuels the loss of muscle tissue!

Sleep Deprivation

The majority of us fail to prioritize sleep, but women are especially guilty of putting sleep on the back burner, as evidenced by the 2007 National Sleep Foundation Poll, which focused only on the sleep habits of women. Half of those polled reported that sleep and exercise are the first activities they sacrifice when they are pressed for time. The same percentage admitted they reach for foods high in sugar or carbohydrates when they feel sleepy during the day. And the cycle of weight gain and insulin imbalance continues.

This poll provides incredible insight into women's health. The findings reveal that women are not only sleep deprived or experiencing sleep disorders but are also carrying around excess weight. In fact, more than half the women surveyed were either overweight or obese. Women who reported experiencing sleep problems nightly were significantly more likely to be classified as obese, compared to women who experienced sleep problems only a few nights a month. So, which comes first? Improper sleep or weight gain?

Go back to Chapter 5 if you need to refresh your mind on the benefits of sleep for beating carb cravings, along with great tips on healthy sleep habits for optimal insulin balance.

Yo-yo Dieters Beware

When your caloric intake bounces up and down like a yo-yo, your metabolism suffers through a dangerous series of highs and lows. The end result of this havoc includes weight gain (exactly what you did *not* want), mood changes, cravings, the loss of precious metabolically active muscle tissue and, ultimately, a damaged metabolism. Remember, less muscle means increased risk for higher insulin release. *The more you have dieted in the past, the more carb sensitive you will surely be now.*

The short-term victories achieved with a drastic cut in calories followed by a return to your old ways are *always* followed with rebound weight gain. This is caused by the loss of muscle and, whether we like it or not, our hormones, like leptin, kicking in to return the body to status quo.

Furthermore, the increase in stress hormones caused by excessive caloric restriction is highly destructive and will actually cause you to want to eat and eat—and eat some more—while you continue to lose more muscle. Here's the really scary part: Repeatedly losing and gaining weight is also linked to cardiovascular disease, stroke, diabetes and altered immune function. This type of caloric restriction can ravage both your hormonal balance and your metabolism.

Remember, your body and your hormones are programmed to work *against* you by increasing your appetite and slowing your metabolic rate when you slash your calories. When your metabolism drops, you gain weight and feel tired and sluggish. On the other hand, when you use the right weight-loss techniques, your metabolism gets an energizing boost that leaves you feeling brighter and looking your best.

Fatty Liver Disease and Obesity = More Metabolic Disruption
Most of us begin life with a healthy liver. As we gain weight and experience more metabolic imbalance, the liver becomes fatty, a condition commonly referred to as fatty liver disease. Some sources say it is the first sign of metabolic disease and, at the same time, perpetuates the cycle of metabolic disease as the liver cells fail to process insulin and fats properly. The same is true for obesity. The fatter we are, the more inflamed, insulin resistant and obese we become.

All the factors I've described in this chapter play a large role in contributing to metabolic damage, the end results of which include carb sensitivity and increased insulin resistance. Regardless of the cause, you *can* repair your metabolism with the Metabolic Repair Program I have outlined for you in the coming chapters.

"When I first came to Dr. Turner I was suffering from PCOS and I was frustrated that nothing seemed to work—I was constantly chasing quick fixes and getting nowhere, fast. Dr. Turner started to teach me about customizing nutrition for my body type as opposed to a cookie-cutter nutrition program. I was also on metformin, the birth control pill, and Aldactone in an attempt to balance my hormones, stabilize my mood swings and combat adult acne. Today, I am not only off both those medications, I feel great! Even my endocrinologist couldn't believe it. I lost weight—and even better, I lost it off the areas that count!"

SUSAN, 54

STATS	BEFORE	AFTER
Weight	151 lb	139 lb
Body Fat	39%	34%
BMI	29.4	27

INITIAL CHIEF COMPLAINTS:

1. Weight
2. Hormonal imbalance
3. PCOS

CHAPTER 10

YOUR METABOLIC REPAIR DIET
AND METABOLIC REPAIR SUPPLEMENTS

I don't believe you have to be better than everybody else.
I believe you have to be better than you ever thought you could be.

KEN VENTURI

In the last chapter, you learned that improving insulin sensitivity and reducing inflammation are two essential components of metabolic repair. You can achieve these goals by sticking to your Metabolic Repair Diet, and with the help of the supplement prescription outlined in this chapter. The amazingly effective, and totally doable, Metabolic Repair Workout in the next chapter will round out the process.

We all have different degrees of metabolic disruption, which means some of you may need to remain in this phase of the program longer than others. As an initial guideline, however, I suggest sticking with the Metabolic Repair Diet you have been directed to for at least 4 weeks before retrying whichever phase of the CSP you were on. For most people, the supplement and workout prescription for metabolic repair should be continued for at least 3 to 12 months. This will allow for significant improvements in your metabolism at the cellular level.

Determining Your Metabolic Repair Diet

Your individual nutrition prescription will depend on which phase you were in when directed to enter the Metabolic Repair Program. (Go back to Chapter 7 to review the Carb Sensitivity Checklist and CSP flowchart at the end of the phase you have just completed to determine your dietary prescription.) Those of you who have ended up here after Phase One will follow the daily diet beginning on page 139. All other readers will return to the previous phase of the CSP and remain there for 4 weeks before reattempting the phase you were in when the sensitivity symptoms arose. For example, if you failed to lose weight or experienced weight gain in Phase Three, your Metabolic Repair Diet should consist of Phase Two permitted foods. You may follow that particular week's meal plan and recipe ideas, *or any earlier phase's recipes,* for the next 4 weeks.

Once the 4 weeks have passed, you may retry the reintroduction process. Your body will tell you whether your metabolism has improved or if you need to continue with your Metabolic Repair Program. Carrying on with the example above, you would try Phase Three foods again at the 4-week mark. If you gain weight, retain water or experience cravings or an increased appetite, your level of carb sensitivity has not yet improved, and you should return to the same Metabolic Repair Diet and continue with Metabolic Repair Supplements and workout.

If, however, you continue to lose weight and feel energized, your Metabolic Repair Program has been successful. You may carry on with the CSP program, progressing week by week until you have completed all six phases, or until the results of the Carb Sensitivity Checklist direct you otherwise. *You may also choose to remain at a lower phase, if you find that's where you feel your best.*

The Cheat Meal
Regardless of the phase you have been directed to in the Metabolic Repair Program, I have prescribed a weekly cheat meal. Please refer to pages 203–5 for an explanation of the cheat meal.

The Metabolic Repair Diet for Those Who Did Not Progress Beyond Phase One
If you followed the program perfectly in Phase One of the CSP, and failed to experience weight loss or continued to suffer with cravings,

increased hunger, bloating or water retention, your metabolic damage is *severe*. Your diet plan must be very low in starchy carbohydrates in order for you to bring down your insulin levels. For now, this means even the carbohydrates in low–GI fruits must be avoided. It is important to adhere perfectly to this meal outline for the first 2 weeks. It is just as vital to implement a once-a-week cheat meal in weeks 3 and 4, but not before. Remember to follow the rules common to all CSP phases (see pages 108–11) and to avoid constipation (see pages 113–16), which is not uncommon.

The daily meal plan you should follow for the next 4 weeks is outlined on the following pages. The purpose of this specific phase is to remove from your diet the foodstuffs that are causing dramatic surges in blood sugar and insulin, which helps to restore the sensitivity of your insulin receptors so that the CSP can be carried out with success. Consider it your dietary "primer." The order of your meals is unimportant, and one meal may be substituted for another or repeated. Two shakes per day—no more, no less—are required. The meal guidelines for your diet are very basic, but they *must* be followed for the initial 4 weeks of your Metabolic Repair Program. You should feel free to use any recipe in this book that is free of fruit, legumes, grains and starchy vegetables. Many of the Phase One recipes should apply, but the protein content of each will need to be bumped up to meet the required guidelines outlined on the following pages.

With the exception of the once-a-week cheat meal that begins in week 3 of your Metabolic Repair Program, you may consume only carbohydrates sourced from nuts, seeds and nonstarchy (green) vegetables during this phase. The protein amounts listed pertain to *cooked* weight. The nut butters you choose must be all natural, without sugar added. A whey isolate is preferred as your protein powder source. All spices and sugar-free condiments are permitted, including Bragg's Liquid Aminos (which is a sugar-free soy sauce), sugar-free hot sauces and mustards, unsweetened lemon and lime juice, and white or apple cider vinegar (but not balsamic vinegar, which contains sugar).

You may drink water, sodium-free soda water, Perrier, Zevia sugar-free drinks (diet soft drinks), coffee or tea. Four cups of green tea per day is recommended. Coffee and tea should be enjoyed with cream, not milk (milk contains sugar; cream does not). If you need to sweeten your hot drinks, try stevia, a naturally sweet, sugar-free herb. You should eat within 1 hour of rising and every 3 to 4 hours during the day. Do not skip meals.

Remember, there is no cheating on the diet, except during the once-a-week cheat meal, starting in week 3 of the Metabolic Repair Diet. This means no extra nut butters, nuts or additional protein. Strict adherence is essential, but the benefits will pay off!

DAILY MEAL PLANS FOR THOSE WHO DID NOT PROGRESS BEYOND PHASE ONE

MEAL 1

2 (for women) or 4 (for men) whole omega-3 eggs + 4 additional egg whites + 1 to 2 cups chopped nonstarchy vegetables

OR

1 (for women) or 3 (for men) whole omega-3 eggs + 1 tablespoon goat or low-fat cheese + 5 additional egg whites + 1 to 2 cups chopped nonstarchy vegetables or mixed greens

MEAL 2

30 grams (for women) or 40 grams (for men) whey protein isolate mixed with water, 1 level tablespoon of nut butter (almond, hazelnut, cashew), cinnamon to taste and Clear Fiber supplement. The ingredients may be premixed in a shaker cup (you can add the water when you are ready to drink) or you may blend the ingredients with ice.

MEAL 3

5 ounces (for women) or 6 ounces (for men) chicken (or turkey, tilapia, flounder, shrimp, scallops, cod or 1 can of water-packed tuna) + ¼ (for women) or ⅓ (for men) level cup of almonds, cashews or walnuts + 1 to 2 cups of mixed nonstarchy vegetables or a mixed green salad (no tomatoes, carrots or red bell peppers).

MEAL 4

30 grams (for women) or 40 grams (for men) whey protein isolate mixed with water, 1 level tablespoon of nut butter (almond, hazelnut, cashew), cinnamon to taste and Clear Fiber supplement. The ingredients may be premixed in a shaker cup (you can add the water when you are ready to drink), or you may blend the ingredients with ice.

MEAL 5

5 ounces (for women) or 6 ounces (for men) salmon, trout or red meat (e.g., bison, venison, filet mignon, inside round, top round cut, lean ground beef, lean cut sirloin, but try to keep your red meat consumption to once or twice a week) + a mixed green salad (no tomatoes, carrots or red bell peppers) + 1 (for women) or ½ (for men) tablespoons of olive oil

Note: If you find you are overly hungry, increase the serving size of the protein at your meals by 1 ounce. Meal order is unimportant and one meal may be substituted for another.

The Metabolic Repair Supplements

While the dietary aspect of your metabolic repair will focus on limiting insulin release, your cellular sensitivity to insulin must also be restored with the help of the supplements outlined in this chapter and the exercise prescription in the next. These three factors combined are what will ultimately lower your insulin levels and improve your future tolerance for carbs. The great news is, seeing an improvement in your tolerance for processing carbs indicates that your metabolism is being successfully repaired.

The products suggested on the following pages can help do wondrous things to your insulin receptors (in addition to having many other beneficial metabolic effects), but they are by no means a replacement for proper nutrition and exercise. Fortunately, we have many extensively researched and clinically proven options from which to select. Many minerals, including magnesium, calcium, potassium, zinc, chromium, iodine and vanadium, show a beneficial relationship with an improvement of insulin resistance. Amino acids, including L-carnitine, taurine and L-arginine, may also help to improve insulin resistance. Additional nutrients such as coenzyme Q10 and lipoic acid also appear to have therapeutic potential.

The benefits of these nutrients are most noticeable when supplements are taken regularly for at least 3 consecutive months. You certainly do not have to use the Clear Medicine brand of products—the nutrients I recommend are available from different manufacturers at most health-food stores. Also, just like the supplements for the CSP 6-week process, these products are *not* a mandatory part of the program. But the results I have seen in my clinical practice and the research on their effectiveness certainly indicate that they will greatly enhance your metabolic repair and weight loss.

Read on to learn more about the five products I recommend as the Metabolic Repair Supplements. These contain nutrients that can greatly aid your carb sensitivities and your metabolism. Or, just skip to the dosing chart on pages 279–80 if you would like to get started right away.

1. **Metabolic Repair Pack (Clear Medicine)**
   This is my own formula for boosting your metabolism and restoring insulin sensitivity. Just 1 pack twice a day with meals will allow you to obtain therapeutic dosages of several ingredients,

which I have specially selected to improve your metabolism, insulin balance and fat loss. See the Super Insulin-balancing Nutrients textbox (pages 272–78) to learn more about many of the ingredients that make up this powerful product.

Recommended dose:

- Take 1 pack at breakfast and dinner. You should take your second dose at lunchtime if you find the green tea in the product keeps you awake at night.

OR

High-potency Multivitamin

As an alternative to taking the Metabolic Repair Pack, you may take a high-potency multivitamin twice daily, at breakfast and dinner. Although most formulas will not provide the specialized insulin-balancing nutrients that are present in the Metabolic Repair Pack, such as green tea, alpha lipoic acid or coenzyme Q10, a good quality multivitamin will replace many of the deficiencies common with insulin resistance as well as provide a dose of minerals and vitamin C to improve insulin sensitivity. Recommended brands:

- **Clear Essentials—Morning and/or —Evening Pack.**
  Take 1 pack of each daily, with meals. Clear Essentials— Morning contains 2 tablets of the top-rated and most bioavailable multivitamin, a calcium-magnesium tablet (balanced 2:1 with more calcium), a gel cap of mixed vitamin E, and a 400 IU tablet of vitamin D3. Clear Essentials—Evening provides another dose of 2 multivitamins, a lozenge containing 60 mg of coenzyme Q10, two calcium-magnesium tablets (balanced 1:1 with more magnesium to aid sleep) and 1,000 mg of vitamin C. These two daily packs provide all of your required nutrients at the recommended dosage for optimal daily intake.

- **High-potency multivitamin options** (take with meals daily):
  - **UltraNutrient** (Pure Encaps)
  - **Ultra Balance III** tablets with or without iron (Douglas Labs)
  - **MultiThera 1** (ProThera)
  - **Formula Multi 1-2-3** (Jarrow)
  - **Extend Plus** (Vitamin Research Products)

2. **Fish Oil: Omega-3 Fatty Acids**

In Chapter 8, we discussed the numerous studies that support the use of omega-3 fatty acids for weight loss, reduced inflammation and improved cell function. But when it comes to metabolic repair, omega-3s should be a staple in your daily supplement arsenal. A 2010 study published in *Cell Journal* noted that specific receptors found in fat cells are activated and generate a strong anti-inflammatory and an improved systemic insulin-sensitivity effect in the presence of omega-3 fatty acids. A 2011 study conducted at the University of Alberta also revealed the ability of fish oil to preserve lean muscle tissue, even in patients undergoing chemotherapy. The trial involved 16 chemotherapy patients who took 2.2 grams of EPA a day, and 24 patients who did not. The study ran until patients completed their initial treatments, which lasted 10 weeks. Researchers discovered that a whopping 69 percent of patients in the fish oil group gained or maintained muscle mass, while only 29 percent of patients who didn't take fish oils maintained muscle mass. Moreover, most patients in this group *lost* 2.2 pounds of muscle. If you recall that metabolically active lean muscle can improve insulin sensitivity, you will recognize that these recent findings are very exciting—one more reason to include fish oil in your prescription for metabolic repair.

Fish oils were included in the Carbohydrate Sensitivity Program basic 6-week supplement plan, but I recommend increasing the dosage from 2 grams to 3 or 4 grams twice daily for added metabolic repair effects.

Recommended brands:

- **Clear Omega—Extra Strength Fish Oils** (Clear Medicine)
- **o3mega extra strength** (Genuine Health)
- **proDHA Capsules** or **ProEFA** (Nordic Naturals)
- **Super DHA Capsules** or **MedOMEGA Liquid Fish Oil** (Carlson)
- **NutraSea High Potency Capsules** or **Liquid Fish Oil**

3. A High-quality Probiotic

We've learned that healthy bacterial balance within the digestive system is vital for overall health, particularly for the breakdown and elimination of estrogen. Some studies suggest that the bacteria in your stomach can actually impact your weight-loss efforts. Researchers at Emory University found that mice bred to have an altered balance of bacteria in their intestines were 20 percent heavier after 5 months than their counterparts that weren't bred that way. Changes in the concentration of some bacteria may cause inflammation, leading to an increase in appetite and insulin resistance. So, a perfect balance truly comes from the inside out!

While yogurt naturally contains probiotics, supplements are more effective as a concentrated source. All of the probiotic recommended supplements should be refrigerated. During your Metabolic Repair Program, I recommend a probiotic with at least 10 to 15 billion cells per capsule. If you experience bloating when you first begin taking probiotic supplements, simply reduce the dosage and slowly increase it again as your body adapts. Recommended brands:

- **Clear Flora**—2 capsules on rising
- **MultiBiotic 4000** (Douglas Labs)—2 capsules on rising and/or before bed
- **Bio K+**—1 jar (away from food) or 1 capsule per day (with food)
- **Live Probio+ o3mega** (Genuine Health)—1 to 2 capsules on rising

- **Smooth Food 2** or **All Flora** (New Chapter)—2 capsules per day
- **ProbioMax Daily DF** (Xymogen)—1 capsule daily on rising or before bed

4. **Conjugated Linoleic Acid (CLA)**

    CLA is naturally present in dairy products and beef. It has anti-cancer and antidiabetic properties and may be useful in reducing arterial disease, as well as osteoporosis. Data published in the *Canadian Journal of Applied Physiology* (December 2000) reported that CLA is one of only a few supplements proven to reduce body fat and assist in increasing lean muscle mass, even without a change in caloric intake. These powerful effects are due to CLA's insulin-sensitizing properties. CLA also shows anti-inflammatory benefits and seems to reduce fat storage in the fat cells while also increasing fat-burning activity in skeletal muscle. As well, CLA has been shown to increase feelings of fullness and satiety, and decrease feelings of hunger, thereby acting as an appetite suppressant. The minimum dosage is 1,500 mg twice daily with food for at least 3 months. CLA is one of my favorite choices for the treatment of insulin resistance and inflammation. It's also my top choice for preserving precious muscle during weight loss. Recommended brands:
    - **Clear CLA** (Clear Medicine)—2 capsules twice a day with meals
    - **Abs+** (Genuine Health)—2 capsules twice a day with meals
    - **Ultra CLA** (Metagenics)—2 capsules twice a day with meals

5. **Vitamin D3**

    In Chapter 8, we learned that vitamin D has been proven to lower insulin, improve serotonin levels, enhance the immune system, control appetite and even improve fat-loss efforts. Take 4,000 to 5,000 IU daily for optimal results during your Metabolic Repair Program.

Recommended brands:

- **Vitamin D3 drops**—1,000 IU (Pure Encaps)
- **Vitamin D3 capsules**—1,000 IU (Douglas Labs or Metagenics)
- **Solar D Gem** (Carlson)—available in 2,000 or 4,000 IU capsules

Optional but Highly Recommended Products for Added Metabolic Repair, Fat Loss and Insulin Reduction

Combined with a strategic nutrition plan, the right blend of supplements can give your body the tools it needs to shuttle glucose away from your hungry fat cells and into the muscle cells to reduce belly fat and reduce those love handles. A few of my favorites are listed below and on the following pages. They pack a powerful punch when taken consistently over time.

Clear Recovery (Clear Medicine)

Out of all of my formulations, I think this just might be my favorite. Complete with three types of L-glutamine, creatinine, branched-chain amino acids (BCAAs), resveratrol, berry extracts, minerals and loads of antioxidants, Clear Recovery aids recovery after exercise, and reduces postworkout soreness and the production of growth hormone. It contains tons of nutrients that reduce inflammation and stress, as well as others that help with insulin balance and the maintenance of healthy skin! Take 1 serving in water after exercise or enjoy it as a midafternoon snack with a serving of whey protein for an energy boost. If you are extremely athletic, you can take 2 servings during or after weight-training sessions or endurance exercise.

Glyci-Med Forte—Insulin Balancing Formula (Clear Medicine)

This is my blend of a rich source of antioxidants and monounsaturated oils, including olive and avocado oils, to assist with fat loss.

Recent studies have shown olive oil improves insulin balance, shrinks the size of fat cells, reduces the harmful effects of high carbohydrate intake and increases weight loss, especially when consumed at breakfast. Almost every patient reports that this supplement cuts their cravings and helps to shrink belly fat. Take 2 capsules with a meal, preferably breakfast.

Resveratrol

A number of studies show this natural red wine extract assists with weight loss. Have you heard of the French paradox—the fact that the French seem to eat and drink what they want but still remain slim? This may be due to the resveratrol from all that red wine! Now we have access to this in a bottle, and it's not a wine bottle. Data published in *Nature* (November 2006) showed that resveratrol protected mice from the harmful effects of a high-calorie diet, including heart disease, weight gain and diabetes. Resveratrol appears to act on adiponectin and also possesses natural anti-inflammatory properties. Adiponectin is produced by our fat cells but actually helps us lose fat by improving our insulin sensitivity. Resveratrol also provides plenty of antioxidant protection. Take 200 to 500 mg a day. Look for Resveratrol Extra from Pure Encapsulations, which, I have found, seems to offer a good dosage or Clear Resveratrim (Clear Medicine); a form of methylated resveratrol, which increases the absorption eight fold.

Whey Protein Isolate

Go back to Chapter 8, page 225, if you need a refresher on the wonderful benefits of whey for balancing insulin and improving metabolism. Recommended brands:

- **Dream Protein**—This is a favorite of our patients and readers. In fact, many mention that this is the best-tasting protein supplement they have ever tried.
- **Proteins +** (Genuine Health)—This is a 100 percent whey protein isolate that is free of sugar and artificial sweeteners.

A Fiber Supplement to Toss into Your Smoothies

A hypoallergenic source of fiber is a must-have in your regimen because it is so difficult to obtain my suggested 35 grams of fiber on a carb-conscious diet. If you need a refresher on the benefits of fiber for insulin balance see page 221. Otherwise, select one of the brands I have suggested here to help your metabolic repair:

- **Clear Fiber** (Clear Medicine)
- **Gentle Fibers** (Jarrow)
- **Fiber-Tastic!** (Renew Life)
- **Organic Clear Fiber** (Renew Life)

THE SUPER INSULIN-BALANCING NUTRIENTS

Many nutrients have a proven track record for improving insulin resistance and thereby increasing the odds of fat loss.

MAGNESIUM

Magnesium is involved in more than 300 physiological processes in the body, from the action of the heart muscles, to the formation of bones and teeth, to the relaxation of blood vessels and the promotion of proper bowel function. Magnesium also plays an important role in carbohydrate metabolism and may influence the release and activity of insulin, which in turn helps control blood sugar levels. As a result, there is a strong link between magnesium deficiency and insulin resistance. In fact, *most insulin-resistant, overweight and type 2 diabetic patients have a deficiency of magnesium,* as reported in a recent article published in *Clinical Nutrition Journal* (January 2011). This deficiency not only affects healthy blood sugar and insulin balance but also is linked to increases in blood pressure and hypertension.

Several clinical studies have examined the positive impact that magnesium supplementation can have on type 2 diabetes. In one such study, published in *Diabetes Care* (2003), 63 subjects with below-normal serum magnesium levels received 300 mg elemental magnesium per day or a placebo. At the end of the 16-week study period, those who received the magnesium supplement had improved control of their diabetes. Magnesium improves our cellular response to insulin, stabilizes blood sugar, prevents cravings and reduces anxiety. To treat and prevent constipation, try increasing the dosage to 400 to 800 mg per day, to bowel tolerance (i.e., the point at which you experience loose stools).

CALCIUM

We all know the importance of calcium for healthy bones, but the latest research shows that calcium can improve weight loss and insulin sensitivity. A 2-year study completed at Purdue University (1999) found that adequate amounts of calcium slowed weight gain, possibly by accelerating the burning of fat for energy. The researchers found that the women who consumed at least 780 mg of calcium either had no increase in body fat or lost body fat over the 2-year period. A separate study published in the journal *Hypertension* (1997) evaluated the effect of calcium supplementation on blood pressure, carb metabolism and insulin resistance in patients with high blood pressure. Researchers found that the high-calcium group showed decreased insulin levels and a significant increase in insulin sensitivity.

ZINC

Zinc is involved in more than 200 enzymes in the body, yet insufficient zinc is one of the most common mineral deficiencies I find in my clinical practice. A deficiency of zinc will not only leave you susceptible to colds and infections, but it can also drop your testosterone levels, reduce your lean muscle mass and compromise your body's response to insulin. In fact, according to a study published in the journal of the *American Journal of Physiology* (1986), rats who were fed a zinc-deficient diet demonstrated a resistance to insulin within just 8 days. A quick way to detect a zinc deficiency is to crush a zinc tablet to powder and mix with ¼ cup of water. Slosh the mixture around your mouth for 10 seconds and then spit or swallow it. People who notice no taste or who notice a mineral-type taste *are likely to be deficient* in zinc. Those who notice a strong, unpleasant taste are *not likely to be deficient* in this mineral.

IODINE

Iodine is an essential trace element that has a whole lot to do with the master of your metabolism, your thyroid. All cells in the body need iodine for proper functioning, while major glands such as your adrenals and your thyroid require iodine for the proper production of hormones. Dr. David Brownstein, a strong advocate for using iodine in the treatment of hypothyroidism and hyperthyroidism, believes that iodine deficiency is a major cause of breast cancer and other diseases of the reproductive organs, as well as prostate cysts and cancers.

Although I was familiar with these benefits of iodine, I was amazed when I found new research published in the Ukrainian journal *Lik Sprava* (January 2010) that suggests iodine insufficiency plays a major role in type 2 diabetes and insulin control. A dosage of 150 to 200 mcg per day has been found to reduce the amount of insulin a diabetic patient may require. Another study published in the *European Journal of Endocrinology* (2009) found a link between metabolic syndrome and iodine deficiency.

Interestingly, in Japan, most people consume about ⅕ ounce of seaweed—an excellent source of iodine—per day and experience a low incidence of metabolic syndrome, also known as pre-diabetes. The people of Okinawa, Japan, in particular, enjoy one of the lowest mortality rates and one of the longest life expectancies in the world—a relatively high percentage of Okinawans live to 100 years of age! Besides being a source of iodine, seaweed is known to contain a large amount of fucoidans, which are believed to strengthen the immune system and to regulate glucose and insulin levels. Keep in mind that more is not better in this case:

Too much iodine can aggravate the thyroid in certain individuals with an autoimmune disease known as Hashimoto's.

CHROMIUM

Chromium is a key mineral involved in regulating the body's response to insulin. As such, a chromium deficiency may lead to insulin resistance. A 2006 pilot study published in *Diabetes Technology & Therapeutics* found that supplementation with a combination of 600 mcg a day of chromium and 2 mg a day of biotin in patients with type 2 diabetes improved glucose management and several lipid measurements.

The influence of chromium on blood sugar and insulin levels is well documented. Together with the recommended insulin-sensitizing superfoods listed in Chapter 6, chromium can have a substantial impact on blood-test markers linked to diabetes and heart disease *and* your waistline.

The signs of chromium deficiency are similar to those of metabolic syndrome, and supplemental chromium has been shown to improve all related health indicators. In a 2008 study conducted at the Beltsville Human Nutrition Research Center, researchers demonstrated that long-term glucose control, insulin and cholesterol improved in patients with type 2 diabetes following chromium supplementation. Overall, chromium can aid the loss of body fat and help raise good cholesterol (HDL) while assisting in the retention of lean muscle mass, especially in conjunction with a carb-sensitizing nutrition program. Select chromium picolinate or polynicotinate, the most absorbable forms of chromium. Prediabetic people or patients with type 2 diabetes often benefit from 600 mcg per day, which is close to the amount you receive while taking the Metabolic Repair Pack.

POTASSIUM

Potassium, an important electrolyte, helps maintain the balance between the contents of a cell and the fluid surrounding it. The effect of insulin on potassium is clinically important, since high insulin can also cause an influx of potassium into the cells and, in turn, suppress potassium concentrations in the blood. As you now know, a high-carbohydrate diet eventually decreases the sensitivity of our cells to insulin. This leads to increased blood sugar, which then uses up our stores of potassium and magnesium.

COENZYME Q10

Coenzyme Q10, also known as CoQ10, plays a critical role in the function of your cells. It is a compound found naturally in the energy-producing center of the cell, known as the mitochondria. CoQ10 is involved in making adenosine triphosphate (ATP), which serves as the cell's major energy source and drives a number of biological processes, including muscle contraction and the production of protein. Unfortunately, CoQ10 decreases with age and tends to be low in patients with certain chronic conditions such as heart disease, muscular dystrophy, Parkinson's disease, cancer, diabetes and HIV/AIDS. Supplementation with CoQ10 may not only improve your energy but also your heart health, blood sugar balance and nervous system function. It can also help to manage high cholesterol and high blood pressure in individuals with diabetes. Keep in mind that the role of CoQ10 with regard to insulin resistance is more about protecting the cardiovascular system from the effects of diabetes versus reversing the disease itself. According to a study published in *Hypertension,* oral treatment with 120 mg of coenzyme Q10 daily was shown to lower blood sugar and fasting insulin levels, reduce blood pressure and improve blood cholesterol. Supplementation also resulted in improvements in blood levels of the antioxidant vitamins A, C, E and beta carotene.

ALPHA LIPOIC ACID (ALA)

ALA is a potent antioxidant capable of enhancing the activity of other antioxidants including vitamin C, vitamin E, glutathione and coenzyme Q10. ALA is known to assist with diabetes, blood sugar control and cellular energy. Often referred to as R+ lipoic acid, ALA plays a key role in the processing of proteins, carbohydrates and fats. It also influences the balancing of blood sugar levels by enhancing glucose uptake. In type 2 diabetics, ALA has been shown to inhibit glycosylation (the abnormal attachment of sugar to protein) and has been used to improve diabetic nerve damage. Basically, ALA acts as a coenzyme, or partner, in the production of energy by converting carbohydrates into energy. A study published in *Hypertension* (2002) investigated the effects of ALA on insulin resistance, hypertension and free radical stress. Researchers found that ALA reduced blood pressure and prevented insulin resistance in rats who were fed sugar water by preventing an increase in oxidative stress (which is typical after a high-sugar or -carb meal).

VITAMIN C

Vitamin C is one of the most widely used supplements today, but many of us don't realize that it plays a key role in our blood sugar levels. A study published in the *Indian Journal of Medical Research* (2007) looked at 84 patients with type 2 diabetes who randomly received either 500 mg or 1,000 mg of vitamin C daily for 6 weeks. The researchers discovered that the group supplementing with 1,000 mg of vitamin C experienced a significant decrease in fasting blood sugar, triglycerides, cholesterol (LDL) and insulin levels. The dose of 500 mg of vitamin C, however, did not produce any significant changes (which is why each Metabolic Repair Pack contains 1,000 mg of vitamin C).

Vitamin C has also shown promise in preventing complications associated with metabolic disorders. Researchers at the Harold Hamm Oklahoma Diabetes Center discovered they could halt blood vessel damage caused by type 1 diabetes by combining insulin and vitamin C. By reducing or stopping the damage, patients with diabetes could avoid some of the painful and potentially fatal consequences of diabetes, including heart disease, reduced circulation (which can lead to amputation), kidney disease and diabetic retin-opathy (which can lead to blindness). At the same time, high-carbo-hydrate foods can diminish levels of vitamin C in the body because they compete with the same receptors as glucose. So, if you eat a lot of simple sugars, less vitamin C can be absorbed. In return, there is less resistance to stress (the adrenal glands process vitamin C) and a compromised immune system. Avoiding these outcomes are two of the main benefits of daily vitamin C use. And since vitamin C is similar in cellular structure to glucose, cravings for sweet foods are often an indicator of a need for vitamin C.

GREEN TEA

Recent research has found that the catechin antioxidants in green tea help to increase fat burning, while also reducing the risk of cancer, high cholesterol and diabetes. Besides its natural anti-inflammatory effects, green tea may also lower blood sugar by inhibiting enzymes that allow starch and fat absorption from the intestine. The most important bioactive substance in green tea, EGCG (epigallocatechin gallate), prompts muscle cells to absorb more glucose. Think of your muscle cells as sponges that can absorb excess sugar, making less of it available to feed your fat cells. Weight training, which builds mus-cle, also enhances this effect. After an intense strength workout, you are more sensitive to the carbs you ingest, and your muscle tissue readily absorbs the glucose created. This is why weight training trumps aerobic activity when it comes to insulin-sensitizing benefits. The typical dosage is 3 to 4 cups of green tea a day, or a 300 to 400 mg capsule of green tea extract 1 to 3 times daily.

Dosing Chart for the Metabolic Repair Supplements

Though this seems like a lot of information to take in, I have created the following simple dosing chart to guide you. This is the exact same format my patients receive when they come for an office visit. If you'd like a printable version of this chart, please visit the Book Extras section of my Web site: www.carbsensitivity.com.

TIME OF DAY	SUPPLEMENT	BENEFIT
Upon rising (empty stomach)	2 Clear Flora (Clear Medicine) Alternative: • See page 268	Probiotic supplements reduce inflammation, aid estrogen detoxification, improve digestion and immunity and, according to the latest research, promote healthy insulin balance.
	Optional recommendation: 2 caps resveratrol • Resveratrol Extra (Pure Encaps) or • Clear Resveratrim (Clear Medicine)	Resveratrol promotes weight loss and insulin balance, and gives anti-inflammatory and antiaging support. Just as a side note, Suzanne Somers recommends this as one of the top three supplements along with fish oils and vitamin D3.
Breakfast	Metabolic Repair Pack (Clear Medicine) or high-potency multivitamin or multimineral Alternative: • See page 265–67	This is a mixture of beneficial oils and antioxidants that promote insulin balance, reduce cravings and aid appetite control.
	3 Clear Omega (Clear Medicine) Alternative: • See page 268	Omega-3 oils reduce inflammation and improve insulin sensitivity. They also reduce cravings and aid fat loss, especially when combined with exercise.
	4,000–5,000 IU vitamin D3	Vitamin D3 aids insulin balance, serotonin activity in the brain (important for mood and craving control) and immunity.
	2 Clear CLA (Clear Medicine) Alternative: • See page 269	CLA aids fat loss, preserves muscle and improves insulin sensitivity. Clear CLA also contains green tea extract, which has been found to aid weight loss.
	Optional recommendation: 2 Glyci-med Forte (Clear Medicine)	This pack contains a mixture of vitamins, minerals and other nutrients that work synergistically to improve insulin and blood sugar balance.

(continued)

TIME OF DAY	SUPPLEMENT	BENEFIT
Postworkout or with midafternoon snack (combined with ½ serving of whey protein)	Clear Recovery (Clear Medicine) Alternative: • Select a low-sugar content postworkout drink high in antioxidants and avoid energy drinks	Clear Recovery contains a mixture of amino acids, creatine and antioxidants that aid energy, exercise recovery, insulin balance and cellular repair. So far, this is my favorite formulation of the entire Clear Medicine brand. It's amazing for preventing soreness after exercise.
Dinner	1 Metabolic Repair Pack (Clear Medicine) or high-potency multivitamin or multimineral Alternative: • See page 265–67	This pack contains a mixture of vitamins, minerals and other nutrients that work synergistically to improve insulin and blood sugar balance. Take the metabolic repair pack at lunch if the green tea keeps you awake at night.
	2 Clear CLA (Clear Medicine) Alternative: • See page 269	CLA aids fat loss, preserves muscle and improves insulin sensitivity. Clear CLA also contains green tea extract, which has been found to aid weight loss.
	3 Clear Omega (Clear Medicine) Alternative: • See page 268	Omega-3 oils reduce inflammation and improve insulin sensitivity. They aid fat loss—especially when combined with exercise—and reduce cravings.
Before bed	200 to 600 mg (or until bowel tolerance is reached) magnesium glycinate or citrate	This improves sleep, digestion, cravings and blood sugar balance, reduces blood pressure, prevents muscle cramps or spasms, and calms the nervous system.

Although I have recommended some specific brands, don't feel you have to purchase these exact products. Products with similar ingredients should be fine, provided they are from a reputable company. Ask the staff at your local health-food store for advice. If you do wish to try the Clear Medicine products listed, they are available online at www.carbsensitivity.com. The CSP Metabolic Repair Kit includes my custom formulations: the Metabolic Repair Pack; Clear Flora, Clear

Omega and Clear CLA—Metabolic Enhancement Formula (although you may add or remove any product from the kit to create your own). Like the Basic Six CSP Program Kit, this kit also contains a 30-day supply (provided two bottles of the Metabolic Repair Pack are included in your order). You may add protein, low-glycemic protein bars, a fiber supplement, vitamin D3 or additional magnesium if you do not have similar products on hand and wish to include them in your Metabolic Repair Program. Please note that you do not need to take everything I've listed. Select the supplements you feel resonate most with your particular issue(s). After all, you know your body best.

THE IMPORTANCE OF DIETARY SALT: KUDOS FOR CELTIC!

Think twice before completely removing salt from your diet. Yes, I realize this is a shocking statement considering the high prevalence of hypertension, often a complication of insulin resistance, in our society. But recent studies summarized in the *Portuguese Journal of Endocrinology and Metabolism* (July 2009) have revealed sodium intake restrictions may *increase* insulin resistance and induce changes on inflammation markers characteristic of metabolic syndrome.

It appears a moderate dietary sodium reduction *may* lower blood pressure without adverse effects on blood sugar metabolism in patients with high blood pressure, but salt restriction *does not* improve insulin resistance in those same patients. In fact, evidence seems to suggest that a severe reduction of salt may contribute to increased cholesterol and insulin levels *and* a deterioration of insulin sensitivity in both healthy volunteers and patients with hypertension.

Table salt, however, is not the best option when it comes to keeping a healthy level of salt in your diet. I encourage you to use Celtic sea salt instead. Unlike table salt, which is stripped of all minerals and trace elements except sodium and chloride during processing, Celtic sea salt contains between 80 and 90 live elements found in seawater, with no added chemicals or pre-servatives. Among the minerals and trace elements it contains are calcium, iron, magnesium, manganese, potassium, zinc and iodine. It is also alkalizing and is touted to improve healthy saliva production. You can purchase Celtic sea salt at most health-food stores.

Thyroid Hormone and Your Metabolism

No discussion about your metabolism is complete without mention-ing the thyroid. This hormone regulates our metabolism and organ function and directly affects heart rate, cholesterol levels, body weight, energy, muscle contraction and relaxation, skin and hair texture, bowel function, fertility, menstrual regularity, memory and mood—so many of the factors that deeply affect how we look and feel. Without enough thyroid hormone, attaining your perfect weight is almost impossible.

That is why any program for metabolic repair must take thyroid function into consideration. An underactive thyroid keeps your body from burning fat and shedding pounds. The symptoms of underac-tive thyroid disease, also known as hypothyroidism, can vary, and not all individuals will present in the same way, but the following are symptoms to watch for:

- Frequently feeling cold or having an intolerance of cold temperatures
- Dry skin, brittle hair and splitting nails
- Lack of or diminished ability to sweat during exercise
- Hair loss or thinning at the outer half of the eyebrows
- Irregular menses or heavy menstrual bleeding
- Poor memory
- Depression
- Decreased libido

- Constipation
- Unexplained fatigue or lethargy
- Unexplained weight gain or an inability to lose weight
- Associated iron-deficient anemia and/or high cholesterol

In Appendix A, I have outlined the tests you may want to request from your doctor to fully assess the condition of your thyroid. Thyroid disease is diagnosed with blood tests. Four tests—for TSH, Free T3, Free T4 and thyroid antibodies—should be completed to get the most accurate picture of your thyroid health.

One important note on testing: In my practice, I often find that thyroid antibodies register as abnormal long before the other three parameters. Many health-care providers also share concerns about the currently accepted normal reference ranges for TSH. In the United States the normal range is 0.35 to 4.7. Health professionals in the United States have recently reduced the upper range to 3. However, many integrated health practitioners feel it should be less than 2.0, and I agree.

Supplement options for a high-performing thyroid include:

- **Clear Metabolism.** This formulation is complete with specific herbs and nutrients to boost thyroid hormone and, therefore, metabolism. L-tyrosine is a major component in thyroid hormones. Minerals such as zinc, iodine and selenium are also essential to healthy thyroid function, as they are required for the intracellular conversion of thyroid hormone to its most potent form. Selenium is required in the transport of thyroid hormones into our cells, while the herb ashwagandha may enhance blood levels of thyroid hormone. The herb coleus aids thyroid function by increasing thyroid hormone production and release. I recommend 3 capsules on rising, before breakfast. You may take this product if you are currently on prescription medicine for hypothyroidism.

- **Ashwagandha.** This supplement may increase both thyroxine (T4) and its active counterpart, T3. Both ashwagandha and gugulipids appear to boost thyroid function without influencing the release of the pituitary hormone TSH (thyroid stimulating hormone), indicating that these herbs work directly on the thyroid gland and other body tissues. That's good news, since thyroid problems most often occur within the thyroid gland itself or in the conversion of T4 into T3 in tissues outside the thyroid gland. Take 750 to 1,000 mg twice a day.
- **L-tyrosine.** This amino acid is necessary for the production of thyroid hormone in the body. The recommended dose is 1,000 mg on rising, before breakfast. *Do not take this supplement if you have high blood pressure.*

The Good News Is . . .

For most of us, metabolic damage or insulin resistance is the cumulative result of a lifetime of poor choices. Factors that have likely contributed to the health issues that led you to pick up this book include poor diet, lack of exercise, smoking, sleep deprivation and stress, just to name a few. Although there are certainly genetic factors contributing to your overall metabolic state, "lifestyle" factors are all modifiable. This means your metabolism *can* be repaired and your degree of insulin resistance is potentially *preventable* and *reversible.*

Even for those of us who may be genetically predisposed to metabolic challenges, the appropriate lifestyle, dietary and supplement choices outlined in this chapter can play a huge role in reversing that situation. By making the effort to heal your metabolism, you can also reduce your risk for almost every disease associated with aging—and also look and feel your best every day!

CSP SUCCESS STORY: JENNIFER

"For years I was obsessed with the scale. I overexercised and underate and despite all my efforts the pounds kept on piling on. I met with Dr. Natasha Turner and she started me on the Carb Sensitivity Program. Within 2 weeks I noticed that my energy levels improved, my cravings for carbs started to reduce and I *finally* started losing weight. I couldn't believe it! It felt like I was eating more than I used to and exercising less and yet I was seeing results. More so, my digestion improved and I was no longer plagued with symptoms of IBS, which I have battled with ever since I was 19. I am so grateful—thanks Dr. T!"

JENNIFER, 38

STATS	BEFORE	AFTER
Weight	171 lb	138 lb
BMI	27.6	22.3

INITIAL CHIEF COMPLAINTS:

1. Weight gain
2. Digestive problems
3. Bloating

CHAPTER 11

THE METABOLIC REPAIR WORKOUT

All life is an experiment.
The more experiments you make, the better.

RALPH WALDO EMERSON

Since we now know that insulin resistance is caused by genetics, environmental influences *and* what you put in your mouth, learning that it can be improved or even reversed by what you do in the gym should be music to your ears. Your Metabolic Repair Workout will include three types of activities: circuit-style strength training, interval cardio and yoga. All of these activities specifically enhance the one bodily function we need to get firing on all cylinders again: your insulin sensitivity.

As we learned in Chapter 2, insulin causes the speedy uptake of glucose in cells of the liver, muscle and fat tissue, wreaking havoc in a healthy body. Sugar is then stored as glycogen (an energy source) in the liver and muscle tissue. Consequently, what *feeds* the muscle also helps to *build* and *maintain* it. As such, insulin plays a large role in increasing your metabolic rate via muscle tissue. It is therefore very difficult to gain lean muscle without insulin.

Imagine finishing a gut-wrenching workout and not having the ability to shuttle nutrients into the muscle cells that in turn help build and maintain muscle tissue—all that effort would be futile. Depending on your frame, every extra pound of muscle burns 30 to 50 calories—even at rest!

Why Strength Matters

To understand the importance of weight training to insulin sensitivity, it's valuable to know that muscle cells and fat cells are both strongly influenced by insulin's actions. While fat cells store excess food energy for later use, muscle cells enable movement, breathing and structural support. Together they account for two-thirds of all cells in the human body. When insulin is released into the bloodstream, it shuttles glucose (which originated as the carbohydrates on your plate), amino acids (protein) and fats into the cells where they are needed. If these nutrients are delivered effectively into the muscle cells, muscles grow and body fat does *not* accumulate. If the nutrients are escorted into the fat cells instead, muscles do not grow and body fat increases. Insulin resistance leads to the latter situation—not good! With chronically elevated levels of insulin, the ability of muscle cells to store nutrients is compromised, which in turn leads to muscle wasting and increased fat storage.

The solution? *Boost* insulin sensitivity in the muscle cells, *reduce* sensitivity in the fat cells and control insulin release throughout the day. The Metabolic Repair Workout in this chapter involves a lot of resistance training, which helps improve insulin sensitivity and reduce the rise of type 2 diabetes. Ultimately this will enable you to add a little more variety to your dinner plate as your body increases its ability to handle certain carbohydrates. Cardio plays only a small part. Before your jaw drops and you wonder how you will wean yourself off the treadmill, let's review the benefits of weight training and discuss how we will manipulate traditional methods to increase your heart rate to alternate between the cardio and fat-burning zones while also incorporating a host of other functional benefits.

There is a plethora of research to support the use of exercise to enhance insulin sensitivity and to improve many of the risk factors associated with metabolic syndrome. Before we get into the actual exercise prescription you must follow in order to repair your metabolism, let's quickly summarize some of the science behind the specific workouts I have put together here with the help of a top strength and conditioning expert.

We now know that resistance training improves diabetes and insulin resistance through a variety of mechanisms:

- It increases the uptake of glucose into the muscle cells.
- It improves the storage of glucose as glycogen, for release as energy when needed.
- It makes it easier for the body to use insulin more effectively, thereby reducing insulin resistance.
- It increases metabolism and provides that wonderful "after burn" that boosts your metabolic rate for extended periods.
- It decreases total fat and intra-abdominal fat (the fat around your organs that contributes to cardiovascular disease).
- It primes your body to burn 50 calories per pound of lean muscle while actively moving throughout your day.

A study published in *Archives of Physical Medicine and Rehabilitation* (August 2005) compared the effects of a 4-month strength-training program versus aerobic endurance training on muscle control, muscle strength and cardiovascular health in subjects with type 2 diabetes. The results of this experiment may give all you cardio bunnies out there a big surprise: When it came to blood values, strength training encouraged a *significant* improvement in overall blood sugar levels and insulin sensitivity, whereas *no* changes were observed in the group who did only aerobic activity. Baseline levels of total cholesterol, LDL cholesterol and triglycerides also dropped, while HDL cholesterol levels (the "good" cholesterol) increased in the strength-training group only. Moreover, overall strength *and* metabolically active muscle tissue also increased in the weight-training group. Weight loss was similar in both groups; however, the participants in the weight room lost more than 9 percent of their body fat, while their counterparts on the treadmill lost an average of just 3 percent. An important lesson to be learned here is that the number on your scale is not always a good indicator of your success. While those who strength train will likely notice fat loss, their weight may not drop significantly because they are *gaining* healthy muscle in the process. At the same time, those of you who are aerobically inclined will not see many, if any, of these benefits.

A similar study published in the *International Journal of Medical Science* (2007) confirmed these findings in older adults and high-risk populations. Researchers found that strength training improved muscle quality and whole-body insulin sensitivity. Decreased inflammation and increased adiponectin levels were also associated with improved metabolic control. High blood levels of adiponectin are linked with a reduced risk of heart attack, while low levels are often found in people who are obese—and at *increased* risk of heart attack.

The metabolic equation is very simple: The more muscle tissue you have, the better your insulin sensitivity, and the more calories you will burn (even while at rest). Even the process of breaking down and repairing your muscles postworkout increases your metabolism. Miriam Nelson, a Tufts University researcher, showed that a group of women who followed a weight-loss diet *and* did weight-training exercises lost 44 percent more fat than those who only followed the diet.

While aerobic activity can help burn calories during the activity, building muscle via strength training means you will continue to burn more calories, even while you sleep. And doing your cardio sessions right after your strength training will render even better results. A new study from the College of New Jersey confirms that pumping iron or even lifting your own body weight can make your cardio workout more effective. Participants who performed an intense weight workout before riding a stationary bike burned more fat during their cardio session than those who pedaled but skipped the weights. So, remember to do your cardio sessions either immediately after your weight training or on a separate day, never before and not for too long.

It has long been established that the *right* exercise increases insulin's ability to transport sugar into the tissues versus letting it build up in the blood. This effect can be seen even in previously sedentary adults, which is great news for those of you who are not currently exercising. In fact, according to an article published in the *New England Journal of Medicine* (1996), a single session of moderate-intensity exercise can improve blood sugar balance by at least 40 percent. This impact isn't permanent, however, since the effects of exercise diminish within 48 to 72 hours. *This research, therefore, supports my recommendation of a program that includes resistance training 3 days a week, with only 1 to 2 days of cardio. This regimen will have a profound impact on your level of insulin sensitivity—not to mention your body composition.*

Sweat Science: Interval Cardio and Fat Burning

I don't want to leave you with the impression that cardiovascular exercise has no value. At least one cardio session a week is required for metabolic repair. In a randomized controlled trial published in the *Annals of International Medicine* (September 2007), researchers found that *both* aerobic and resistance exercise improved blood sugar control in people with type 2 diabetes. The greatest improvements, however, came from *combined* aerobic and resistance training.

While it's pretty clear that resistance training is a must-have tool in our arsenal against insulin resistance, the right type of cardio boosts insulin sensitivity in a different way. Increased insulin sensitivity will result in greater levels of carbohydrates being absorbed into the muscle cells, versus into fat cells, and will lead to more muscle growth. Basically, GLUT4 (glucose transporter 4) receptors draw glucose into the muscle.

Luckily, there are many forms of these receptors. Cardio training tends to improve a different receptor than resistance training, so the combination of cardio and weights provides a potent tool for increasing overall insulin sensitivity. Not all cardio is the same, however, and contrary to popular belief, when it comes to losing weight—and turning your body into an insulin-sensitive powerhouse—more is *not* necessarily better. People who do short bursts of high-intensity running will retain more muscle mass than their counterparts who perform lower-intensity cardio over a much longer period. Readers of *The Hormone Diet* will remember that lengthy cardio sessions also boost your stress hormones, which can end up *reducing* your hard-earned muscle mass. On the Carb Sensitivity Program, as in my previous books, I strongly recommend using interval cardio sessions, which give you more bang for your exercise buck, in half the time.

Body Composition: Sprinter or Marathoner?

To see the benefits on body composition of short, intense-interval cardio compared to low intensity long-distance cardio, you need look no further than a marathoner versus a sprinter. The latter is often leaner, with more metabolically active muscle—a great prescription for improving carb sensitivity! An interval is a short burst of exercise performed at a higher intensity for a specific, usually brief, period of time. Each interval is separated from the next by a short rest or period of lighter activity. To truly benefit from interval training, you must be willing to shake the mind-set that endless (and boring!) cardio training is the key to weight loss. Brief, intense bursts of exercise at 70 to 95 percent of your maximum heart rate, interspersed with recovery interludes during which your heart rate slows to 60 percent of your maximum or lower, burn more calories than long bouts of steady, less-intense cardio. They also improve performance. For instance, cyclists doubled their endurance after just 2 weeks of sprint-interval training, according to a study in the *Journal of Applied Physiology.* Interval-training principles may also apply to running, stair climbing, rowing and circuits.

With interval training, 25 minutes of running can be more effective than 40. How? You will burn more fat during and after your workout if you run for 10 minutes at a steady pace, then alternate 1 minute of sprinting with 1 minute at a slower pace for the next 10 minutes, then finish at the slower pace for the last 5 minutes to cool down. Even though you're exercising for a shorter period, you'll still see greater fat loss using this method, and a 2001 study conducted at East Tennessee State University showed this to be the case. It demonstrated that high-intensity interval sessions increased resting metabolic rate (RMR) for a full 24 hours due to boosting the "after burn," or the calories expended after an exercise session.

Alternating intense cardio with moderate cardio is also a great way to expend calories without risking repetitive injury. Best of all, this type of exercise can be done on any cardio machine or even just by hitting the pavement. And you get to be creative with your cardio routine, as there are many ways to modify the timing and intensity. For example, sprinting for 30 seconds then walking for 60 seconds is considered high-intensity interval training. While the actual timing you decide upon doesn't matter, the goal is to alternate between a more-intense, faster effort and a lower-intensity, moderate period of exercise.

Yoga Is of the Essence

It's no secret that I am a big fan of yoga, and not just for its ability to lower your stress hormones and boost your flexibility. A study published in *Diabetes Research and Clinical Practice* (January 1993) looked at the impact of yoga therapy on 104 patients with type 2 diabetes. All participants showed significant improvements in their blood sugar levels after 40 days of yoga and were able to reduce the medications they were on to maintain normal blood sugar levels.

Yoga is also a terrific stress reliever. Numerous studies, including one completed in 2003 by the Center for Integrative Medicine of Thomas Jefferson University, in collaboration with the Yoga Research Society, have shown that yoga can lower blood cortisol levels in healthy men and women. It is also known to reduce adrenaline and stimulate the calming brain chemical GABA. Research from Boston University School of Medicine and McLean Hospital, published in the *Journal of Alternative and Complementary Medicine* (May 2007), suggests yoga should be explored as a possible treatment for disorders often associated with low GABA levels, such as depression and anxiety.

Recall from my prescription for carb addiction presented in Chapter 5 that achieving optimal GABA levels will indirectly aid fat loss because of the beneficial effects of GABA on sleep, mood, and reduction of stress and tension. And anything that reduces stress hormones also curbs cravings and, in turn, halts our desire to raid the fridge late at night.

Yoga's benefits extend even further. A study at Ohio State University and published in *Psychosomatic Medicine* (January 2010) indicates that yoga may reduce inflammation. In this trial, 50 subjects were divided into two groups: those who regularly participated in yoga and a group of yoga beginners. Researchers assessed blood samples from each of the subjects and found that those in the beginners' group had 41 percent higher levels of an inflammatory compound called interleukin-6 compared to their more advanced peers.

There are many types of yoga. My favorites are ashtanga, anusara and hatha, but find the practice that suits you best. Ashtanga is often called power yoga, while hatha is a less-intense workout. Anusara is my favorite because I feel it falls nicely between the two.

THE HEART RATE MONITOR ADVANTAGE

A heart rate monitor (HRM) can serve as a key tool in assuring your fitness gains and success. An HRM uses the science of telemetry, which means it works very similarly to the electrocardiograms used in hospitals to monitor patients' hearts. There are many advantages to using an HRM.

1. **Safety.** These monitors never lie. If you have a health issue, tracking your heart rate is a strong indicator of the effect of exertion on your body.

2. **Motivation.** Once you set your target heart rate, the alert system will beep to indicate whether you are overdoing it or falling short. This "coaching aspect" of the monitor keeps you on track and allows you to explore higher levels of fitness as you adapt.

3. **Efficiency and results.** The monitor provides a valuable link between how your heart rate affects your body and which energy system (aerobic/anaerobic/fat burning, etc.) is being used. Using the monitor can, therefore, give you the cues to manipulate different energy resources as you work toward your desired results.

4. **Discover your best starting point.** Using the monitor to gauge your changing fitness level can help to provide a sense of security, if you are concerned about pushing yourself too hard at the start. It can also provide a sense of your starting point as you ease into your metabolic training program and should eliminate the myth of "no-pain no-gain" with regular training.

5. **Increased body awareness.** The monitor is a wonderful educational tool that provides invaluable information about your body. It does this by allowing you to visualize how certain exercises or routines affect your heart rate. Although your perceived exertion is still one of the best ways to indicate how hard you are exercising, tracking your heart rate will let you identify which routines best suit your fitness level at any given point in time.

6. **You can monitor your heart anywhere, any time.** A monitor is good to use at home, in the gym or even on vacation. At home it can be an excellent tool when you are mowing the lawn or shoveling snow. These are activities we take for granted as everyday chores, but they tax the body immensely and can put you at risk. You can also use a monitor to make sure your walking, running, circuit-training or golfing routine is at the right intensity to offer the best results for the effort and time you put into your training. And remember, if you have a health issue, a monitor may give you an excellent indication of what you should and should not be doing.

The Metabolic Repair Workout:
Rules, Tools of the Trade,
Weekly Schedule and Daily Routines

The philosophy behind the Metabolic Repair Basic Workout is similar to the philosophy behind the workout presented in *The Hormone Diet*: It is the perfect combination for maintaining hormonal balance and strength while simultaneously preventing the stress of overexercising. Keep in mind that whether we engage in strength training or aerobic activity, cortisol is released in proportion to the intensity of our effort. Both high-intensity and prolonged exercise cause increases in cortisol, which can remain elevated for several hours following a vigorous workout. Numerous studies have proven that this rise in cortisol tends to occur with very strenuous exercise and when we exercise for longer than 40 to 45 minutes. Repeated strenuous workouts without appropriate rest between sessions can also result in chronically elevated cortisol.

We know that persistently high cortisol can cause muscle breakdown, suppress our immune function and contribute to stubborn abdominal fat. Researchers at the University of North Carolina have also linked strenuous, fatiguing exercise to higher cortisol *and* lower thyroid hormones. Remember: Thyroid hormones stimulate your metabolism, so depletion is definitely not a desired effect of exercise! The same study found thyroid hormones remained suppressed even 24 hours after recovery, while cortisol levels remained high throughout the same period.

So, as you can see, *more is not always better* when it comes to exercise. Overexercising can lead to loss of muscle, frequent colds and flus, stress, an increase in free radicals, poor recovery after exercise, and slower gains from your workout efforts. Plus, your risk of illness and injury increases as your metabolic rate slows. Certainly these are not the effects you were looking for when you joined the gym! So, I need you to stick to the rules listed on the next page.

1. **Keep it short and sweet.** All your workouts, with the exception of yoga sessions, are 30 minutes (maximum 40 minutes).

2. **Give every workout your all.** High intensity and maximal effort—to the point where you just can't squeeze out one more rep—is a *must* for effective fat burning and hormonal benefits. If you find you are not at the point of fatigue at the end of the suggested repetitions, you can increase the resistance slightly. For instance, increase your weight (but by no more than 5-pound increments at a time). When you're pushing yourself hard in the gym (or wherever you exercise), remember that your workout is short, and it will all be over soon!

3. **Work in a little rest between each circuit.** Circuit training (which involves moving from one exercise to another with little to no rest between exercises) keeps your heart rate high throughout your workout. When you use this method, you get your cardio workout and resistance training all in one shorter session. Circuit training is also the best type of workout for improving insulin response, boosting testosterone and stimulating growth hormone. You'll spend less time exercising but will realize even more benefits.

4. **Work multiple muscle groups with each strength-training session.** You will see in the Metabolic Repair Program that many exercises are hybrids—moves that have been combined to give you maximum metabolic benefit. This approach is designed to increase growth hormone and stimulate several muscle groups at once. It also lets you complete more work in less time and ensures your muscles get the proper recuperation time they need *between* sessions.

5. **Keep cardio sessions short and use intervals.** Intervals are a series of shorter periods of intense exercise separated by periods of brief rest or lighter activity. This method of training

offers the most fat-burning potential and the greatest health benefits. It increases the intensity of your training too, which once again means greater benefits with less time spent exercising. Even cardiac patients can use interval training to improve their fitness.

6. **Use a heart rate monitor.** A heart rate monitor is an excellent tool to keep yourself in check and safe. It helps to ensure you are not over- or underexerting, according to your current fitness level and health status. In addition, the monitor is a great motivator. You will literally watch your cardiovascular fitness improve, as your heart rate recovers faster and remains lower compared to when you first began exercising. Turn to page 293 to learn more about the advantages of a heart rate monitor.

7. **Use yoga for its hormone-enhancing effects.** Besides challenging and stretching your muscles, yoga can lower blood cortisol levels, reduce adrenaline and stimulate brain-calming GABA. Although there is a common misconception that yoga is not a "real" workout, I can assure you it is a stellar choice when it comes to building your strength and increasing muscle tone. And it is definitely not just for girls.

8. **Consume the right stuff before and after your workouts for optimal hormonal effects.** Always consume a CSP meal or snack about 1 hour before your resistance-training sessions. Within the 45 minutes following your session, enjoy a higher carb and protein meal, such as a shake made with fruit juice or frozen fruit and whey protein (but no added oils or fats). This combination is proven to stimulate more growth hormone release and encourage more muscle gain. You can do cardio on an empty stomach (though you don't have to), but eat your snack of protein and carbs (again no fat) within 45 minutes of finishing your workout. Drink only water during your workouts—no sports drinks allowed!

Tools of the Trade

Whether you choose to work out in the gym, outside or at home, you will need a few key pieces of equipment to get the job done. Most gyms provide these items for you. Otherwise, you may want to purchase them for yourself. Here's all the equipment you will need to complete your weekly exercise routine:

- **A stability ball (SB).** These come in different sizes, so be sure to purchase/use the proper one for your height.
- **A set of dumbbells (DB).** Women will need 3, 5, 8, 10, 12 and 15 pounds; men will need 10, 15, 20, 25 and 30 pounds.
- **A support bench.** A weight bench or other stable bench is helpful. A bench is not essential if you have a stability ball.
- **A medicine ball (MB).** If you do not want to buy one, you can use a dumbbell instead.
- **Options for indoor cardio.** A stationary bike, treadmill, stepper or elliptical machine. (You can also walk, skip, bike or run outside when weather permits.)
- **Music.** Listening to your favorite tunes while you work out can be a great motivator, so have your iPod or other player on hand.
- **A heart rate monitor (HRM).** This is optional but recommended (see page 293).

Suggested Weekly Workout Schedule

For maximum health and hormonal benefits, I recommend that you exercise 6 days a week. You will complete three types of workouts each week:

1. Three days a week you will perform 30 minutes (maximum of 40) of circuit training.
2. Once or twice a week you'll do interval cardio for 20 to 40 minutes. Choosing an additional session—a walk, an active game or another fun, heart-pumping activity that you enjoy weekly— is also recommended.

3. Once or twice a week you'll do yoga for 30 to 90 minutes. A yoga class or yoga DVDs to complete at home are both excellent options. As far as the type of yoga is concerned, I prefer anusara, but hatha, vinyasa or ashtanga are fine too. You can decide which you like best.

One day per week you should rest and do *no* exercise. Whew! Your weekly workout schedule may look something like this:

MON.	TUES.	WED.	THURS.	FRI.	SAT.	SUN.
Day 1 Circuit workout	Day 2 Circuit workout	Yoga or Cardio	Day 3 Circuit workout	Cardio	Yoga	Rest or go for a walk or do an activity you enjoy

Two things to keep in mind:
- If you wish to do cardio and weights on the same day, split them into two different workouts (e.g., cardio in the morning and weights in the afternoon) so you can avoid the stress of exercising too long in one session. If your schedule doesn't permit splitting the workouts this way, then always do your cardio *after* your weight training—never before.
- Avoid doing your yoga on the same day as your weights to limit undue stress on your muscles.

Now let's get to your actual weekly daily routine. Since hormonal health—not exercise—is my area of expertise, I have recruited one of the best fitness specialists I know to help me build this program. Don Hunter is not only one of my closest and dearest friends (we have known each other since grade school!) but also an expert in circuit training, sports-specific training and postinjury rehab. He is also the cofounder of Slim Gyms Fitness Limited, a facility founded upon Don's principles of training. I am very grateful for his contributions to this book, and I know that you will feel the same way once you start doing this workout. It is guaranteed to transform your body and your metabolism in very little time!

The best thing about this workout is that you can continue to modify and adapt it for years, no matter your fitness level. For instance, you can begin by completing as much or as little of the daily exercise routine as you can handle. Whether you complete a full round of the three groups of exercises with a moderate amount of weight or just one round of one of the group of exercises with very light weights, you can continue to build from your starting point. You can increase the intensity of the workout by:

- Increasing the number of reps you do for each exercise to the maximum recommended
- Increasing the number of times you complete the exercise groups
- Increasing the weights you use for each exercise
- Increasing the tempo in which you do the workout. You can do this by moving faster through the repetitions of each individual exercise (but be sure to always maintain proper exercise form) or through the entire workout by taking less rest.

Your three strength-training routines are outlined on the following pages. For better reference and quick guidance during your workouts, I have also created the **Carb Sensitivity Program Metabolic Workout poster**, which clearly displays all three days of circuit-training exercises and provides space for you to record up to 3 months of your training habits at a time. It's available to purchase through www.carbsensitivity.com. On your yoga workout day, you can attend a class in your area or use a DVD at home. I have also included a few suggestions for your cardio day.

Each workout follows a pattern designed to eliminate confusion and to help you quickly become familiar with the routine and easily flow through the circuits. Almost all exercises have been created to combine two to three motions into one move. This allows maximum metabolic benefit in the least amount of time. Ultimately, this style of training creates, without a doubt, the critical solution for metabolic repair. In this workout, you will find yourself moving in all directions, engaging all joints and touching on all planes of movement, without setting yourself up for the risk of repetitive injury. Full-body routines like these are not only the best for metabolic effects but also the next revolution in fitness for a time-crunched society. Like Dr. Turner, I believe this is the most effective approach for encompassing all paradigms of training, as your overall strength, core strength, cardiovascular fitness, fat burning, coordination and balance are all enhanced within a single training session.

Each day's program comprises three groups of four exercises. At the beginning, you will likely be able to complete each group only once in your workout for the day. Eventually you will become more familiar with the exercises, and your endurance, strength and fitness will increase. This will allow you to complete each circuit of four exercises up to three times. You may also mix it up by completing the first circuit three times and the second and third circuit of the day twice. The possibilities are endless—yet another benefit of this style of training.

Each exercise has a suggested maximum number of reps. Keep in mind that reaching the maximum reps is *less* important than maintaining your form. You should complete the exercise with perfect form to failure (i.e., until you just can't do another rep), whether it is only 1 rep or 15. The format of this workout will allow you to easily keep modifying and adapting to keep your strength, fitness and, most important, your metabolism progressing. Here are a few key suggestions:

- Keep breathing: Breathe at the exertion (i.e., the push/pull) portion of the exercise.
- Stay strong: Your core should be engaged *at all times* throughout all moves. This will tighten and strengthen those abs, obliques and lower back, which will help support your body not only during your workout but also in your day-to-day life.
- Keep your knees in check: Make sure that your knees never go past the plane of your big toes during all lunges and squats. This will help you avoid injury or undue strain on your knees.

I have included a faster-paced exercise—a move Dr. Turner has labeled the Metabolic Move of the Day—as the final exercise in the third circuit of each strength-training routine. This power move gets your heart pumping and your whole body moving. Why speed things up at the end of each routine? Why not? It not only gets your heart pumping but also boosts your metabolism and helps your body burn calories for a longer period of time after your workout.

I encourage you to be patient with yourself. Many of these moves require focus and coordination. When pertinent, I have included beginner and advanced modifications to allow you to match each exercise to your abilities at any point in time. You need to remind yourself that you really can do anything! It just requires commitment and a bit of repetitive learning. Have fun with it. Trust your body. Take breaks when you need to, *and hydrate*. Start with easier, lighter weights and track your progress so that you can increase the weight as you adapt.

Before you begin, a warmup is important. Warming your body just 2 to 3 degrees allows the muscles to prepare for contraction, increases bloodflow and also increases the elasticity of your soft tissues and ligaments. Doing so enhances performance, flexibility and the engagement of your muscles. Your warmup should be dynamic, not static, meaning that you do not hold stretches but rather move lightly in and out of the stretch position. I use this simple approach with all of my clients not only to increase the effectiveness of their training but also—and more importantly— to keep them injury free and less sore after the workout. I do not want you to perform your warmup in a vigorous manner. The goal is simply to warm your body as you prepare for the more intense workout to follow.

At the end of your routine, a static, full-body stretch is important to keep the body from tightening after all the intense activity and muscle contractions. The benefits of postworkout stretching include staving off delayed-onset soreness and potential injury, as well as shaping the body by elongating the muscle. Keep in mind that the longer you stretch, the more long-term benefits you will experience. From 40 seconds to 2 minutes is ideal. The longer hold will benefit not only soft tissue (e.g., muscles, tendons, ligaments) but also other tissues such as the myofascial layer, which provides support and structure throughout the human body. Over time our body will deal with stress-related diseases, trauma, overuse, infections, even inactivity, all of which can distort and twist this fascia, inevitably leading to alignment issues throughout the entire body.

To see exactly what you should be doing, watch me complete the warmup and cooldown stretch routine online via the link posted on www.carbsensitivity.com.

Enjoy your workout!

Day 1 Strength-Training Routine: Full Body

Begin by completing each circuit once. Add a second and/or third set of Group 1, 2 and/or 3 as you become more familiar with the workout and your fitness improves.

CIRCUIT GROUPING	EXERCISE	#REPS TO STRIVE FOR	RESISTANCE	MODIFICATIONS B=BEGINNER ADV=ADVANCED
Group 1	Standing squat/press	12–15	DB or MB	Adv: Add calf raises as you stand up from the squat and press the DBs above your head.
	SB abdominal reach	15	Adv: DB or MB	Adv: Use the suggested resistance to stress core engagement.
	SB hamstring curl	12–15	None	Adv: Split the reps between doing single leg curls during the same circuit, instead of completing the exercise with both legs at once.
	Alternating lateral lunge with single DB front raise	8–10 on each side	DB	Adv: With each side lunge, raise both arms at the same time.

Begin by completing one round of Group 1. Gradually work toward completing two or three rounds before taking a break. Once you have completed Group 1, take a minute before moving to Group 2. Remember to hydrate and trust your body!

Note: DB = dumbbells; MB = medicine ball; SB = stability ball

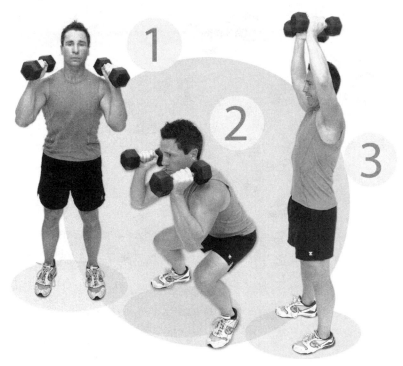

Standing Squat/Press: Remember to always keep the DB directly above your shoulders and close to your body as you move into the squat position. This will ensure the resistance is not being applied to the lower back area.

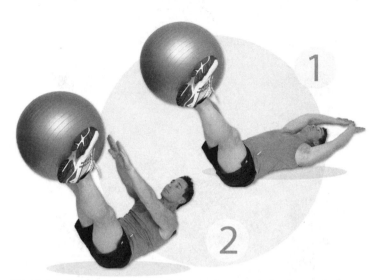

SB Abdominal Reach: If your abdominal strength limits you from getting much range as you reach, use the momentum of your arms to swing as much as you can as you lift from position 1 to 2.

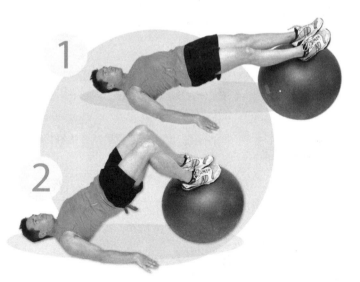

SB Hamstring Curl: Make sure your glutes and core remain fully elevated during the curl motion. This ensures correct alignment and maximum benefits. If you find yourself wobbling or unstable, create more stability by stretching your arms out in line with your shoulders, with your palms pressing on the floor.

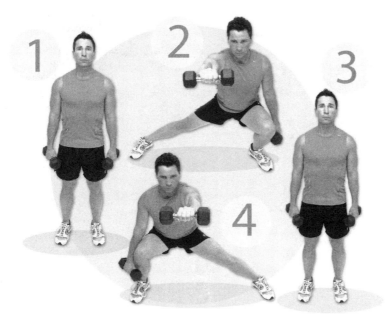

Alternating Lateral Lunge with Single DB Front Raise: With each lunge and front raise, engage your core to protect your lower back.

CIRCUIT GROUPING	EXERCISE	#REPS TO STRIVE FOR	RESISTANCE	MODIFICATIONS B=BEGINNER ADV=ADVANCED
Group 2	Weighted stepup (left leg) with high knee (right leg)	10–15	DB or MB	Adv: Add a bicep curl once in the top position of the stepup on the bench.
	Plank with leg raise (right) and glute flex	15	None	B: If you have a back issue or find this overly taxing, do the exercise from your knee.
	Alternating T-bar pushup	5–10 (each side)	Adv: DB	B: If you cannot do a pushup, you may try doing a partial one or eliminate the pushup and move into the T-bar on each arm from the beginning pushup position. Adv: Add a straight arm lift using a DB.
	Alternating lunge rotate low to high	8–10 (each leg)	DB or MB	B: Do this without the resistance but still move your arms the through rotation.

Begin by completing one round of Group 2. Gradually work toward completing two or three rounds before taking a break. Once you have completed Group 2, take a minute before moving to Group 3. Remember to hydrate and trust your body!

Note: DB = dumbbells; MB = medicine ball; SB = stability ball

Group 2

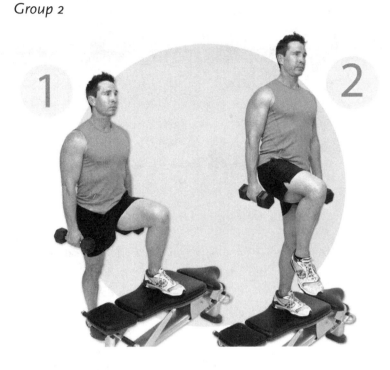

Weighted Stepup LEFT with High Knee RIGHT: Always make sure your heel is well planted on the step and that your weight transfers from your heel as you step up. Your left leg remains stationary on the bench. This will engage all aspects of the legs, including the calf, glute, hamstring and quadriceps. When you step back down with your right leg, make sure to bring your foot back to the floor with control and as lightly as possible to absorb the momentum with your knees. This will also protect your Achilles tendon and lower back from excessive impact.

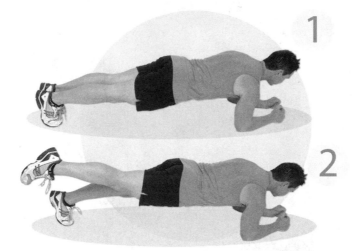

Plank with Leg Raise RIGHT and Glute Flex: Engage your core throughout the whole move to protect your lower back. Make sure your neck
is aligned with your spine and that your breathing is normal, as many
people tend to hold their breath.

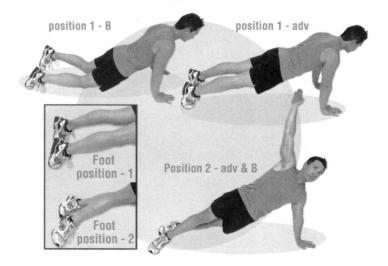

position 1 - B

position 1 - adv

Foot
position - 1

Position 2 - adv & B

Foot
position - 2

Alternating T-bar Pushup: It is imperative to shift your feet sideways,
with your toes pointing toward whatever side or arm you are lifting.
Your arm should remain straight through the lift and the rotation of

your body to maximize the effort from your core, while bringing the arm to the top extended position.

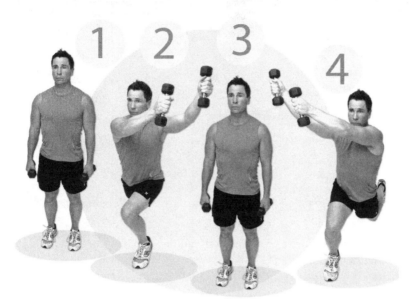

Alternating Lunge Rotate Low to High: As you lunge, avoid added neck strain by making sure you slightly rotate your head to keep your neck in line with your spine and rotation. Lunging back immediately rather than hesitating will allow you to maximize the power and energy built up in your legs and Achilles tendon.

CIRCUIT GROUPING	EXERCISE	#REPS TO STRIVE FOR	RESISTANCE	MODIFICATIONS B=BEGINNER ADV=ADVANCED
Group 3	Weighted stepup (right leg) with high knee raise (left leg)	10–15	DB or MB	Adv: Add a bicep curl once in the top position of the stepup on the bench.
	Plank with leg raise (left) and glute flex	15	None	B: If you have a back issue or find this overly taxing, do the exercise from your knees.
	Lying chest press with leg bicycle	15	DB or MB	B: Hold legs stationary with a 90-degree bend without bicycle to eliminate stress if you find leg movement stressful on lower back. Adv: Scissor straight leg up and down.
	METABOLIC MOVE OF THE DAY: Split leg jump with crossing rotation	20–30	MB or single DB	B: Hold the MB in front of your chest and let your legs meet in the middle before going back into the leg split.

Begin by completing one round of Group 3. Gradually work toward completing two or three rounds before taking a break. Remember to stay hydrated and trust your body!

Note: DB = dumbbells; MB = medicine ball; SB = stability ball

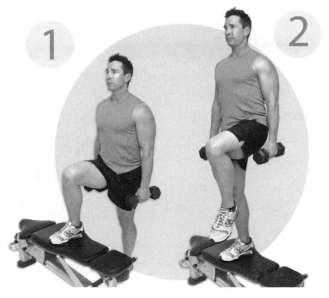

Group 3

Weighted Stepup RIGHT with High Knee LEFT: Refer to the description in Group 2, **Weighted Stepup LEFT with High Knee RIGHT.**

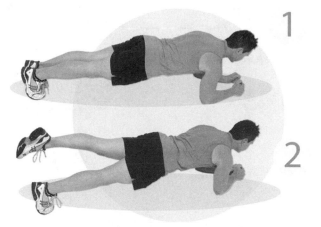

Plank with Leg Raise LEFT and Glute Flex: Refer to the description in Group 2, **Plank with Leg Raise RIGHT and Glute Flex.**

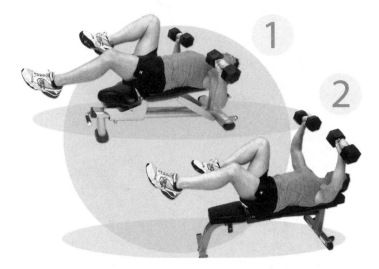

Lying Chest Press with Leg Bicycle: As you bicycle your legs, keep your core engaged. Your heels should remain no more than 3 inches above the bench or surface you are lying on.

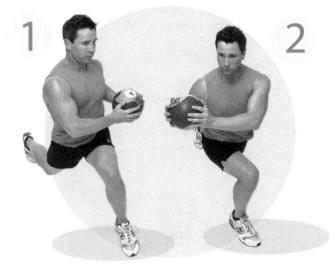

Split Leg Jump with Crossing Rotation: Your beginning position should always have the MB or DB rotated across whichever leg is forward. As this is the Metabolic Move of the Day, perform this movement at a fast pace.

Day 2 Strength-Training Routine: Full Body

Begin by completing each circuit once. Add a second and third set of Group 1, 2 and 3 as you become more familiar with the workout and your fitness improves.

CIRCUIT GROUPING	EXERCISE	#REPS TO STRIVE FOR	RESISTANCE	MODIFICATIONS B=BEGINNER ADV=ADVANCED
Group 1	Three-point lunge (right leg)	4–8 (consider all 3 angles as 1 rep)	Adv: MB or single DB	B: Keep the resistance centered in front of your chest. B: Keep your arms above your head the whole time, without adding the suggested resistance.
	SB alternating chest press	10–15 (each arm)	DB	B: Lower your hips closer to the floor. Adv: Bring your feet closer together on the floor to increase the workload on your core as you perform the motion.
	SB alternating ab crossover (hand to knee)	10–15	None	Adv: Try to touch your toe, but be careful! It takes time to gain coordination and you may want to work with a trainer to spot you while teaching you this advanced move.
	Hamstring stretch (right) row/twist/ press	10–15	DB or MB	B: Keep your foot/toes planted for better balance. B: Do this without the resistance.

Begin by completing one round of Group 1. Gradually work toward completing two or three rounds before taking a break, then once you have completed Group 1 take a minute before moving to Group 2. Remember to hydrate and trust your body!

Note: DB = dumbbells; MB = medicine ball; SB = stability ball

Group 1

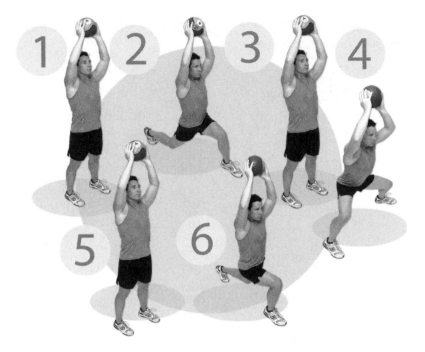

Three-Point Lunge RIGHT: As you move through each lunge position, always engage your core. If you feel any discomfort, drop your hands to your sides until your core is conditioned enough to advance. For those with knee issues: Lunge down only to the point where you remain pain free and feel comfortable. These moves definitely call for a high level of balance and require support around the knee.

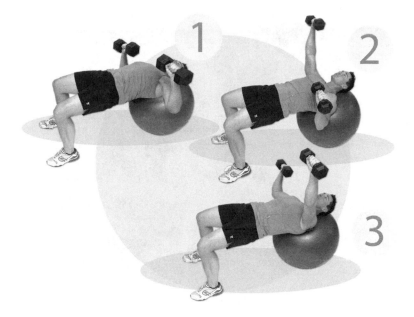

SB Alternating Chest Press: Have your head and upper back lying on the ball, with your hips raised and parallel to the floor. Your feet should be a minimum shoulder-width apart. You must flex your glutes, tighten your core and breathe through each lift to feel your chest and core work while perfecting this great move.

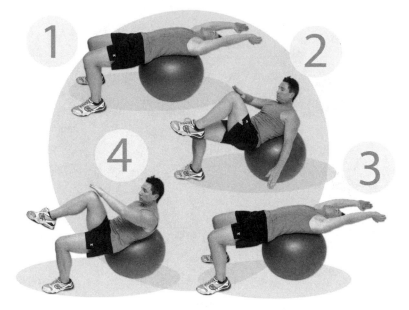

SB Alternating Ab Crossover (hand to knee): Take your time to slowly gain the coordination for this move by remaining centered on the ball as you crunch to touch your hand to the opposite knee.

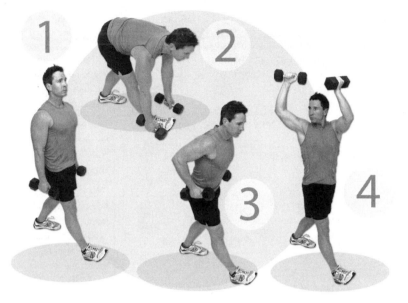

Hamstring Stretch RIGHT Row/Twist/Press: When performed properly, with protection for the lower back, this move will not only strengthen your normal daily movements but also help you develop new capabilities. It combines the best elements of full-body strengthening, rotation, balance and flexibility into one steady, flowing move. Again, keep your core tight and your back straight, and make sure the position of your back leg keeps your hips pulled back through the bending motion so your knee does not extend past the plane of your toes.

CIRCUIT GROUPING	EXERCISE	#REPS TO STRIVE FOR	RESISTANCE	MODIFICATIONS B=BEGINNER ADV=ADVANCED
Group 2	Three-point lunge (left leg)	4–8 (consider all 3 angles as 1 rep)	Adv: MB or single DB	B: Keep your arms above your head the whole time, without adding the suggested resistance.
	Isolated squat with concentration biceps curl (right)	10–15	DB	Adv: Alternate between a regular curl and a hammer curl.
	SB alternating shoulder press	8–10 (each arm)	DB	Adv: Start with your palms facing you and twist to a neutral grip as you raise the resistance.
	Hamstring stretch (left) row/press/ twist	10–15	DB or MB	B: Keep your foot/ toes planted for better balance. B: Do this without the resistance.

Begin by completing one round of Group 2. Gradually work toward completing two or three rounds before taking a break. Once you have completed Group 2, take a minute before moving to Group 3. Remember to hydrate and trust your body!

Note: DB = dumbbells; MB = medicine ball; SB = stability ball

Group 2

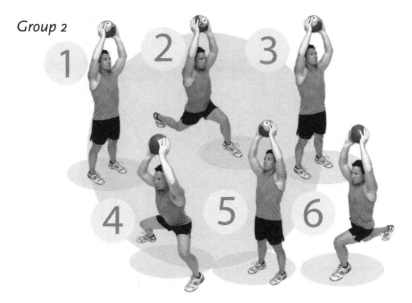

Three-Point Lunge LEFT: Follow the same sequence of lunges as in the **Three-Point Lunge RIGHT** in Group 1.

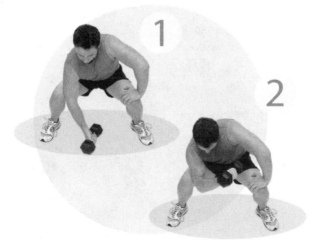

Isolated Squat with Concentration Biceps Curl RIGHT: Remember to squat down far enough to allow your elbow to be positioned on your inner thigh while still allowing you to keep your back upright and straight. Keep your core tight.

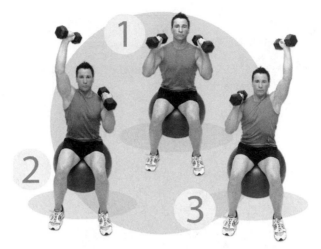

SB Alternating Shoulder Press: Your neck should be aligned with your spine, and your core drawn tight. Breathe through each lift as you alternate between each arm. Remember, the closer your foot stance, the more you work your core and balance.

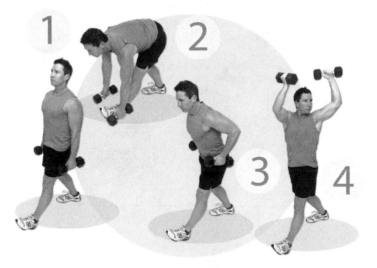

Hamstring Stretch LEFT Row/Twist/Press: Follow the description from Group 1 for **Hamstring Stretch RIGHT Row/Twist/Press**.

CIRCUIT GROUPING	EXERCISE	#REPS TO STRIVE FOR	RESISTANCE	MODIFICATIONS B=BEGINNER ADV=ADVANCED
Group 3	Wide stance alternating shoulder lateral/front raise	10 (each direction)	DB	
	Isolated squat with concentration bicep curl (left)	10–15	DB	Adv: Alternate between a regular curl and a hammer curl.
	SB alternating triceps extension	10 (each arm)	DB	Adv: Try different grips to isolate other areas of the triceps, such as with palms facing the body or facing away from the body.
	METABOLIC MOVE OF THE DAY: Prison jacks	15	None	

Begin by completing one round of Group 3. Gradually work toward completing two or three rounds before taking a break. Remember to stay hydrated and trust your body!

Note: DB = dumbbells; MB = medicine ball; SB = stability ball

Group 3

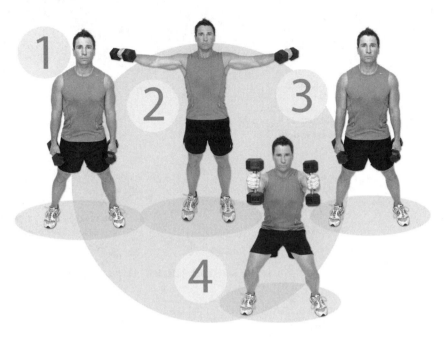

Wide Stance Alternating Shoulder Lateral/Front Raise: Keep your knees slightly bent and your core tight, and begin with a light weight to avoid potential stress on your lower back especially during the front raise. Your grip should have your palms turned toward your body for the lateral raise and facing each other during the front raise.

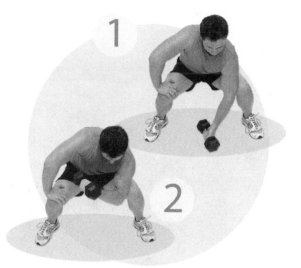

Isolated Squat with Concentration Bicep Curl LEFT: Follow the description from Group 2 for **Isolated Squat with Concentration Biceps Curl RIGHT**.

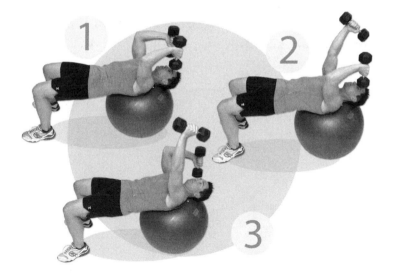

SB Alternating Triceps Extension: To isolate your triceps, keep your elbows in close to your chin as you simultaneously raise one arm while the other goes down.

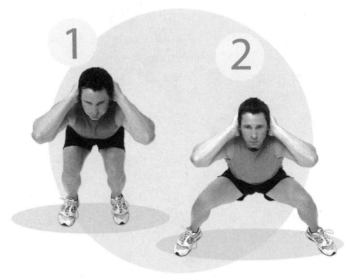

Prison Jacks: This move will raise your heart rate and increase the burn you feel in your leg muscles. Keep your hands beside your head and not locked behind your neck to avoid neck strain. Keep your body from bouncing upward as you move your legs in and out. As this is the Metabolic Move of the Day, perform this movement at a fast pace.

Day 3 Strength-Training Routine: Full Body

Begin by completing each circuit once. Add a second and third set of Group 1, 2 and 3 as you become more familiar with the workout and your fitness improves.

CIRCUIT GROUPING	EXERCISE	#REPS TO STRIVE FOR	RESISTANCE	MODIFICATIONS B=BEGINNER ADV=ADVANCED
Group 1	Duck squat with front shoulder raise	10–15	DB or MB	Adv: Alternate arms as you squat up and down.
	SB pushup stance with drawing knees to chest	10–12		Adv: Add a pushup in between, drawing knees to chest.
	Lying triceps extension with bent knees	10–15	DB	Adv: Add a straight leg raise as you extend through the triceps move. Adv: Alternate extending one arm at the same time as the opposite leg, then switch.
	Standing hammer biceps curl into 90-degree lateral raise	10–12 (each move)	DB	

Begin by completing one round of Group 1. Gradually work toward completing two or three rounds before taking a break. Once you have completed Group 1, take a minute before moving to Group 2. Remember to hydrate and trust your body!

Note: DB = dumbbells; MB = medicine ball; SB = stability ball

Group 1

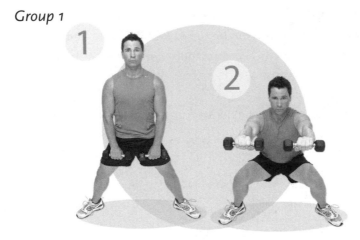

Duck Squat with Front Shoulder Raise: Keep your toes turned out as you take a comfortable wide stance. Remember to keep your core firm as you squat low and raise the weights.

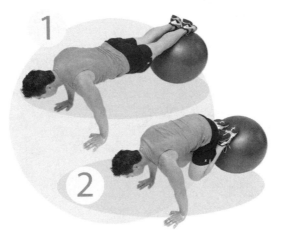

SB Pushup Stance with Drawing Knees to Chest: Start this move by holding a pushup stance and draw your abs in as you bring your knees toward your chest. Take your time, adding a pushup between each rep of drawing knees to chest, since simply steadying your upper body on the floor requires substantial strength. Consider asking a trainer to guide you through this move until you master it.

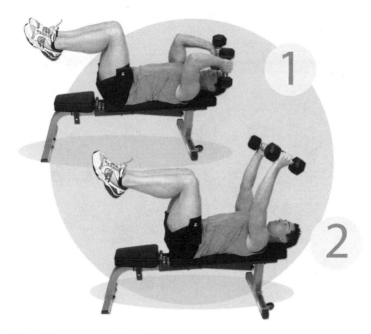

Lying Triceps Extension with Bent Knees: Simply holding the bent-knees position while working your arms activates your core. Therefore, if you progress to one of the advanced modifications, it's important to keep your core engaged to avoid stress on your lower back while you extend your legs. If you have a lower-back issue, you should avoid trying the advanced move.

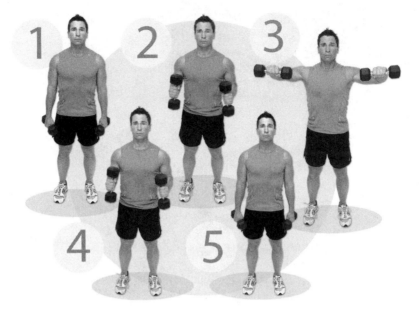

Standing Hammer Biceps Curl into 90-degree Lateral Raise: As you do the lateral raise, the weights and your hands should come to be in line with your shoulders. Maintain the 90-degree bend as you complete the lateral raise motion.

CIRCUIT GROUPING	EXERCISE	#REPS TO STRIVE FOR	RESISTANCE	MODIFICATIONS B=BEGINNER ADV=ADVANCED
Group 2	Standing single leg (right) balance with single arm press (right)	12–15	Single DB	Adv: Add DB to the arm opposite the working leg.
	SB alternating back row and reverse back fly	8–10 (of each exercise)	DB	
	Side plank (left) with lateral arm raise (right)	8–12	DB	B: Raise your upper body only, with your knees on the ground and your lower legs tucked in toward your glutes. Use no resistance. Adv: Raise your upper leg as you raise your arm and body.
	Alternating lunge with biceps curl	10 (each leg)	DB or MB	

Begin by completing one round of Group 2. Gradually work toward completing two or three rounds before taking a break. Once you have completed Group 2, take a minute before moving to Group 3. Remember to hydrate and trust your body!

Note: DB = dumbbells; MB = medicine ball; SB = stability ball

Group 2

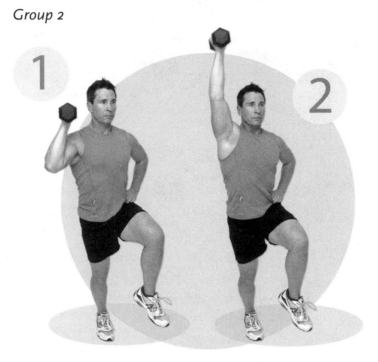

Standing Single Leg RIGHT Balance with Single Arm Press RIGHT:
Your core must be engaged throughout this exercise in order to aid
your balance and resistance as you press upward. Keep your free hand
on your waist for balance and remind yourself to keep your core tight.

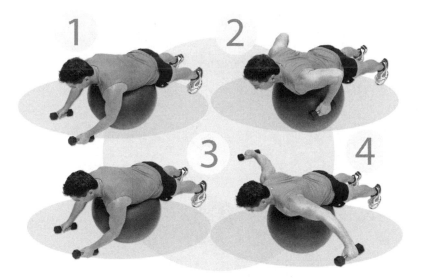

SB Alternating Back Row and Reverse Back Fly: Lie down with the ball between your chest and abdominal area, and your feet spread apart to stabilize you. If you find your feet sliding, simply place them against a wall. Your arms should be extended in the beginning position, as well as between the row and fly. You will find that you are stronger with the row than the fly; therefore, try increasing the pace of the row portion of the movement. It will increase the force of pounds-per-square-inch and enhance the fatigue factor to your muscles. Note that some people find this exercise uncomfortable or hard to do while lying on the SB. If you find this to be the case, try a bent-over stance with a straight back position.

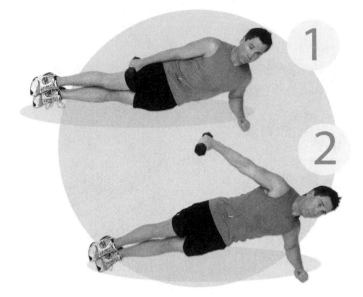

Side Plank LEFT with Lateral Arm Raise RIGHT: If it is too difficult for you to maintain your balance with your feet stacked one on top of the other, separate your feet and place them in a scissor position on the floor.

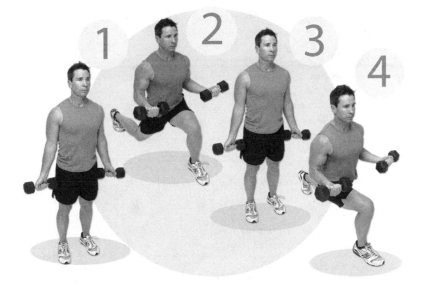

Alternating Lunge with Biceps Curl: This is a fantastic move to really engage the full body. As you lunge the leg forward, curl the weights at the same time; then bring the weights back to the starting position as you move out of the lunge. Repeat with the alternate leg. If you have enough space, a walking lunge can be performed. Simply turn around at the halfway point of the determined repetitions.

CIRCUIT GROUPING	EXERCISE	#REPS TO STRIVE FOR	RESISTANCE	MODIFICATIONS B-BEGINNER ADV-ADVANCED
Group 3	Standing single leg (left) balance with single arm press (left)	12–15	DB	Adv: Add a DB to the arm opposite the working leg.
	Horizontal up/out, in/ down	8–12 (Consider the full cycle of moving up/ out and down/ in as 1 rep)	None	Adv: Complete the move in an up/out, down/in pattern.
	Side plank (right) with lateral arm raise (left)	8–12	Single DB	B: Raise your upper body only, with your knees on the ground and your lower legs tucked in toward your glutes. Use no resistance. Adv: Raise your upper leg as you raise your arm and body.
	METABOLIC MOVE OF THE DAY: Floor or step mountain climbers	15 (each leg)	None	Adv: As you bring your knees toward your chest, don't let your feet touch the floor—you will feel the extra abdominal burn.

Begin by completing one round of Group 3. Gradually work toward completing two or three rounds before taking a break. Remember to stay hydrated and trust your body!

Note: DB = dumbbells; MB = medicine ball; SB = stability ball

Group 3

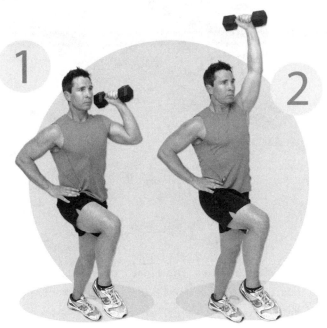

Standing Single Leg LEFT Balance with Single Arm Press LEFT: Refer to the description from Group 2 for **Standing Single Leg RIGHT Balance with Single Arm Press RIGHT**.

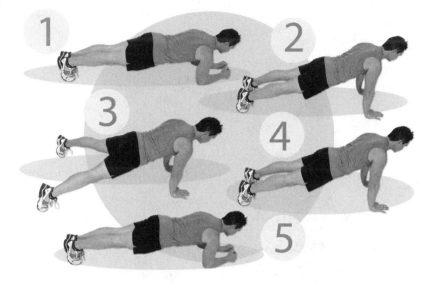

Horizontal Up/Out, In/Down: This move requires a lot of coordination. To reduce confusion, start with the arm movement "up," followed by the leg movement "out." Then bring the legs back "in" and, lastly, bring the arms "down." This simple pattern of arms-legs-legs-arms will keep you flowing through a full-body move while your core and lower back are forced to stabilize your center of gravity.

Another point regarding the arm motion is to try alternating the arm you use to begin this exercise. Most people tend to start with the same arm each time, which can cause an imbalance in strength—one always ends up doing the majority of the work during lifting. Always keep this in mind when doing exercises that involve alternating limb lifts or raises.

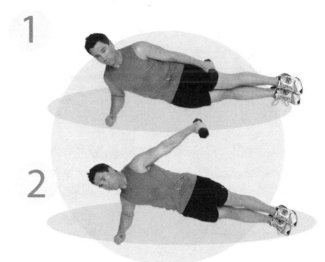

Side Plank RIGHT with Lateral Arm Raise LEFT: Refer to the description from Group 2 for **Side Plank LEFT with Lateral Arm Raise RIGHT**.

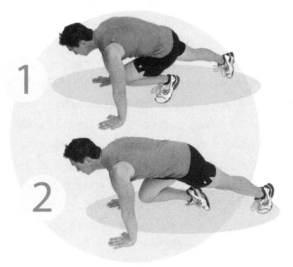

Floor or Step Mountain Climbers: You can make this move easier by placing your hands on a step or on any raised surface that keeps your upper body higher than your feet. As this is the Metabolic Move of the Day, perform this movement at a fast pace.

Options for Interval Cardio Training

We all know that sticking to a regular exercise routine can be tough. Choosing an activity you enjoy—one you know you'll keep up with consistently—is always your best cardiovascular fitness option. Remember, short bursts of exercise not only improve your cardiovascular fitness but also your fat-burning capacity, even during low- or moderate-intensity workouts.

Do not rush into interval training if you have heart disease, high blood pressure or joint problems, or if you are over the age of 40. If you fit into any one of these categories, you should definitely consult your health-care provider first.

Four Examples of Interval Training

If you are not familiar with the concept of interval training, here are a few examples to choose from. You'll do cardio at least once a week for 20 to 30 minutes. A second cardio workout, one that could include a sport or an activity that you enjoy, is optional.

1. Steady-pace intervals of walking, jogging, running, cycling, etc.
   - Complete a 5-minute warmup at a gentle or moderate pace.
   - Start with 30 to 60 seconds at a fast pace or high intensity followed by 60 to 90 seconds at a moderate or walking pace. Alternate 5 to 8 times.
   - Complete a 5-minute cooldown at a gentle or moderate pace.

2. Intervals that increase in speed or intensity throughout the workout.

   This example applies to running on a treadmill. However, a similar approach could be taken by changing the tension or pedaling faster on a stationary bike, by increasing the level or moving faster on your elliptical machine, or by walking on the treadmill while increasing the speed or incline.
   - 5-minute warmup at 5.5 mph
   - 1 minute at 7 mph
   - 1 minute at 6 mph
   - 1 minute at 7.5 mph
   - 1 minute at 6 mph
   - 1 minute at 8 mph
   - 1 minute at 6 mph
   - 1 minute at 8.5 mph
   - 1 minute at 6 mph
   - 1 minute at 9 mph
   - 5-minute cooldown

3. Intervals that vary by duration with 1-minute, low-intensity sessions between each interval.

   Rather than increasing the speed or intensity, your intervals can range in duration, for example:

- 30 seconds
- 60 seconds
- 90 seconds
- 60 seconds
- 30 seconds

4. Advanced option: sprinting (only 15 minutes or so).
- Warm up with a light jog for 5 to 10 minutes.
- Sprint 50 to 100 yards and lightly jog or walk back. Repeat 10 times.
- Cool down with a light jog for another 5 to 10 minutes.

You could also use this approach on hills by running (or speed-walking) up the hill and jogging down.

———

You've reached the end of the CSP. I hope that you will use my suggestions and the support tools I've included to keep you metabolically young and hormonally balanced for a lifetime. Please share your questions, comments and success stories at www.carbsensitivity.com or on www.facebook.com/carbsensitivity.

"Dear Dr. Turner, I wanted to thank you for helping me turn my health around. I just came back from my physician and he said that my blood pressure and cholesterol levels are now within the normal range. While I have a big frame in general, I knew that my health was slowly deteriorating, and I was starting to feel 'old.' I was low in energy, gaining weight, my joints hurt and my doctor was concerned over my recent round of blood work. After a short time on the Carb Sensitivity Program I have lost weight and I feel more energetic. Not only that, but I don't even feel like I am dieting or deprived."

JOHN, 46

STATS	BEFORE	AFTER
Weight	229 lb	210 lb
Body Fat	33%	25%

INITIAL CHIEF COMPLAINTS:

1. Weight gain (around the middle)
2. High blood pressure
3. Joint and muscle pain

PART FOUR

TIME-SAVING TIPS FOR THE KITCHEN AND CSP RECIPES

Act as if what you do makes a difference.
It does.

WILLIAM JAMES

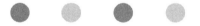

TOP TIME-SAVING TIPS
FOR THE KITCHEN

If you can dream it, you can do it.

WALT DISNEY

Believe it or not—despite the assortment of mouthwatering, appetite-satisfying and carb-sensitizing recipes in this book—I don't spend a lot of time in the kitchen. Like many of you, my busy schedule just doesn't permit it, which is why many of these recipes are quick and easy, regardless of your culinary aptitude. Whether balancing work, school or family life (or all of the above), we all have the same 24 hours in a day, and often it feels like that's not enough. This can be a hard hurdle to clear when starting a new program—especially one that requires preparation and consistency to succeed. The good news is that there are some time-saving tips that will make preparing and sticking to the CSP a whole lot easier.

Purchase a portable blender. While I love my powerful Vitamix blender, I like to keep a smaller, inexpensive blender (such as the Magic Bullet) at work and at my cottage, along with the key ingredients for a perfect smoothie. My selection includes whey protein isolate, frozen berries, a package of ground flaxseed or chia seeds, and a selection of sugar-free nut butters. If you don't have access to a fridge or freezer, you can bring in fresh (or frozen) berries as needed, or skip them altogether. Although ground flaxseed and chia seeds should be kept in the fridge, most fiber alternatives can be stored at room temperature.

Double up on recipes. Although the recipes listed in this book range from single servings to family size, you can always double or even triple the ingredients and freeze extras for later. The great thing about this program is that the caloric breakdown of the meals is fairly equal, so dinners can become lunches and breakfasts can even become dinners (just be sure to follow the "allowed" food lists of the particular phase that you are in).

Purchase a shaker cup and glass containers. Out of all my must-have diet essentials, a good shaker cup tops the list. Shaker cups can be purchased at almost any health-food store for under $10. If I know that I will be out of the house all day, I will put a scoop of whey protein isolate in my shaker cup along with a little bit of cinnamon, a serving of chia seeds or Clear Fiber, and 1 tablespoon of almond butter. When I am ready for a meal, I just add water, shake well and drink. The almond butter becomes a tasty little "cookie" at the bottom of the shaker that can be eaten separately. I also recommend having an assortment of glass containers in which to store and carry your meals so you aren't tempted to stray from the program. Although plastic containers are cheaper and lighter to carry, they can leach chemicals into your food, especially if reheated.

Prepare snack options in bulk. You can be diligent in preparing your meals, but if you skip a snack you may find yourself being pulled to the vending machine at work once that midday slump hits. Since the snack options I recommend are so easy to prepare, you may find it helpful to put together several servings and separate them into baggies or small glass containers that are easy to grab on the go. If you are storing your snacks at work, be sure to replenish your inventory regularly. I usually keep a box of protein bars, a large bag of tamari almonds, and a selection of low-fat cheeses and/or Greek yogurt at the clinic for easy access.

Cook protein in batches, twice weekly. Many of the CSP recipes allow you to select a source of protein, whether it's chicken, turkey, tofu, shrimp or even lean organic steak (preferably once a week only). Since most proteins will remain fresh once cooked for 3 or 4 days, I find it helpful to cook protein twice weekly in larger batches using either the oven, the barbecue or the stove. Given that Sundays and Wednesdays are my slower days, I set aside a bit of time on these days to prepare the powerful protein punch that will top my lunches and keep my metabolism revving.

RECIPES PERMITTED
IN ALL PHASES OF THE PROGRAM

Breakfast Recipes
Chocolate Hazelnut Coffee Smoothie (Serves 1)

¾   serving whey protein isolate (chocolate)

¾   cup unsweetened almond milk (chocolate)

½   cup fresh or frozen berries, or ½ banana, chopped

2   tablespoons Fage Total 0% yogurt, plain

1   tablespoon hazelnut butter

1   tablespoon organic coffee, ground

4–6   ice cubes

Place all ingredients in a blender and blend on high speed until smooth and creamy. Add extra water if desired.

Calories 289 | Protein 29 g | Fat 11 g | Carbohydrates 23 g | Fiber 5 g

Apricot Yogurt Smoothie (Serves 1)

¼   serving whey protein isolate (vanilla)

1   cup Fage Total Classic yogurt, plain

3   dried apricots, chopped

1   tablespoon slivered almonds

2–3   ice cubes

Place all ingredients in a blender and blend on high speed until smooth and creamy. Add extra water if desired.

Calories 282 | Protein 27 g | Fat 11 g | Carbohydrates 21 g | Fiber 2 g

Chocolate Hazelnut
Coffee Smoothie

Apricot Yogurt
Smoothie

Berrylicious Iron-booster Smoothie (Serves 1)

-   1   serving whey protein isolate (vanilla)
-   ½   cup unsweetened almond milk
-   ½   cup water
-   ½   cup fresh or frozen mixed berries
-   ½   small fresh or frozen banana, chopped
-   ½   cup chopped spinach leaves
-   1   tablespoon chia seeds
-   3–4   ice cubes

Place all ingredients in a blender and blend on high speed until smooth and creamy. Add extra water if desired.

Calories 265 | Protein 28 g | Fat 8 g | Carbohydrates 29 g | Fiber 9 g

Chocolate Banana Smoothie (Serves 1)

-   1   serving whey protein isolate (chocolate)
-   ½   cup unsweetened soy milk
-   ½   cup water
-   ½   small fresh or frozen banana, chopped
-   1   tablespoon almond butter
-   ½   teaspoon vanilla extract
-   2–3   ice cubes

Place all ingredients in a blender and blend on high speed until smooth and creamy. Add extra water if desired.

Calories 303 | Protein 31 g | Fat 12 g | Carbohydrates 23 g | Fiber 4 g

Berrylicious Iron-booster Smoothie

Chocolate Banana Smoothie

Mint Chocolate Smoothie (Serves 1)

- ½ serving whey protein isolate (chocolate)
- ½ cup organic pressed cottage cheese
- ½ cup water
- ½ small fresh or frozen banana, chopped
- 1 tablespoon slivered almonds
- ½ tablespoon chopped fresh mint (optional)
- 2–3 drops mint extract
- 2–3 ice cubes

Place all ingredients in a blender and blend on high speed until smooth and creamy. Add extra water if desired.

Calories 289 | Protein 28 g | Fat 11 g | Carbohydrates 20 g | Fiber 4 g

Strawberry Shortcake Smoothie (Serves 1)

- ¾ serving whey protein isolate (vanilla)
- ½ cup unsweetened soy or almond milk
- ½ cup Fage Total Classic yogurt or goat yogurt, plain
- ½ cup fresh or frozen strawberries
- 1 tablespoon chia seeds
- ½ teaspoon vanilla extract
- 3–4 ice cubes

Place all ingredients in a blender and blend on high speed until smooth and creamy. Add extra water if desired.

Calories 311 | Protein 27 g | Fat 12 g | Carbohydrates 31 g | Fiber 10 g

Skinny Banana Split Smoothie (Serves 1)

- 1   serving whey protein isolate (vanilla)
- ¾   cup unsweetened almond milk (vanilla)
- ½   small fresh or frozen banana, chopped
- 1   tablespoon chia seeds
- 1   teaspoon banana extract
- 4–6   ice cubes

Place all ingredients in a blender and blend on high speed until smooth and creamy. Add extra water if desired.

Calories 257 | Protein 28 g | Fat 10 g | Carbohydrates 24 g | Fiber 8 g

Skinny Banana Split Smoothie

Orange Vanilla Shake (Serves 1)

- 1   serving whey protein isolate (vanilla)
- ½   cup water
- ¼   cup orange juice
- 2–3   fresh or frozen strawberries
- ½   small fresh or frozen banana, chopped
- 1   tablespoon almond butter
- 1   teaspoon vanilla extract
      Stevia to taste (optional)
- 4–6   ice cubes

Place all ingredients in a blender and blend on high speed until smooth and creamy. Add extra water if desired.

Calories 325 | Protein 28 g | Fat 11 g | Carbohydrates 34 g | Fiber 6 g

Orange Vanilla Shake

Breakfast Cooler Smoothie (Serves 1)

1	serving whey protein isolate (vanilla)
½–¾	cup water
1	ripe plum, pitted and chopped
2	tablespoons chia seeds or flaxseeds
1	tablespoon fresh lemon juice
	Stevia to taste (optional)
4–6	ice cubes

Place all ingredients in a blender and blend on high speed until smooth and creamy. Add extra water if desired.

Calories 273 | Protein 29 g | Fat 10 g | Carbohydrates 29 g | Fiber 9 g

Wild Berry Breakfast (Serves 1)

1	serving whey protein isolate (vanilla)
¼	cup unsweetened soy or almond milk
½	cup fresh or frozen raspberries
½	cup fresh or frozen blueberries
1	tablespoon almond or hazelnut butter
	Stevia to taste (optional)
4–6	ice cubes

Place all ingredients in a blender and blend on high speed until smooth and creamy. Add extra water if desired.

Calories 303 | Protein 31 g | Fat 12 g | Carbohydrates 22 g | Fiber 10 g

Cinnamon Apple Smoothie (Serves 1)

   1   serving whey protein isolate (vanilla)
   ½   cup unsweetened soy or almond milk
½–¾   cup water
   1   small apple, peeled and chopped
   1   tablespoon almond butter
   ½   teaspoon ground cinnamon
        Stevia to taste (optional)
 4–6   ice cubes

Place all ingredients in a blender and blend on high speed until smooth and creamy. Add extra water if desired.

Calories 294 | Protein 30 g | Fat 11 g | Carbohydrates 27 g | Fiber 3 g

Cinnamon Roll Smoothie (Serves 1)

   1   serving whey protein isolate (vanilla)
   ¾   cup unsweetened almond milk
   1   tablespoon almond butter
   ½   teaspoon vanilla extract
   ¼   teaspoon ground cinnamon
        Stevia to taste (optional)
 4–6   ice cubes
   1   small apple, peeled and chopped

Place all ingredients except the apple in a blender and blend on high speed until smooth and creamy. Add extra water if desired. Enjoy with apple on the side.

Calories 286 | Protein 25 g | Fat 11 g | Carbohydrates 21 g | Fiber 4 g

Root Beer Float Smoothie (Serves 1)

- 1 serving whey protein isolate (vanilla)
- 1 can Zevia All Natural Ginger Root Beer
- ½ cup fresh or frozen berries
- 1½ tablespoons chia seeds
- ½ teaspoon vanilla extract
  Stevia to taste (optional)
- 4–6 ice cubes

Place all ingredients in a blender and blend on high speed until smooth and creamy. Add extra water if desired. Instead of blending the berries in the smoothie, they can be enjoyed on the side, if preferred.

Calories 261 | Protein 29 g | Fat 8 g | Carbohydrates 29 g | Fiber 10 g

Coco-Vanilla Smoothie (Serves 1)

- 1 serving whey protein isolate (vanilla)
- ¼ cup Fage Total Classic yogurt, plain
- ½ cup water
- ¼ small fresh or frozen banana, chopped
- 1 tablespoon ground flaxseed
- ½ teaspoon coconut extract
- 4–6 ice cubes

Place all ingredients in a blender and blend on high speed until smooth and creamy. Add extra water if desired.

Calories 279 | Protein 31 g | Fat 10 g | Carbohydrates 22 g | Fiber 4 g

Jelly Sandwich Smoothie (Serves 1)

- 1 serving whey protein isolate (vanilla)
- ½–¾ cup water
- ½ cup fresh or frozen strawberries
- 1 tablespoon almond butter
- 1–2 teaspoons no-sugar-added strawberry jam
- 3–4 ice cubes

Place all ingredients in a blender and blend on high speed until smooth and creamy. Add extra water if desired.

Calories 287 | Protein 28 g | Fat 11 g | Carbohydrates 22 g | Fiber 6 g

Piña Colada Smoothie (Serves 1)

- 1 serving whey protein isolate (vanilla)
- ½ can coconut water, or ½ teaspoon coconut extract
- ½ cup water
- ½ small fresh or frozen banana, chopped
- ¼ cup pineapple chunks (fresh, or canned in water and drained)
- 2 tablespoons chia seeds
- 4–6 ice cubes

Place all ingredients in a blender and blend on high speed until smooth and creamy. Add extra water if desired.

Calories 278 | Protein 29 g | Fat 11 g | Carbohydrates 31 g | Fiber 10 g

Alkalizing Breakfast Smoothie (Serves 1)

¾   serving whey protein isolate (vanilla)

½   cup Fage Total Classic yogurt, plain

¼–½   cup water

½   cup spinach, chopped (optional)

¼   small fresh or frozen banana, chopped

1   tablespoon spirulina or greens powder

1   tablespoon ground flaxseed

3–4   ice cubes

Place all ingredients in a blender and blend on high speed until smooth and creamy. Add extra water if desired.

Calories 278 | Protein 33 g | Fat 11 g | Carbohydrates 17 g | Fiber 3 g

Cheesecake Smoothie (Serves 1)

½   serving whey protein isolate (vanilla)

½   cup pressed cottage cheese

½   cup water

½   cup fresh or frozen strawberries or raspberries

1   tablespoon chia seeds

    Stevia to taste (optional)

Place all ingredients in a blender and blend on high speed until smooth and creamy. Add extra water if desired.

Calories 239 | Protein 28 g | Fat 8 g | Carbohydrates 18 g | Fiber 10 g

Sweet Apple Pie Smoothie (Serves 1)

1	serving whey protein isolate (vanilla)
¾	cup unsweetened almond milk
1	small apple, peeled and chopped
1	tablespoon ground flaxseed
½	teaspoon ground cinnamon
½	teaspoon ground nutmeg
	Stevia to taste (optional)
3–4	ice cubes

Place all ingredients in a blender and blend on high speed until smooth and creamy. Add extra water if desired.

Calories 274 | Protein 28 g | Fat 8 g | Carbohydrates 18 g | Fiber 10 g

Sweet Apple Pie Smoothie

Awesome Avocado and Egg Breakfast (Serves 1)

     Olive oil nonstick cooking spray
1   clove garlic, minced
½   medium red onion, diced
     Salt and pepper to taste
2   green onions, sliced
2   cups baby spinach leaves
1   pint grape tomatoes, chopped or halved
1   whole omega-3 egg
½   cup liquid egg whites, or 4–5 egg whites
¼   avocado, sliced

Lightly grease a nonstick skillet with cooking spray, and sauté garlic over medium heat. Add onion and sauté for 4 to 5 minutes, or until softened. Add salt and pepper. Stir in green onions, spinach and tomatoes. Cook for another 4 to 5 minutes. Add egg and egg whites, and scramble until set. If you prefer your eggs spicy, you can add chopped jalapeño peppers or hot sauce. Serve with avocado slices.

Calories 361 | Protein 26 g | Fat 11 g | Carbohydrates 27 g | Fiber 4 g

Portobello Mushroom Omelette (Serves 1)

- 1 teaspoon extra-virgin olive oil
- ½ clove garlic, minced
- 1 tablespoon peeled and grated fresh gingerroot
- 2 tablespoons chopped green onions
- 1 cup chopped portobello mushrooms
- 1–2 teaspoons low-sodium soy sauce
- 2 omega-3 eggs
- ½ cup liquid egg whites, or 4 egg whites
- 1 apple or orange

In a nonstick skillet, heat olive oil over medium-high heat. Sauté garlic, ginger and green onions until fragrant. Add mushrooms and soy sauce, and cook for 2 to 3 minutes. Set aside on a plate. Add eggs and egg whites to the skillet and scramble over medium heat. Before the eggs are completely cooked, return the vegetable mixture to the skillet and stir together. Serve with apple or orange.

Calories 298 | Protein 29 g | Fat 12 g | Carbohydrates 24 g | Fiber 5 g

Salmon and Dill Omelette (Serves 1)

- 1 tablespoon extra-virgin olive oil
- ¼ small red onion, finely chopped
- 1 small handful baby spinach leaves
- 2 ounces smoked salmon, coarsely chopped
- ½ teaspoon finely chopped fresh dill
- ½ cup liquid egg whites, or 4 egg whites
- 1 apple or pear

In a nonstick skillet, heat olive oil over medium-high heat. Sauté onion until softened. Add spinach and sauté until wilted. Add salmon and dill. Pour in egg whites and stir. Let mixture set, then fold over and cook until the whites are completely solid. Serve with apple or pear.

Calories 293 | Protein 30 g | Fat 17 g | Carbohydrates 26 g | Fiber 5 g

Pepper and Spinach Omelette (Serves 1)

- 1 cup cooked fresh or frozen spinach
  Salt and pepper to taste
  Olive oil nonstick cooking spray
- ¼ cup diced onion
- ¼ cup chopped red bell pepper
- ¼ cup chopped yellow bell pepper
- 2 whole omega-3 eggs
- ½ cup liquid egg whites, or 4 egg whites
- 1 small orange, peeled and separated

Drain spinach, pressing out any excess water. Season with salt and pepper. Place on a serving plate and set aside. Lightly grease a nonstick skillet with cooking spray and sauté onion and bell peppers over medium heat until softened. Add eggs and egg whites and scramble until set. Top the spinach with the eggs. Enjoy with orange segments.

Calories 315 | Protein 29 g | Fat 11 g | Carbohydrates 29 g | Fiber 6 g

Breakfast Salsa Dish (Serves 1)

2	teaspoons extra-virgin olive oil, divided
2	slices turkey bacon
¼	cup chopped Vidalia onion
¼	cup chopped red bell pepper
1	whole egg
¼	cup liquid egg whites
	Salt and pepper to taste
½	teaspoon finely chopped fresh parsley, or dried
2–3	tablespoons no-sugar-added salsa
½	cup chopped green apple

In a nonstick skillet, heat 1 teaspoon olive oil over medium heat. Cook turkey bacon, then remove from the pan, break into small pieces, and set aside. Rinse the pan, then add 1 teaspoon of olive oil and place over low heat. Sauté onion and bell pepper until softened. Add the reserved turkey bacon, egg, and egg whites, and scramble until the eggs are set. Add salt and pepper. Place on a serving plate and top with parsley and salsa. Enjoy with apple on the side.

Calories 271 | Protein 29 g | Fat 9 g | Carbohydrates 25 g | Fiber 6 g

Lunch and Dinner Recipes

Blueberry Chicken Salad (Serves 2)

2 boneless, skinless chicken breasts (approximately 4 to 5 ounces each)

Salt and pepper to taste

Olive oil nonstick cooking spray

2 teaspoons extra-virgin olive oil, divided

¼ cup diced red onion

4–6 cups baby spinach leaves

2 tablespoons apple cider vinegar

1–2 tablespoons finely chopped fresh parsley

1 cup fresh blueberries

1–2 ounces goat cheese, crumbled

Preheat oven to 375°F. Generously season each chicken breast with salt and pepper. Lightly grease a large oven-safe skillet with cooking spray, and sear the chicken over high heat for 2 to 3 minutes on each side or until lightly golden. Place the skillet in the oven and bake the chicken until cooked through, about 15 minutes.

While the chicken is cooking, heat 1 teaspoon olive oil in a large skillet over medium heat, and sauté onion until softened, 3 to 4 minutes. Add spinach and toss until wilted. Season with salt and pepper, and transfer to a large platter or divide evenly between two plates.

Wipe out the skillet and heat 1 teaspoon olive oil and the vinegar. Stir in parsley. Arrange the cooked chicken breasts on the spinach and top with the parsley dressing. Sprinkle with blueberries and goat cheese.

Calories 312 | Protein 32 g | Fat 11 g | Carbohydrates 21 g | Fiber 4 g

Mexican Summer Salad (Serves 3)

1	purple eggplant, thinly sliced
2	tablespoons extra-virgin olive oil
4	small zucchini, sliced
3	ripe plum tomatoes, seeded and diced
¼	cup fresh roasted or canned green chilies, chopped
1	tablespoon chopped jalapeño pepper, to taste
2–3	tablespoons fresh lime juice
4–5	cloves garlic, minced
2	pinches ground cumin
	Salt and lemon pepper to taste
3	tablespoons chopped fresh cilantro
3	servings of protein from "allowed" list
	Lime wedges

Cut out the excess seeds of the eggplant slices. Lay eggplant slices on a rack set over a baking sheet. Season with salt and let stand 15 minutes. Pat dry with paper towels. In a large nonstick skillet or wok, heat olive oil over medium-high heat. Sauté the eggplant and zucchini for 3 to 4 minutes, until slightly tender. Add tomatoes, green chilies, jalapeño, lime juice, garlic, cumin, salt and lemon pepper; stir to combine. Cover and cook until the vegetables are tender, about 15 minutes. Add a few tablespoons of additional liquid if needed to avoid scorching the pan. To serve, stir in fresh cilantro and top with your choice of allowed protein. Serve with lime wedges.

Calories 311 | Protein 27 g | Fat 13 g | Carbohydrates 25 g | Fiber 7 g

Ahi Tuna Steak and Salad (Serves 4)

- 4 fresh ahi tuna steaks (approximately 4 to 5 ounces each)
- 3 tablespoons extra-virgin olive oil, divided
  Salt and pepper to taste
- 2 green onions, thinly sliced
- 2 tablespoons fresh lime juice
- 2 tablespoons low-sodium soy sauce (or gluten-free tamari sauce)
- 1 tablespoon unpasteurized wasabi paste
- 4–6 cups baby greens
- 2 small cucumbers, thinly sliced
- ½ pint grape tomatoes, halved
- 2–3 tablespoons rice vinegar

Brush tuna steaks with 1 tablespoon olive oil and sprinkle with salt and pepper. In a nonstick skillet over high heat, combine green onions, lime juice, soy sauce and wasabi. Add tuna steaks and sear for approximately 2 to 3 minutes; remove from heat when done. Remember to not over-cook the tuna (it's best served medium rare). Meanwhile, prepare the salad by tossing together baby greens, cucumbers, tomatoes, 2 table-spoons olive oil, and rice vinegar. Top salad with the tuna and serve.

Calories 364 | Protein 40 g | Fat 16 g | Carbohydrates 13 g | Fiber 6 g

Miso Salad (Serves 1)

4–5	cups baby spinach leaves
1	cucumber, chopped
1	tomato, chopped
½	avocado, sliced
2	tablespoons fresh lemon juice
1	tablespoon unpasteurized miso paste
1	clove garlic, minced
	Salt and pepper to taste
1	serving of protein from "allowed" list

In a large bowl, toss together spinach, cucumber, tomato, avocado, lemon juice, miso paste, garlic, and salt and pepper until the dressing coats the spinach. Top with chosen protein source and enjoy.

Calories 342 | Protein 34 g | Fat 15 g | Carbohydrates 25 g | Fiber 7 g

Grilled Mediterranean Salad (Serves 4)

1   small eggplant, cut into ¼-inch-thick rounds
     Salt
2   medium zucchini, cut into ¼-inch-thick rounds
1   fennel bulb, trimmed and cut into 8 wedges
1   red onion, cut into ¼-inch-thick slices (rings kept intact)
1   lemon, sliced
4   tablespoons goat feta, crumbled
8   Kalamata olives, pitted and halved
     Pepper to taste
4   servings of protein from "allowed" list

Cut out the excess seeds of the eggplant. Lay eggplant slices on a rack set over a baking sheet. Season with salt and let stand 15 minutes. Pat dry with paper towels. Place the eggplant, zucchini, fennel, onion and lemon slices on greased grill over medium-high heat, and cook in batches if necessary, turning often, until browned and tender. (The fennel will take 4 to 5 minutes per side; the eggplant, zucchini and onion 2 to 3 minutes per side; and the lemon 1 to 2 minutes per side.) Transfer the vegetables to a large, shallow serving dish. Toss gently with the dressing. Garnish the salad with feta, olives and a grinding of pepper. Top with chosen protein source and enjoy.

Dressing

2   plum tomatoes, seeded and coarsely chopped
3   tablespoons lemon juice
3   tablespoons reduced-sodium chicken broth
2   tablespoons extra-virgin olive oil
1   tablespoon oregano, fresh or dried
     Salt and pepper to taste

In a blender or food processor, combine tomatoes, lemon juice, broth, olive oil and oregano; blend or process until smooth. Season with salt and pepper.

Calories 300 | Protein 28 g | Fat 16 g | Carbohydrates 16 g | Fiber 4 g

Garlic Chicken and Asparagus (Serves 2)

2 boneless, skinless chicken breasts (approximately 4 to
      5 ounces each)
   Olive oil nonstick cooking spray
1 teaspoon garlic powder
1 teaspoon onion powder
   Salt and pepper to taste
2 tomatoes, sliced
1 tablespoon extra-virgin olive oil
1 ounce Cabot 75% reduced-fat Cheddar cheese or low-fat
      Jarlsberg cheese, sliced or grated
3 cups cooked chopped asparagus

Preheat oven to 375°F. Lightly grease a small casserole dish with cooking
spray. Sprinkle each chicken breast with garlic powder, onion powder,
and salt and pepper, and place in the baking dish. Lay tomato slices on
each chicken breast and drizzle with 1 tablespoon olive oil. Bake for 20
minutes. Top the chicken breasts with cheese and return to oven for
another 5 minutes or until cooked through. Serve with asparagus.

Calories 312 | Protein 33 g | Fat 13 g | Carbohydrates 23 g | Fiber 9 g

Feta Cheese Meatballs with Grilled Vegetables (Serves 4)

- 1 pound ground lamb or beef (organic, grass fed)
- 4 tablespoons goat feta cheese, crumbled
- ½ cup green or black olives, pitted and chopped
- ½ cup finely chopped fresh parsley
- 2 tablespoons finely chopped onion
- 2 whole eggs
- 1 teaspoon Italian seasoning
- 4–6 cups cooked vegetables (e.g., asparagus, zucchini and eggplant)

In a large bowl, gently combine lamb, feta, olives, parsley, onion, eggs and Italian seasoning with your hands. Form 20 meatballs (golf-ball sized) and place on a baking sheet. Put oven rack at the highest position and place the baking sheet in the oven on broil. When meatballs are brown, after approximately 3 to 6 minutes, flip them over and continue to broil the other side until cooked through. Serve with vegetables.

Calories 304 | Protein 31 g | Fat 12 g | Carbohydrates 15 g | Fiber 3 g

Apricot-glazed Chicken and Kale (Serves 2)

- 2 tablespoons apricot spread (no sugar added)
- 2 tablespoons low-sodium soy sauce
- 1 tablespoon apple cider vinegar
- 2 teaspoons Dijon mustard
- Stevia to taste
- Olive oil nonstick cooking spray
- 2 boneless, skinless chicken breasts (approximately 4 to 5 ounces each)
- 2 tablespoons chia seeds
- 1 tablespoon extra-virgin olive oil
- 2 cups chopped kale
- 2 cups chopped bok choy
- 1 Vidalia onion, thinly sliced
- Salt and pepper to taste

Preheat oven to 350°F. In a small bowl, combine apricot spread, soy sauce, apple cider vinegar, Dijon mustard and stevia. Lightly grease a baking dish with cooking spray and place chicken in the dish. Pour apricot sauce over chicken, top with chia seeds and bake for 45 to 60 minutes or until cooked through. Heat olive oil in a skillet over medium heat, and add kale, bok choy and onion. Season with salt and pepper, and sauté until kale is cooked.

Calories 306 | Protein 34 g | Fat 15 g | Carbohydrates 20 g | Fiber 8 g

Cucumber and Cottage Cheese Salad (Serves 1)

- 1 large cucumber, diced
- 2 small tomatoes, seeded and diced
- 1 tablespoon garlic powder
- 1 tablespoon dried dill weed
- ¾ cup Western 0.1% pressed cottage cheese
  Salt and pepper to taste
- 1 tablespoon pine nuts or slivered almonds

In a bowl, toss the cucumber, tomatoes, garlic powder and dill. Add cottage cheese and salt and pepper, and stir together lightly. Sprinkle with nuts.

Calories 327 | Protein 28 g | Fat 15 g | Carbohydrates 28 g | Fiber 7 g

Sautéed Shrimp and Green Beans (Serves 2)

- 1½ tablespoons extra-virgin olive oil or macadamia nut oil
- 1 pound fresh green beans
- 1 large Vidalia onion, thinly sliced
- 8 ounces cooked baby shrimp
  Salt and pepper to taste

In a large skillet or wok, heat olive oil over medium heat. Sauté green beans until they start to brown, 4 to 6 minutes. Add onion and sauté until softened and golden. Add shrimp and cook until heated through. Season with salt and pepper.

Calories 341 | Protein 32 g | Fat 12 g | Carbohydrates 32 g | Fiber 11 g

Immunity-boosting Ginger Chicken (Serves 2)

2   boneless, skinless chicken breasts (approximately 4 to
      5 ounces each)
     Salt and pepper to taste
1   tablespoon sesame oil
1   teaspoon peeled and grated fresh gingerroot
1   large cucumber, thinly sliced
2   medium-sized tomatoes, chopped
1   bunch watercress, chopped
½   small onion, diced
2   tablespoons fresh lemon juice
1   tablespoon extra-virgin olive oil

Place chicken in a small pot with enough water to cover; add salt and pepper. Bring to a simmer over medium heat and poach until cooked through, approximately 15 minutes. Drain and set chicken aside.

In a small bowl, combine sesame oil and ginger. Pour over the chicken. In a separate, larger bowl, toss together cucumber, tomatoes, watercress, onion, lemon juice, olive oil, and salt and pepper. Divide the salad between two plates and top each with a chicken breast.

Calories 336 | Protein 27 g | Fat 17 g | Carbohydrates 24 g | Fiber 5 g

Baby Bok Choy and Chicken (Serves 2)

- 2 tablespoons sesame oil
- 2 cups sliced yellow bell pepper
- 2 cups chopped broccoli
- 4 green onions, chopped
- 1 pound baby bok choy, chopped
- 1 tablespoon sesame seeds
- 2 boneless, skinless chicken breasts (approximately 4 to 5 ounces each), cooked and sliced, or 2 servings of protein from the "allowed" list

In a nonstick skillet, heat oil over medium-high heat. Add bell peppers, broccoli and green onions, and cook, stirring occasionally, until lightly browned. Lower the heat and add bok choy. Stir well. Cook only until the bok choy has wilted and the thicker, white ends are still somewhat crisp. Add sesame seeds and stir. Divide between two plates and top each with chicken or chosen protein source.

Calories 328 | Protein 30 g | Fat 14 g | Carbohydrates 28 g | Fiber 7 g

Selenium-boosting Shrimp and Salsa (Serves 1)

Salsa

½	cup diced Granny Smith apple (unpeeled)
¼	cup diced red onion
¼	cup diced red bell pepper
2	tablespoons chopped fresh cilantro
2	tablespoons red wine vinegar
2	tablespoons apple cider vinegar
	Pinch chipotle powder

In a glass bowl, combine all ingredients thoroughly and refrigerate for at least 1 hour.

Shrimp

4	tablespoons mild paprika
2	tablespoons pepper
½	teaspoon salt
1	tablespoon chili powder
12	small shrimp
1	tablespoon extra-virgin olive oil

In a small bowl, combine paprika, pepper, salt and chili powder. Add shrimp and toss with the spice mixture. In a nonstick pan, heat olive oil over medium heat and add the shrimp. Cook for approximately 1 minute on each side or until the shrimp are cooked through. Serve with the salsa.

Calories 362 | Protein 25 g | Fat 15 g | Carbohydrates 35 g | Fiber 8 g

Curry Chicken Soup (Serves 2)

1   tablespoon coconut oil
1   clove garlic, minced
1   teaspoon peeled and grated fresh gingerroot
1   teaspoon chili powder
2   tablespoons curry powder
1   bay leaf
2   cups low-sodium chicken broth
2   boneless, skinless chicken breasts (approximately 4 to
       5 ounces each), diced
       Salt to taste
2   tablespoons Fage Total 0% yogurt, plain

In a medium saucepan, heat coconut oil over high heat. Sauté garlic, ginger, chili powder, curry powder and bay leaf until fragrant. Add chicken broth and bring to a boil. Add chicken, reduce the heat to a simmer, and cook until chicken is cooked through, approximately 8 to 15 minutes. Remove from the heat and season with salt. Just before serving (either hot or cold), top each bowl of soup with 1 tablespoon of yogurt.

Vegetables

1   tablespoon extra-virgin olive oil
2   cups chopped broccoli
2   cups chopped cauliflower
1   cup chopped red bell pepper
1   clove garlic, minced
       Salt and pepper to taste
1   tablespoon slivered almonds or pine nuts

In a nonstick skillet, heat olive oil over medium-high heat. Add vegetables and sauté until tender. Top with almonds and serve with the soup.

Calories 357 | Protein 32 g | Fat 16 g | Carbohydrates 19 g | Fiber 5 g

Perfect Peppercorn Fish (Serves 4)

- 2 tablespoons extra-virgin olive oil
- 3 zucchini, thinly sliced
- 2 large tomatoes, diced
- 1 Vidalia onion, sliced
- 2 tablespoons low-sodium soy sauce
- 1½ tablespoons rice vinegar
- 1 tablespoon sesame oil
- 1 clove garlic, minced
- 4 fillets whitefish (cod, halibut or tilapia, 4 to 5 ounces each)
- 1 teaspoon black peppercorns, crushed
- Salt and pepper to taste
- 4 mandarin oranges

In a nonstick wok or skillet , heat olive oil over medium-high heat. Sauté zucchini, tomatoes and onion until softened. In a separate bowl, combine soy sauce, rice vinegar, sesame oil and garlic.

Heat an ovenproof skillet over medium heat and cook fish with approximately half of the sauce. After 3 to 4 minutes, flip the fish and add the remaining sauce. Put oven rack at the highest position. Just before the fish is completely cooked, approximately 4 to 7 minutes, top with crushed peppercorns and transfer to the oven. Broil for 3 to 4 minutes or until slightly crispy. Season with salt and pepper. Serve fish with vegetables and mandarin oranges.

Calories 302 | Protein 28 g | Fat 14 g | Carbohydrates 19 g | Fiber 3 g

Crispy Chicken and Lettuce Wraps (Serves 1)

- 1 small green apple, diced (unpeeled)
- ¼ cup diced red bell pepper
- ¼ cup diced cucumber
- 1 tablespoon finely chopped red onion
- 1 boneless, skinless chicken breast (approximately 4 to 5 ounces each), cooked and diced
- ¼ cup Fage Total Classic yogurt, plain
- 2 teaspoons extra-virgin olive oil
  Salt and pepper to taste
- 1 small head of lettuce (4–5 leaves)

In a bowl, combine all ingredients except for the lettuce, and chill for 1 hour.

Place the chicken mixture inside each lettuce leaf, roll into cylinders and serve.

Calories 325 | Protein 34 g | Fat 13 g | Carbohydrates 26 g | Fiber 5 g

Wasabi Whitefish with Almond Crust (Serves 2)

- 2   fillets of whitefish (halibut, tilapia, bass or sole, 4 to 5 ounces each)
- 1   tablespoon salt, divided
- 1   tablespoon white pepper, divided
- ½   cup almond flour
- 2   tablespoons wasabi powder
- 1   tablespoon chopped fresh gingerroot
- 2   egg whites

  Olive oil nonstick cooking spray

Rinse fish in cold water then pat dry with a paper towel. Sprinkle ½ tablespoon each of the salt and white pepper evenly on both sides of the fish. Refrigerate for 30 to 60 minutes. In a small bowl, combine almond flour, wasabi powder, ginger, and ½ tablespoon each of the salt and white pepper; pour onto a plate. In a separate bowl, beat egg whites. Dip the fillets into the egg whites, coating entire surface, then into the almond flour mixture, coating the fish entirely.

Lightly grease a small skillet with cooking spray, and cook fillets over medium heat for approximately 3 to 4 minutes, depending on thickness, flipping halfway through the cooking. Serve with sautéed vegetables or a large salad.

Calories 369 | Protein 36 g | Fat 18 g | Carbohydrates 19 g | Fiber 6 g

Salmon with Spinach and Strawberry Salsa (Serves 2)

  2   salmon fillets, skin removed (approximately 4 to 5 ounces
        each)
  ½   lemon, sliced
  1   tablespoon extra-virgin olive oil, divided
  1   cup fresh strawberries, diced
  1   kiwi, peeled and diced
  1   cucumber, diced
        Juice from ½ fresh lemon
  2   cloves garlic, minced
  4   cups baby spinach leaves, rinsed but not dried

Preheat oven to 350°F. Place salmon fillets on a baking sheet and top
each with one slice of lemon and 1 teaspoon olive oil. Bake for 15 to 18
minutes or until cooked through.

In a separate bowl, add strawberries, kiwi, cucumber and lemon
juice; toss to combine. In a large skillet, heat 1 teaspoon olive oil over
medium heat and sauté garlic for 3 minutes. Add spinach and stir for
30 seconds to wilt. Remove from pan and top with salmon and fruit
salsa. Serve with lemon slices.

Calories 275 | Protein 25 g | Fat 12 g | Carbohydrates 23 g | Fiber 8 g

Cauliflower and Kale Soup (Serves 2)

1	tablespoon extra-virgin olive oil
½	cup diced Vidalia onion
1	tablespoon minced garlic
1	head cauliflower, cored and chopped
3	cups vegetable stock
1	cup kale, thinly sliced
1	teaspoon chopped fresh tarragon
1	teaspoon salt
1	teaspoon pepper
2	servings of protein from "allowed" list

In a large saucepan, heat olive oil over medium-high heat. Sauté onion and garlic until the onions are translucent. Add the cauliflower and vegetable stock. Bring to a boil. Reduce the heat to low and simmer until the cauliflower softens, approximately 15 to 20 minutes. Add kale and simmer for another 5 minutes. Let mixture cool completely, then transfer to a blender and purée until smooth. Return the soup to the saucepan and bring to a simmer. Add tarragon, salt and pepper. Remove from heat and serve with chosen protein source.

Calories 356 | Protein 40 g | Fat 12 g | Carbohydrates 29 g | Fiber 10 g

Tuna Waldorf Salad (Serves 1)

- 1   medium apple, chopped
- 1   tablespoon fresh lemon juice
- 1   can tuna packed in water, drained
- 1   cup chopped celery
- 1   cup diced cucumbers
- 1   tablespoon chia seeds
- 1   tablespoon olive oil mayonnaise
     Salt and pepper to taste
- 2–3   cups mixed greens

In a bowl, toss apple with lemon juice. Add tuna, celery, cucumbers and chia seeds and toss to combine. Add mayonnaise and stir well. Season with salt and pepper. Refrigerate for 1 hour and serve over mixed greens.

Calories 364 | Protein 33 g | Fat 12 g | Carbohydrates 31 g | Fiber 4 g

Spicy Pepper Salmon with Pear Salsa (Serves 2)

2   fresh salmon or trout fillets (approximately 4 to 5 ounces each)
    Juice of 1 lemon
2   small pears, diced
1   red bell pepper, chopped
½   medium red onion, finely chopped
¼   cup chopped fresh cilantro
2   tablespoons fresh lime juice
1   tablespoon extra-virgin olive oil
    Salt and pepper to taste
½   teaspoon chipotle powder

Preheat oven to 400°F. Line a baking sheet with a large sheet of aluminum foil. Place fish on the aluminum foil. Sprinkle lemon juice over the fish and set aside. In a medium bowl, combine pears, bell pepper, red onion, cilantro, lime juice and olive oil; season with salt and pepper. Rub the fish with salt, pepper and chipotle powder. Bake the fish for 15 to 20 minutes, or until the fish flakes easily with a fork. Top the fish with the pear salsa and serve.

Calories 322 | Protein 25 g | Fat 12 g | Carbohydrates 31 g | Fiber 7 g

PHASE TWO RECIPES

Scrumptious Edamame Salad (Serves 4)

2–3 cups of shelled edamame, defrosted
1 cucumber, diced
1 cup celery, diced
3–4 green onions, thinly sliced
3 large radishes, thinly sliced
1 cup loosely packed chopped fresh cilantro leaves
4 chicken, turkey or fish fillets, cooked (approximately 4 to 5 ounces each)

In a large bowl, combine edamame, cucumber, celery, green onions, radishes and cilantro. Pour dressing over edamame mixture, and toss to coat. Cover and chill for 30 minutes before serving. Serve ½ cup of edamame salad per person along with chosen protein source. Accompany with steamed or stir-fried mixed vegetables.

Dressing

¼ cup rice wine vinegar
Juice of 1 lemon
1 tablespoon extra-virgin olive oil
⅛ teaspoon pepper
¼ teaspoon salt

In a small bowl, whisk together ingredients.

Calories 331 | Protein 34 g | Fat 16 g | Carbohydrates 14 g | Fiber 5 g

Chilled Dill and Beet Salad (Serves 4)

- 4 medium beets, peeled and thinly sliced
- 1 red onion, halved and thinly sliced
- ⅓ cup fresh lemon juice
- 4 tablespoons extra-virgin olive oil
- 1 small bunch fresh dill, stemmed and minced
- ½ teaspoon salt
- ¼ teaspoon pepper
- Lemon slices
- 4 servings of protein from "allowed" list

Steam the beets until tender, and let cool. In a large bowl, combine the beets with onion and carefully toss. In a separate bowl, whisk together lemon juice, olive oil, dill, salt and pepper. Pour over vegetables and gently stir to coat. Adjust seasonings. Set aside to marinate for 1 to 2 hours. Serve chilled or at room temperature, garnished with lemon slices. Top with chosen protein source and enjoy.

Calories 314 | Protein 25 g | Fat 18 g | Carbohydrates 17 g | Fiber 4 g

Carrot and Ginger Soup (Serves 2)

- 1 tablespoon extra-virgin olive oil
- ½ cup diced onion
- 1 tablespoon peeled and grated gingerroot
- 1 cup peeled and chopped carrots
- 3 cups vegetable stock
- ¼ teaspoon dried thyme
- ¼ teaspoon minced garlic
- ¼ teaspoon pepper
- 2 boneless, skinless chicken breasts (approximately 4 to 5 ounces each), grilled or baked

In a large saucepan, heat olive oil over low heat. Sauté onions until they are translucent. Add ginger, and continue to cook until the onions start to turn golden brown, 10 minutes. Add carrots, stock, thyme, garlic and pepper. Cover and simmer until the carrots are soft, 10 minutes. Let mixture cool, then transfer to a blender and purée until smooth. Serve with the grilled or baked chicken and a side of mixed vegetables.

Calories 340 | Protein 36 g | Fat 11 g | Carbohydrates 22 g | Fiber 6 g

Summer Squash and Sesame Chicken (Serves 4)

- 4 cups chopped summer squash
  Salt and pepper to taste
- 1 tablespoon extra-virgin olive oil
- 4 boneless, skinless chicken breasts (approximately 4 to
  5 ounces each), chopped
- 2 tablespoons white sesame seeds
- 1 tablespoon black sesame seeds
- 1 tablespoon salt
- 2 tablespoons sesame oil

Preheat oven to 450°F. Season squash with salt, pepper and a touch of olive oil. Place in a baking dish lightly greased with olive oil. Bake for 15 minutes, until browned.

While the squash is cooking, prepare the chicken. In a bowl, combine white and black sesame seeds and salt and sprinkle over chicken. In a large skillet, heat sesame oil over medium heat, and sauté chicken until golden brown and cooked through, 5 to 6 minutes. Serve chicken with summer squash and a side of mixed green salad or vegetables.

Calories 294 | Protein 27 g | Fat 12 g | Carbohydrates 22 g | Fiber 7 g

Warm Beet and Goat Cheese Salad (Serves 1)

- 3 medium-sized beets, unpeeled
- 2 cups mixed greens
- ¼ teaspoon basil
- ½ teaspoon chopped fresh cilantro
- 1 ounce Cabot 75% reduced-fat Cheddar cheese or low-fat Jarlsberg cheese, diced
- 2 ounces goat cheese, crumbled
  Salt and pepper to taste

Preheat oven to 425°F. Wrap beets in a double sheet of aluminum foil and bake for 45 to 50 minutes, or until tender. Peel beets and cut into small cubes. In a bowl, toss together mixed greens, basil, cilantro, beets, and the dressing. Top with cheeses, salt, and pepper.

Dressing

- 4 tablespoons white wine vinegar or fresh lemon juice
- 1 tablespoon Dijon mustard

In a small bowl, whisk together vinegar and mustard.

Calories 338 | Protein 25 g | Fat 16 g | Carbohydrates 28 g | Fiber 9 g

Curried Pumpkin and Green Beans (Serves 2)

1½   tablespoons extra-virgin olive oil

1   medium onion, sliced

1   clove garlic, minced

1   tablespoon curry powder
     Salt and pepper to taste

1   medium pumpkin, peeled, seeded and cut into 1-inch cubes

1½   cups low-sodium chicken broth

1   cup green beans
     Fresh cilantro

2   servings of protein from "allowed" list

In a large nonstick skillet, heat olive oil over medium-high heat. Sauté onion until golden, about 5 minutes. Add garlic and sauté 1 minute more. Stir in curry powder, salt and pepper. Add pumpkin and cook for 5 minutes, stirring frequently. Pour in broth, cover and reduce heat to medium. After 15 minutes, add green beans. Replace the cover and continue to cook until the pumpkin is tender, 5 to 10 minutes more. Garnish with cilantro. Divide between two plates and serve with your choice of protein.

Calories 337 | Protein 30 g | Fat 14 g | Carbohydrates 25 g | Fiber 9 g

Summerlicious Squash with Yogurt Chicken (Serves 2)

½   cup Fage Total 0% yogurt, plain
2   teaspoons ground cumin
1   teaspoon fresh lime juice
    Salt and pepper to taste
2   boneless, skinless chicken breasts (approximately 4 to
      5 ounces each), cooked
1   zucchini, diced
1   yellow summer squash, diced
2   onions, chopped
¼   cup chopped fresh cilantro
2   tablespoons balsamic vinegar
1   tablespoon extra-virgin olive oil

In a medium bowl, combine yogurt, cumin, lime juice and salt. Add cooked chicken and coat entirely with the yogurt mixture; marinate for 15 minutes at room temperature. Transfer the chicken to a plate; sprinkle with additional salt and pepper if desired. Place the chicken breasts on a hot grill and cook for 7 to 8 minutes on each side. In a large bowl, toss together zucchini, squash, onions, cilantro, balsamic vinegar and olive oil. Divide between two plates. Top with cooked chicken.

Calories 334 | Protein 35 g | Fat 11 g | Carbohydrates 27 g | Fiber 5 g

PHASE THREE RECIPES

Curried Red Lentils with Shrimp or Tofu (Serves 4)

- 2 cups red lentils
- 2 tablespoons extra-virgin olive oil
- 1 large Vidalia onion, diced
- 1 clove garlic, minced
- 2 tablespoons curry paste
- 1 tablespoon curry powder, mild or hot
- 1 teaspoon ground turmeric
- 1 teaspoon ground cumin
- 1 teaspoon chili powder
- 1 teaspoon salt
- ½ teaspoon pepper
- 1 can (14.25 ounces) tomato purée
- 1 package (14 ounces) firm tofu or 36 cooked baby shrimp

Rinse the lentils well in cold water. Place the lentils in a saucepan, cover with water (1–2 cups) and simmer, covered, until lentils are tender, approximately 30 minutes. If needed, add more water. Drain lentils and set aside.

Meanwhile, in a large skillet, heat olive oil over medium heat. Sauté onion and garlic until softened. In a small bowl, combine curry paste, curry powder, turmeric, cumin, chili powder, salt and pepper. Add the curry mixture to the onions, and continue cooking over high heat for 1 to 2 minutes. Add the tomato purée and reduce the heat. Stir in tofu or baby shrimp and the lentils, and simmer for approximately 5 minutes. When lentils are heated through, divide between four dishes and serve.

Calories 338 | Protein 24 g | Fat 14 g | Carbohydrates 29 g | Fiber 3 g

Lovely Lemongrass Tofu (Serves 3)

- ¼ cup low-sodium tamari soy sauce
- ¼ cup low-sodium vegetable stock
- ½ cup chopped green onions
- ¼ cup finely chopped lemongrass
- 2 tablespoons minced garlic
- 1 tablespoon sesame oil
- 10 ounces firm organic tofu, sliced
- 1½ cup cooked lentils
- 1 tablespoon finely chopped fresh parsley

In a deep baking dish, combine tamari, stock, green onions, lemongrass, garlic and sesame oil. Marinate the tofu slices in the tamari mixture for 2 hours, turning after 1 hour. Remove the marinated tofu and place on a grill or nonstick pan over high heat for 1 minute on each side. Serve with ½ cup of lentils per person, topped with parsley and any desired spices.

Calories 343 | Protein 29 g | Fat 15 g | Carbohydrates 21 g | Fiber 5 g

Halibut and Rapini in Portobello Mushroom Sauce (Serves 4)

- 4 fillets of halibut or whitefish (approximately 4 to 5 ounces each)
- 1 cup portobello mushroom caps, diced
- 1 cup broccoli, chopped
- ¾ cup water
- 2 tablespoons extra-virgin olive oil, divided
- 1 tablespoon low-sodium tamari soy sauce
- 2 cloves garlic, minced
- 1 bunch rapini, chopped coarsely
- Garlic salt to taste
- ½ fresh lemon
- 2 cups canned black beans, rinsed, drained and warmed

Place the fillets in a shallow dish. In a separate bowl, combine mushrooms, broccoli, water, 1 tablespoon olive oil, tamari and garlic. Pour over the fish and place in the fridge for 1 to 3 hours, turning the fillets and spooning the sauce over them occasionally. Set the oven on broil. Remove the fish and vegetables from the dish and place on a broiling pan. Broil approximately 4 minutes on each side.

Meanwhile, in a nonstick skillet, heat 1 tablespoon of olive oil over medium heat. Sauté rapini and garlic salt approximately 3 to 4 minutes.

Remove the fish from the oven when it flakes easily with a fork and squeeze fresh lemon juice over the fillets. Serve fish fillet over ½ cup of warmed black beans.

Calories 351 | Protein 40 g | Fat 12 g | Carbohydrates 26 g | Fiber 7 g

Summer Tomato Lentils (Serves 4)

3	cups cherry tomatoes
1	tablespoon extra-virgin olive oil, divided
1	teaspoon minced garlic
2	cups lentils
1½	cups water
3–4	tablespoons goat cheese
	Zest and juice of 1 lemon
2	large shallots, thinly sliced
1	tablespoon Dijon mustard
	Pepper to taste
⅓	cup chopped basil
⅓	cup finely chopped chives
	Salt to taste
4	butter lettuce leaves
4	servings of protein from "allowed" list

Preheat oven to 325°F. Cut the tomatoes in half and toss with ½ table-spoon olive oil and garlic. Place the tomatoes, cut side up, on a baking pan and roast for 30 minutes.

Rinse and drain lentils. In a medium saucepan, bring the water to a boil. Add the lentils, reduce the heat and simmer for about 20 minutes, adding more water if necessary. When the lentils are tender, drain and place in a large bowl. Crumble in goat cheese, add lemon zest and juice, and toss to combine.

While the lentils are cooling, prepare the shallots. In a small sauce-pan, heat ½ tablespoon olive oil over medium heat. Add the sliced shal-lots and sauté for about 15 minutes, until they are golden brown. Gently fold the shallots, Dijon mustard, pepper, basil, chives and roasted toma-toes into the lentil mixture. Season with salt. Serve in a butter lettuce leaf and top with desired protein source.

Calories 346 | Protein 36 g | Fat 12 g | Carbohydrates 24 g | Fiber 3 g

Beautiful Bean and Protein Salad (Serves 2)

Vinaigrette

4	tablespoons wine vinegar
1	tablespoon extra-virgin olive oil
1	clove garlic, minced
1	teaspoon dried oregano
¼	teaspoon salt
¼	teaspoon pepper

In a large bowl, whisk together vinegar, olive oil, garlic, oregano, salt and pepper, and set aside.

Salad

2	cups chopped green beans
1	red bell pepper, seeded and finely chopped
½	cup canned chickpeas, drained and rinsed
½	cup canned kidney beans, drained and rinsed
¼	cup chopped fresh parsley or cilantro
1	tablespoon minced jalapeño pepper
2	servings of protein from "allowed" list

In a saucepan of boiling water, add green beans, cover and cook until crisp-tender, approximately 5 minutes. Drain and add to the vinaigrette. Add bell pepper, chickpeas, kidney beans, parsley and jalapeño and toss to coat. Refrigerate for 30 minutes. Divide between two plates and top with chosen protein source.

Calories 371 | Protein 35 g | Fat 11 g | Carbohydrates 33 g | Fiber 10 g

Fresh Mint Chickpea Salad (Serves 4)

- 2 cups canned chickpeas, drained and rinsed
- 2 stalks celery, diced
- 1 green bell pepper, seeded and diced
- 1 red bell pepper, seeded and diced
- 4–6 green onions, diced
- 4 servings of protein from "allowed" list

In a medium-sized bowl, add chickpeas, celery, bell peppers and green onions. Pour dressing over chickpea salad and stir gently. Serve with chosen protein source and enjoy.

Dressing

- 3 tablespoons red wine vinegar
  Juice from ½ fresh lemon
- 2 tablespoons extra-virgin olive oil
- 1 tablespoon finely chopped fresh parsley
- 1 teaspoon finely chopped fresh mint
- 1 teaspoon ground cumin (optional)
  Salt and pepper to taste

In a small bowl, whisk together vinegar, lemon juice, olive oil, parsley, mint, cumin and salt and pepper.

Calories 357 | Protein 31 g | Fat 13 g | Carbohydrates 32 g | Fiber 9 g

Bison Chili and Beans (Serves 5)

1½	pounds ground bison or organic lean ground beef
1	red bell pepper, seeded and diced
1	onion, diced
2	cloves garlic, minced
1	tablespoon chili powder
1	teaspoon ground turmeric
1	teaspoon dried oregano
2	cans (15 ounces) black beans, drained and rinsed
2	cans (15 ounces) diced tomatoes
1	can (14 ounces) low-sodium beef broth
1	teaspoon pepper
¼	teaspoon salt

In a large saucepan, cook the ground bison, bell pepper, onion and garlic until no longer pink, 5 to 6 minutes. Add chili powder, turmeric, oregano, beans, tomatoes, broth, salt and pepper. Increase heat and bring to a boil. Reduce heat and simmer for 20 minutes, or until chili achieves desired thickness.

Calories 353 | Protein 37 g | Fat 10 g | Carbohydrates 32 g | Fiber 7 g

Spicy Lentil Burgers (Serves 3)

- 3 cups cooked black lentils
- 4 large eggs
- ½ cup grated carrots
- ½ teaspoon salt
- 1 onion, finely chopped
- 1 teaspoon ground turmeric
- 5 tablespoons ground flaxseed
- 1 tablespoon extra-virgin olive oil
- Salt and pepper to taste
- 3–4 cups mixed greens

In a large bowl, combine lentils, eggs, carrots and salt, and mix for 1 minute. Stir in onion and turmeric. Add flaxseed, stir, and let sit for a couple of minutes so that the flaxseed absorbs some of the moisture. In a heavy skillet, heat oil over medium-low heat. Form 6 small patties, place in the skillet, cover, and cook for 7 to 10 minutes, until the bottoms begin to brown. Flip the patties and cook the second side for 7 minutes, or until golden. Serve with a large mixed green salad or vegetables on the side.

Calories 332 | Protein 27 g | Fat 12 g | Carbohydrates 33 g | Fiber 4 g

PHASE FOUR RECIPES

Breakfast Cereal Smoothie (Serves 1)

1	serving whey protein isolate (vanilla)
¾	cup Kashi GoLean cereal or Fiber One
1	tablespoon almond butter
½	teaspoon vanilla extract
½–¾	cup water
3–4	ice cubes

Place all ingredients in a blender and blend on high speed until smooth and creamy.

Calories 336 | Protein 32 g | Fat 12 g | Carbohydrates 32 g | Fiber 7 g

Quinoa Salad with Orange, Walnuts and Mint (Serves 4)

2	cups water
1½	cups quinoa
¼	cup chopped walnuts
1	handful fresh mint leaves, chopped
2	oranges, peeled and chopped
	Juice of 1 lime
2	tablespoons extra-virgin olive oil
	Salt and pepper to taste
4	servings of protein from "allowed" list

In a medium saucepan, bring water to a boil. Place the quinoa in a sieve and rinse under running water until water runs clear. Add quinoa to boiling water, bring back to a boil and cover. Simmer for 12 minutes, or until the quinoa has absorbed the water. Remove from the heat, fluff with a fork, cover and let stand for 10 minutes. Toast walnuts in a non-stick skillet until lightly golden, or use raw if preferred. Add the walnuts, mint, oranges, lime juice and olive oil to the quinoa and stir. Season with salt and pepper, and top with your choice of protein.

Calories 352 | Protein 28 g | Fat 16 g | Carbohydrates 26 g | Fiber 4 g

Turkey Bacon Scallops (Serves 2)

- 3 slices turkey bacon
- 6 large scallops
- 1 tablespoon extra-virgin olive oil
  Salt and pepper to taste
- 1 teaspoon finely chopped fresh parsley
- 1 cup cooked kasha or chickpeas

Preheat oven to 425°F. Cut turkey bacon in half lengthwise. Pat scallops dry with paper towel. Wrap a piece of bacon around each scallop and secure with a toothpick; place on a baking sheet. Drizzle olive oil over the scallops. Season with salt and pepper, sprinkle with parsley and place in the oven. Bake for approximately 12 to 15 minutes, turning once and draining excess fluid if necessary. The bacon should be browned and crispy, but be careful not to overcook the scallops: They should be just firm and opaque when done. Serve 3 scallops with ½ cup cooked kasha or chickpeas for each serving (or with Fresh Mint Chickpea Salad, page 397).

Calories 385 | Protein 32 g | Fat 11 g | Carbohydrates 25 g | Fiber 4 g

Quick Cinnamon Quinoa (Serves 2)

- ½ cup organic quinoa
- 1 cup water
- 1 cup fresh berries
- 2 tablespoons chopped pecans, toasted
- ¼ cup almond milk, unsweetened
- ½ teaspoon ground cinnamon
- 1½ cups pressed cottage cheese

Place quinoa in a sieve and rinse under running water until water runs clear. Combine the quinoa and 1 cup water in a medium saucepan. Bring to a boil over high heat. Reduce heat to medium-low, cover and simmer for 10 minutes, or until most of the liquid is absorbed. Turn off heat; let stand, covered, for 5 minutes. Top with berries, pecans, almond milk and cinnamon. Serve with cottage cheese.

Calories 321 | Protein 24 g | Fat 13 g | Carbohydrates 23 g | Fiber 5 g

Cherry Tomato Salmon in Wine Broth (Serves 4)

¼ cup quinoa, cooked

¾ cup low-sodium chicken broth

2 tablespoons dry white wine (sauvignon blanc), or rice wine vinegar

4 salmon fillets (approximately 4 to 5 ounces each)

12 cherry tomatoes, halved

½ teaspoon dried parsley or basil

In a medium saucepan, bring water to a boil. Place quinoa in a sieve and rinse under running water until water runs clear. Add quinoa to ¼ cup boiling water, bring back to boil and cover. Simmer for 12 minutes, or until the quinoa has absorbed the water. Remove from heat, fluff with a fork, cover and let stand for 10 minutes. Set aside.

In a skillet, heat chicken broth over medium-high heat. Add wine and bring to a boil. Place salmon in the pan. Reduce the heat to a simmer, cover and cook for 10 minutes, or until the fish flakes easily with a fork. Remove the salmon from the pan and place on a serving dish. Increase the heat to high and bring the broth mixture to a boil. Add tomatoes and cook for 2 minutes. Pour the tomatoes and sauce over the salmon, and top with parsley or basil. Serve with quinoa.

Calories 333 | Protein 36 g | Fat 9 g | Carbohydrates 32 g | Fiber 6 g

Apple, Arugula and Chicken Salad (Serves 4)

- 2 tablespoons extra-virgin olive oil, divided
- 1 large shallot, sliced
- 4 boneless, skinless chicken breasts (approximately 4 to 5 ounces each), cubed
  Salt and pepper to taste
- 4–6 cups arugula leaves
- 1 green apple, thinly sliced (unpeeled)
- 2 tablespoons chopped walnuts, toasted
- 1 tablespoon goat cheese, crumbled
  Fresh lemon juice to taste
- 1½ cups cooked quinoa or other grain

In a nonstick skillet, heat 1 tablespoon olive oil over medium heat. Sauté shallot for 3 to 5 minutes; remove from pan. Add 1 tablespoon olive oil and cook chicken, stirring occasionally, until just cooked through, approximately 5 minutes. Season with salt and pepper. Remove the chicken from the pan and set aside.

In a large serving bowl, toss together the shallots, chicken, arugula, apple, walnuts and goat cheese. Drizzle with lemon juice. Serve with quinoa.

Calories 377 | Protein 32 g | Fat 16 g | Carbohydrates 24 g | Fiber 4 g

Ezekiel Crumb-coated Chicken (Serves 2)

- 2 slices Ezekiel bread
- 1 tablespoon salt-free herb mixture
- 1 teaspoon salt
- 2 boneless, skinless chicken breasts (approximately 4 to 5 ounces each)
  Nonstick cooking spray
- 2 cups mixed vegetables, steamed or stir-fried
- 1 tablespoon extra-virgin olive oil

Preheat oven to 350°F. Toast bread until dry and flaky. In a bowl or food processor, break the toast into small pieces or crumbs. Add herb mixture and salt. Press the bread crumb mixture onto each chicken breast and place on a baking sheet lightly greased with cooking spray. Bake for 30 to 40 minutes, or until cooked through. Serve with vegetables, drizzled with olive oil.

Calories 372 | Protein 33 g | Fat 11 g | Carbohydrates 30 g | Fiber 6 g

Chicken with Bulgur and Mushrooms (Serves 2)

- ½ cup bulgur
- 2 cups sliced mushrooms
- 2 green onions, finely chopped
- ½ cup finely chopped fresh parsley
- 2 tablespoons slivered almonds
- 2 boneless, skinless chicken or turkey breasts (approximately
     4 to 5 ounces each), grilled or baked

In a saucepan, combine bulgur, mushrooms, onions, parsley and enough water to cover (approximately 2–3 cups). Bring to a boil. Reduce heat and simmer, covered, for 15 minutes or until the liquid is absorbed and the bulgur is cooked. Stir in almonds and serve with chicken.

Calories 352 | Protein 33 g | Fat 11 g | Carbohydrates 30 g | Fiber 8 g

Grilled Chicken Skewer Wraps (Serves 4)

- ⅓ cup fresh lemon juice
- 2 teaspoons fresh lemon zest
- 2 teaspoons dried oregano
- 2 teaspoons dried basil
- 2 teaspoons dried rosemary
- 1 teaspoon Dijon mustard
- 1 clove garlic, minced
- 2 tablespoons extra-virgin olive oil
- 4 boneless, skinless chicken or turkey breasts (approximately 4 to 5 ounces each), cubed
  Mixed vegetables for grilling (e.g., sliced red, yellow and green bell peppers—six bell peppers in total)
- 1–2 cups lettuce or mixed greens
- 4 Ezekiel wraps
  Salt and pepper to taste

In a large resealable plastic bag, add lemon juice and zest, oregano, basil, rosemary, mustard, garlic and olive oil. Seal the bag and shake to combine. Add chicken, seal the bag and shake thoroughly. Let chicken marinate for approximately 20 minutes. Thread chicken onto skewers, alternating with vegetables.

Place the chicken and vegetable skewers on a grill over high heat and cook for about 5 minutes per side, or until cooked through. Remove from the grill. Place lettuce on each Ezekiel wrap. Remove chicken and vegetables from skewers and distribute among the wraps. Roll up the wraps and use a toothpick to secure if necessary.

Calories 369 | Protein 29 g | Fat 14 g | Carbohydrates 31 g | Fiber 7 g

PHASE FIVE RECIPES

Berries and Oats Breakfast Smoothie (Serves 1)

- 1   serving whey protein isolate (vanilla)
- 1   cup unsweetened almond milk
- ½   cup water
- ¼   cup steel-cut oats or oat bran (measured dry)
- ¼   cup fresh or frozen mixed berries
- 1   tablespoon chia seeds
- 2–3   ice cubes

Place all ingredients in a blender and blend on high speed until smooth and creamy. Add extra water if desired.

Calories 295 | Protein 30 g | Fat 10 g | Carbohydrates 27 g | Fiber 9 g

Choco-Berry Breakfast (Serves 1)

- ½ cup liquid egg whites
- ¼ cup steel-cut oats or oat bran (measured dry)
- ¼ cup water
- ½ scoop (15 grams) whey protein isolate (chocolate)
- 2 tablespoons unsweetened cocoa powder
- 1 tablespoon slivered almonds
  Stevia to taste (optional)
- ½ cup fresh or frozen berries

In a saucepan, combine egg whites, oats, water, whey protein isolate, cocoa, almonds and stevia. Cook over medium heat, stirring occasionally, until oatmeal thickens, approximately 3 to 4 minutes. Add the berries, stir and serve immediately.

Calories 340 | Protein 33 g | Fat 11 g | Carbohydrates 32 g | Fiber 8 g

Banana Bread Smoothie (Serves 1)

- 1 serving whey protein isolate (vanilla)
- ½–¾ cup water
- ½ fresh or frozen banana, chopped
- ¼ cup steel-cut oats (measured dry)
- 1 tablespoon almond butter
- 1 teaspoon vanilla extract
  Stevia to taste (optional)
- 4–6 ice cubes

Place all ingredients in a blender and blend on high speed until smooth and creamy.

Calories 344 | Protein 30 g | Fat 12 g | Carbohydrates 35 g | Fiber 6 g

Barley and Spinach-stuffed Bell Peppers (Serves 4)

- 1 cup barley
- 3 cups water
- Pinch salt
- 1 teaspoon extra-virgin olive oil
- ¼ teaspoon ground nutmeg
- ¼ teaspoon cayenne pepper
- 1 teaspoon kosher salt, divided
- 1 10-ounce bag fresh spinach leaves
- ¼ cup pine nuts
- ¼ cup finely chopped red bell pepper
- ¼ cup chopped red onion
- 1 egg white
- ¼ cup chopped fresh flat-leaf parsley
- 1 teaspoon dried oregano
- Pepper to taste
- 8 red, yellow or orange bell peppers, tops sliced off, seeds removed
- 6 ounces Cabot 75% reduced-fat Cheddar cheese or low-fat Jarlsberg cheese, sliced
- ⅔ cup balsamic vinegar

In a medium saucepan, combine barley and water with pinch of salt. Bring to a boil. Cover, reduce heat and simmer for 50 to 60 minutes, until liquid is absorbed. Let cool.

Preheat oven to 400°F. Place a nonstick skillet over medium-high heat. Add olive oil, nutmeg, cayenne pepper, ½ teaspoon kosher salt and spinach. Toss to coat spinach evenly. Add pine nuts and toss again. Cook until the spinach is wilted, about 3 minutes. Remove from heat and cool.

In a separate bowl, combine the spinach mixture with the cooked barley, ½ teaspoon kosher salt, bell pepper, onion, egg white, parsley, oregano and pepper. Mix well.

Line a baking sheet with foil. Place peppers, cut-side up, on the baking sheet; fill with barley-spinach mixture. Top each with cheese.

Place on the middle rack in oven for about 20 minutes. Remove and allow to cool.

While stuffed peppers are cooking, heat vinegar in a small saucepan until boiling; reduce heat to medium-high and cook for about 5 minutes, until thickened. Remove from heat and cool slightly. Pour the vinegar over stuffed peppers before serving.

Calories 344 | Protein 22 g | Fat 14 g | Carbohydrates 34 g | Fiber 11 g

Sweet Apple Cinnamon Delight (Serves 1)

¼ cup oat bran
1 serving whey protein isolate (vanilla)
1 cup water
¼ teaspoon vanilla extract
½ cup unsweetened applesauce
½ teaspoon ground cinnamon
  Stevia to taste (optional)
  Nonstick cooking spray
1 tablespoon slivered almonds

Preheat oven to 350°F. In a large bowl, combine oat bran, whey protein isolate, water and vanilla extract. In a small bowl, combine applesauce, cinnamon and stevia. Lightly grease a small baking pan with cooking spray. Pour the applesauce mixture into the baking dish, then pour the oat mixture on top and sprinkle with slivered almonds. Bake for 25 to 35 minutes. Let cool before serving.

Calories 335 | Protein 29 g | Fat 11 g | Carbohydrates 33 g | Fiber 5 g

Honey Chicken and Sweet Potatoes (Serves 2)

- 1 tablespoon extra-virgin olive oil
- 2 boneless, skinless chicken breasts (approximately 4 to 5 ounces each), cubed
-    Salt and pepper to taste
- ¾ cup low-sodium chicken broth, divided
- ½ Vidalia onion, diced
- 2 cloves garlic, minced
- 1 teaspoon peeled and grated fresh gingerroot
- 2 small sweet potatoes, peeled and cubed
- 1 teaspoon ground cinnamon
- ½ teaspoon honey

In a nonstick skillet, heat olive oil over medium-high heat. Cook chicken for approximately 7 to 12 minutes, or until cooked through. Season with salt and pepper and set aside. Rinse the pan and return to medium-high heat, adding 2 tablespoons of broth. Add onion and cook until softened. Add garlic and ginger and stir for 1 minute. Add sweet potatoes, cinnamon, honey and remaining broth. Stir and simmer until the potatoes are tender, approximately 15 minutes. Divide between two plates and top with chicken.

Calories 338 | Protein 24 g | Fat 11 g | Carbohydrates 36 g | Fiber 5 g

Cinnamon Sweet Potato Pancakes (Serves 1)

- 1 small sweet potato
- 1 whole egg
- ½ cup liquid egg whites
- 1 tablespoon Fage Total Classic yogurt or goat yogurt, plain
- 1 tablespoon chia seeds
- ½ teaspoon vanilla extract
- ½ teaspoon ground cinnamon
- Nonstick cooking spray

Bake or boil sweet potato until tender. Cool slightly, and remove the skin with a small knife. In a medium-sized bowl, mash the sweet potato until smooth. Stir in egg, egg whites, yogurt, chia seeds, vanilla and cinnamon; mix well. Lightly grease a skillet with cooking spray and place over medium heat. Using 1 heaping tablespoon of the sweet potato mixture for each pancake, cook pancakes, flipping when bubbles form. Remove from pan when pancakes are firm.

Calories 305 | Protein 27 g | Fat 10 g | Carbohydrates 33 g | Fiber 9 g

Rosemary Salmon Steaks (Serves 4)

- 2   tablespoons extra-virgin olive oil
- 1   tablespoon fresh lemon juice
- ½   teaspoon dried rosemary
- 4   salmon steaks (approximately 4 to 5 ounces each)
- 4–6   cups mixed greens
- 1   cucumber, chopped
      Salt and pepper to taste
- 2   cups brown rice

Preheat oven to 350°F. In a small baking dish, combine olive oil, lemon juice and rosemary. Add salmon steaks and flip to coat. Marinate for 20 minutes. Wrap each steak in aluminum foil and bake for approximately 20 to 25 minutes. Remove from oven and let cool slightly.

In a large bowl, toss mixed greens together with chopped cucumber. Add salt and pepper to taste. Divide among plates and serve with salmon and ½ cup of brown rice per person.

Calories 352 | Protein 25 g | Fat 11 g | Carbohydrates 36 g | Fiber 12 g

Spicy Turkey Muffins (Serves 5)

Olive oil nonstick cooking spray

2   pounds extra-lean ground chicken or turkey

3   egg whites

1   cup quick-cooking oats

1   small onion, finely chopped

2–3   green onions, finely chopped

2   garlic cloves, minced

2   teaspoons dry yellow mustard

2   teaspoons pepper

2   teaspoons chipotle powder

1   teaspoon salt

½   teaspoon ground cumin

½   teaspoon dried thyme

5–6   cups mixed greens

Preheat oven to 375°F. Lightly grease a muffin pan with cooking spray. In a large bowl, combine chicken, egg whites, oats, onions, green onions, garlic, mustard, pepper, chipotle, salt, cumin and thyme. Using your hands, shape the mixture into 8 to 10 balls and place in the muffin pan. Bake for 35 to 40 minutes. Serve with mixed greens salad.

Calories 390 | Protein 40 g | Fat 12 g | Carbohydrates 24 g | Fiber 5 g

Sweet Tooth–satisfying Salmon (Serves 2)

2 medium sweet potatoes, peeled and cut into 1-inch chunks

½ teaspoon ground cinnamon

Stevia to taste (optional)

1 tablespoon extra-virgin olive oil

½ Vidalia onion, finely sliced

2 large salmon fillets, rinsed and skinned (approximately 5
ounces each)*

Salt and pepper to taste

4 lemon slices

Place sweet potatoes in a saucepan, cover with water, bring to a boil and cook until tender, approximately 15 to 20 minutes. Remove from heat, drain and sprinkle with cinnamon. If you like your sweet potatoes sweet, you can add stevia. Mash the sweet potatoes, or whip with a hand mixer, until fluffy. Set aside.

While the sweet potatoes are cooking, heat olive oil in a large skillet over medium-high heat. Sauté onion for 4 to 6 minutes, until softened. Place the salmon fillets in the skillet and cook until the salmon flakes easily with a fork, approximately 10 to 15 minutes. Season with salt and pepper. Serve immediately with the sweet potatoes and lemon slices on the side.

*Note that the salmon can be replaced with another protein source, such as sliced chicken or turkey breast (alter cooking times as necessary).

Calories 328 | Protein 26 g | Fat 12 g | Carbohydrates 30 g | Fiber 5 g

Red Potato and Asparagus Casserole (Serves 1)

2 teaspoons extra-virgin olive oil
1 medium red potato, diced
¼ cup chopped Vidalia onion
    Salt and pepper to taste
6–8 asparagus spears, trimmed and cut into 2-inch pieces
1 whole egg
¾ cup liquid egg whites
1 teaspoon finely chopped fresh basil

Preheat oven to 350°F. In a large nonstick skillet, heat olive oil over medium heat. Add potato and onion and cook until golden brown, approximately 5 minutes. Season with salt and pepper. Add asparagus and continue cooking until tender, another 6 to 7 minutes; transfer to a baking dish.

In a small bowl, whisk the egg and egg whites, and pour over the potatoes and onions. Bake until set in the middle, 20 to 25 minutes. Garnish with basil and serve.

Calories 395 | Protein 34 g | Fat 14 g | Carbohydrates 34 g | Fiber 5 g

SNACK RECIPES—PERMITTED IN ALL PHASES
(UNLESS OTHERWISE MENTIONED)

Carb Sensitivity Shake (Serves 1)

1	serving whey protein isolate (any flavor), or rice, hemp or vegan protein
½–¾	cup water
1	tablespoon almond, hazelnut or pumpkin seed butter
¼	teaspoon ground cinnamon
	Stevia (optional)
3–4	ice cubes (optional)

Place all ingredients in a blender and blend on high speed until smooth and creamy. Alternatively, you can toss all ingredients except water into a protein shaker cup, and add water when ready for a snack. Shake well and drink.

Calories 207 | Protein 27 g | Fat 10 g | Carbohydrates 6 g | Fiber 2 g

Refer to pages 136–38 for additional shake options.

Celery with Tuna Salad (Serves 2)

1	can (5 ounces) tuna, packed in water, drained
1	tablespoon olive oil mayonnaise
½	teaspoon Italian seasoning
¼	teaspoon finely chopped fresh dill (optional)
¼	fresh lemon
2–3	stalks celery, trimmed and chopped into 3 pieces each

In a medium bowl, combine tuna, mayonnaise, Italian seasoning and dill. Squeeze lemon over tuna mixture and stir. Fill celery sticks with the tuna mixture. Serve immediately or store in the fridge for later.

Calories 180 | Protein 21 g | Fat 8 g | Carbohydrates 6 g | Fiber 2 g

Portobello Mushroom Caps (Serves 1)

2   large portobello mushrooms, stems discarded
    Pepper to taste
    Steak seasoning to taste
1   teaspoon extra-virgin olive oil
2   ounces Cabot 75% reduced-fat Cheddar cheese or low-fat
    Jarlsberg cheese, sliced

Preheat oven to 425°F. Gently scrape the gills off the undersides of the mushroom caps with a spoon and discard. Sprinkle the caps with pepper, steak seasoning and olive oil. Place mushroom caps stem-side up on a foil-lined baking sheet. Bake for 10 minutes. Turn the caps over and bake for another 5 minutes. Remove from the oven and top with cheese slices. Serve warm.

Calories 198 | Protein 22 g | Fat 11 g | Carbohydrates 7 g | Fiber 2 g

Not So Devilish Eggs (Serves 2)

    4   eggs
        Salt and pepper to taste
    ½   green onion, finely chopped
    1   teaspoon Dijon mustard
    1   teaspoon olive oil mayonnaise
    ½   teaspoon paprika
    ½   teaspoon dried parsley
    1   green apple, sliced (unpeeled)

In a small pan, cover eggs with room temperature water and a pinch of salt. Cover and bring the water to a boil; simmer for approximately 10 minutes. Drain the eggs and let cool under cold water for 2 minutes. Peel the eggs and cut them in half lengthwise, gently removing the yolks. Set aside egg whites on a plate. Place two yolks in a small bowl, discarding the other two yolks. Add green onion, mustard and mayonnaise to the bowl and mix well until creamy. Fill egg white halves with egg yolk mixture, then sprinkle with paprika, parsley, and salt and pepper. Serve immediately or store in the fridge for later. Serve with apple slices.

Calories 167 | Protein 10 g | Fat 8 g | Carbohydrates 16 g | Fiber 3 g

Mini Turkey Lettuce Wraps (Serves 1)

- 2 slices nitrite-free turkey or chicken breast, cut into strips
- 1 ounce Cabot 75% reduced-fat Cheddar cheese or low-fat Jarlsberg cheese, cut into strips
- 2 large romaine or butter lettuce leaves, cut into 4 strips
- 1 tablespoon walnuts

Roll strips of turkey around cheese, then roll the chicken and cheese in lettuce leaf. Secure with a toothpick if needed. Enjoy with walnuts on the side or included in the wrap.

Calories 167 | Protein 17 g | Fat 8 g | Carbohydrates 8 g | Fiber 5 g

Weightless Wasa Crackers (Serves 2)—Phase Four Only

- 1 tablespoon almond butter
- 3 Wasa crackers
- ½ cup sliced strawberries
- 2 ounces Cabot 75% reduced-fat Cheddar cheese or low-fat Jarlsberg cheese, sliced

Spread almond butter on Wasa crackers. Top with sliced strawberries. Enjoy with Allégro cheese slices on the side.

Calories 158 | Protein 12 g | Fat 7 g | Carbohydrates 15 g | Fiber 4 g

Coconut Almond Butter Protein Bars (Serves 4)—Phase Five Only

1	cup steel-cut oats
2	servings whey protein isolate (chocolate or vanilla)
½	cup liquid egg whites, or 4 egg whites
½	cup unsweetened applesauce
2	tablespoons almond, hazelnut or cashew butter
¼	teaspoon vanilla extract
2	tablespoons grated coconut (unsweetened)

Preheat oven to 350°F. In a large glass bowl, combine large-flake oats, whey protein isolate and egg whites. Add applesauce, nut butter and vanilla and blend well. Lightly grease a small baking dish with cooking spray. Spread the oat mixture in an even layer over the bottom of the dish. Sprinkle grated coconut on top. Bake for approximately 18 to 20 minutes, or until the edge starts to pull away from the sides of the dish. Remove from the oven, let cool and cut into bars.

Calories 242 | Protein 22 g | Fat 8 g | Carbohydrates 22 g | Fiber 4 g

Coconut Almond Butter
Protein Bars

Perfect Balance Banana Bread (Serves 2)

- 2 eggs
- ½–¾ cup water
- ¼ cup Fage Total Classic yogurt or goat yogurt
- 1 serving whey protein isolate (vanilla)
- 1 banana, mashed
- 1 teaspoon baking soda
- ½ teaspoon vanilla extract
- ¼ teaspoon banana extract

Preheat oven to 350°F. Place all ingredients in a blender and blend on high speed until smooth. Pour into a loaf pan and bake for 25 to 30 minutes. Remove and let cool slightly before serving.

Calories 209 | Protein 21 g | Fat 7 g | Carbohydrates 20 g | Fiber 2 g

Spicy Pepper Poppers (Serves 1)

- 4–6 jalapeño peppers
- 1½ ounces Cabot 75% reduced-fat Cheddar cheese or low-fat Jarlsberg cheese
- 1 tablespoon chia seeds
- ¼ cup no-sugar-added salsa

Preheat oven to 375°F. Cut jalapeño peppers in half lengthwise, trim off any stems and scrape out the seeds, being careful not to touch your face and washing your hands immediately after. Arrange on a foil-lined baking sheet. Slice the cheese lengthwise and place inside each pepper. Top each popper with a sprinkle of chia seed. Bake for 10 to 15 minutes. Remove from the oven when the cheese is bubbly and peppers are slightly tender. Serve with salsa.

Calories 201 | Protein 19 g | Fat 10 g | Carbohydrates 19 g | Fiber 10 g

BLOOD TESTS TO ASSESS METABOLIC HEALTH AND INSULIN SENSITIVITY

Live nutty. Just occasionally. Just once in a while. And see what happens. It brightens up the day.

LEO BUSCAGLIA

While you can certainly uncover whether insulin resistance is an issue for you by considering what you have learned in this book, you can also ask your health-care provider for blood tests to definitively assess your metabolism and degree of insulin resistance. As I explained in my last two books, knowing and understanding the medical tests you should ask for puts you in the driver's seat when it comes to managing your own health.

In the pages that follow, you will find a brief outline of the blood tests I feel are helpful for assessing your metabolic profile. Some of you may want to complete these tests before you begin your CSP, though I often find they are most beneficial after the program. Recording values before you start does, however, provide the ability to compare pre- and postprogram values. A table listing all of these tests, which can be conveniently photocopied to take to your doctor, can be found at the end of this appendix.

Whether you request these tests at your annual checkup or when you are going through a particularly symptomatic period, I recommend that you ask for a *copy of your blood test results and keep them in a folder.* It's helpful for you to compare your results yearly, since the goal is to make sure your values remain in the *optimal* ranges I have listed here, and not just within *normal* ranges. Remember, significant changes can occur in your blood work from one year to the next, even without the appearance of obvious physical signs.

- **RBC Magnesium.** Magnesium is important to carbohydrate metabolism, as it may influence the release and activity of insulin. Elevated blood sugar levels increase the loss of magnesium via the urine, which in turn lowers blood levels of magnesium. This explains why low blood levels of magnesium are seen in poorly controlled type 1 and type 2 diabetes. These low levels may also contribute to hypertension, commonly found in diabetics. Evidence suggests that magnesium may play an important role in regulating blood pressure because of its natural muscle relaxant qualities. When blood vessels are relaxed, there is less resistance to the flow of blood and, as a result, lower blood pressure.

  Diets that provide high sources of potassium and magnesium—such as those that are high in fruits and vegetables—are consistently associated with lower blood pressure. The DASH study (Dietary Approaches to Stop Hypertension) suggests that high blood pressure could be significantly lowered by consuming a diet high in magnesium, potassium and calcium, and low in sodium and saturated fat.

- **Liver function tests for AST, ALT and bilirubin.** These tests are used to identify liver disease and function. Your liver is vital for insulin balance, fat loss and wellness. Poor or "sluggish" liver function can interfere with fat loss, cause hormonal imbalance and increase your risk of disease. Normal values are within the laboratory reference range, but lower is better. Milk thistle, dandelion root, turmeric and artichoke are wonderful herbs for supporting the natural processes of the liver. If your levels are abnormal, take Clear Detox—Hormonal Health, which contains many of these herbs along with additional nutrients to support healthy liver function, for at least 3 months. After that point, you should retest your enzymes to see whether your levels have improved.

- **Copper.** Excess vitamin C and zinc interfere with copper availability. A deficiency of copper may result in anemia (indistinguishable from iron deficiency); impaired formation of collagen, elastin and connective tissue proteins; osteoporosis and arterial wall defects. It makes sense, then, to monitor your copper levels closely if you have cardiovascular disease. While deficiencies are harmful, especially for cardiovascular health, it's often more common to have excess copper, mainly due to estrogen dominance, insulin resistance, medication or supplement use, or from the copper that commonly leaches into drinking water from pipes. Symptoms of copper toxicity include depression, acne and hair loss. If you find your copper is low, your multivitamin should provide all that you need. If your copper is too high, take zinc daily to encourage its depletion.

- **Zinc.** Zinc is a cofactor involved in at least 200 different enzymatic reactions in the body. As an essential mineral involved in healthy immunity, blood sugar and insulin balance, thyroid function, collagen production, bone density, tissue healing and repair, antioxidant protection, prostate function and growth hormone and testosterone production, zinc is vital to good health. Zinc depletion is common with use of the birth control pill, corticosteroids and diuretics. Its absorption is greatly compromised when your stomach acid (HCL) levels are low. Zinc deficiency causes decreased senses of taste and smell, poor wound healing, white spots in the fingernails, night blindness, low sperm count, hair loss, behavior or sleep problems, mental sluggishness, impaired immune function and dermatitis. Optimally, your levels should be toward the high end of the laboratory reference range. You may add a supplement of zinc citrate if your zinc is low. Purchase zinc citrate or a chelated form of zinc, which is optimal for absorption. Be sure to take it with food to avoid nausea.

- **Fasting glucose and insulin.** Glucose and insulin are implicated in many age-related diseases, such as type 2 diabetes, hypoglycemia, carbohydrate metabolism, hypertension, heart disease, insulin resistance and stroke. These tests require a fasting blood level, which means a 10- to 12-hour fast is required before the collection of your blood sample. The optimal value for fasting blood sugar is less than 86 mg/dl. A value of less than 5 mU/ml is optimal for fasting insulin. Insulin resistance is associated with a glucose reading greater than 100 mg/dl and fasting insulin greater than 5.

- **2-hour postprandial (pp) glucose and insulin.** During testing day at my clinic, all of our patients arrive fasting and complete their first blood draw. As soon as the blood is drawn, we feed them waffles, maple syrup and orange juice. Then we repeat the glucose and insulin tests 2 hours after they have eaten the high-carb breakfast. The first sign of insulin resistance is elevated insulin *after* a meal, *followed by high fasting insulin*. Insulin tends to be abnormal *long before* blood sugars start to rise, which is typical of the diabetic state. Insulin resistance may be apparent with 2-hour glucose readings of more than 140 mg/dl and insulin levels of more than 30 mU/ml. If either your fasting or your 2-hour test is abnormal, you need to focus on improving your body's sensitivity to insulin with nutrition, stress management, supplements and strength training, as outlined in the Metabolic Repair Program. Depending on the severity of your insulin imbalance, I suggest continuing with the Metabolic Repair Program for 3 to 12 months, and then repeating the test.

- **Fasting triglycerides.** Triglycerides are a type of fat present in our bloodstream that results from the fats or carbohydrates we consume. Calories we ingest that are not used immediately by our tissues are converted to triglycerides and transported to our fat cells to be stored. Then your hormones regulate the release of triglycerides from fat stores to help meet the body's needs for energy between meals. Levels greater than 100 mg/dl are associated with insulin resistance.

- **Fasting cholesterol (total, HDL and LDL).** An optimal level of "good" cholesterol (HDL) should be between 55 and 150 mg/dl. "Bad" cholesterol (LDL) should be between 80 and 120 mg/dl to be safe, and total cholesterol should be less than 150 mg/dl. If your cholesterol is too high, I recommend a product from Integra Nutrition called Cholest-FX. It is the company's best-selling product, and its benefits on cholesterol reduction, without the side effects common to the statins typically prescribed by physicians, are well supported clinically.

- **Uric acid.** Normal levels are less than 5.0 mg/dl. High levels of uric acid cause gout, are linked to increased heart disease risk and are also a sign of insulin resistance.

- **HbA1c levels.** This is an indicator of blood sugar control over the previous 120 days. Ideal levels are between 4 and 6 percent. If the number is higher, your blood sugar control over the last several months has been less than optimal. This is another marker of insulin resistance or poor metabolic function.

- **Fasting homocysteine.** Homocysteine is an inflammatory protein that, if elevated in the blood, is a proven independent risk factor for heart disease, osteoporosis, Alzheimer's disease and stroke. Homocysteine has been found to increase with insulin resistance. The optimal level is less than 6.3. It's useful to test vitamin B12 (optimal value: more than 600) and folic acid (optimal value: more than 1,000) at the same time, since these substances are involved in the metabolic process necessary to reduce homocysteine levels along with vitamin B6 and a compound called trimethylgly-cine. Vitamin B12, found only in animal-source foods, is necessary for the formation and regeneration of red blood cells. It also promotes growth, increases energy, improves sleep and cognition and helps maintain a healthy nervous system. Folic acid helps protect against genetic damage and birth defects. It is needed for the utilization of sugar and amino acids, prevents some types of cancer, promotes healthier skin, and helps protect against intestinal parasites and food poisoning. If your homocysteine is too high, include a complex of vitamin B6, vitamin B12 and folic acid in your daily vitamin regimen for at least 3 months or until your next physical exam.

- **High-sensitivity C-reactive protein.** Hs-CRP is a marker of inflammation and a risk factor for arterial disease. Levels tend to increase as body fat increases and with insulin resistance. An optimal value is less than 0.8 mg/l, although the Life Extension Foundation (check out www.lef.org—it is a leading source for scientific information on antiaging and preventive medicine) recommends less than 0.55 mg/l for men and less than 1.5 mg/l for women. This test is also important for breast cancer survivors and should be completed together with fasting and 2-hour pp insulin levels. High CRP or fasting insulin is associated with increased risk of recurrence of this cancer.

- **Ferritin.** Abnormally high levels of the storage form of iron, called ferritin, can increase the risk of heart and liver disease in both men and women. It also appears to increase inflam-mation. Optimal levels should be close to 70 in women and 100 in men. Low levels of iron are associated with fatigue, hypothyroidism, decreased athletic performance, ADD/ADHD, restless leg syndrome and hair loss. If your ferritin is too high, you should speak to your doctor about the possibility of donating blood to help reduce your levels to a more optimal range. If ferritin is too low, use a supplement of iron citrate with 1,000 mg of vitamin C. The citrate form of iron will not cause constipation.

- **Follicle-stimulating hormone (FSH) and luteinizing hormone (LH).** These hormones are released from the pituitary gland and stimulate the ovaries and testes. High levels are found in menopause, infertility or amenorrhea (lack of menstruation), premature ovarian failure or testicular failure. Low levels indicate pituitary dysfunction. If your FSH or LH is elevated, you will need to replenish estrogen, progesterone and/or testosterone. An excess of LH relative to FSH is common with polycystic ovarian syndrome (PCOS), a condition also commonly linked to insulin resistance.

- **DHEAs.** DHEA is a precursor hormone to estrogen and testosterone. This adrenal hormone tends to naturally decrease as we age. At the same time, it protects against the harmful effects of the stress hormone cortisol. It is also cardioprotective and is crucial for healthy body composition. Most antiaging programs recommend the use of DHEAs, however, I feel they should not be taken unless a true deficiency has been diagnosed via blood work. Follow-up testing should also be completed to ensure there is no excess present. In some cases of PCOS, DHEA may be abnormally high, contributing to hair loss and male pattern balding. Optimal levels should be above 225 mcg/dl or, more specifically, 300 to 400 mcg/dl for men and 225 to 350 mcg/dl for women.

- **Cortisol.** High levels (more than 15 mcg/dl) of cortisol are detrimental for almost every tissue and organ in the body. Excess cortisol causes destruction of muscle, increases calcium loss from bone, accelerates the process of aging and is linked to memory loss, anxiety, depression and low libido, along with an increase in the deposition of fat around the abdomen because of its adverse effects on insulin sensitivity, growth hormones and inflammation. Low levels (less than 9 mcg/dl) indicate adrenal gland burnout.

- **Free and total testosterone.** Many men with insulin resistance, obesity or sleep apnea have low levels of testosterone, which is known to increase the risk of heart disease. This deficiency also influences erectile function, libido, sense of well-being, mood and motivation. Maintaining testosterone levels is crucial for building muscle and losing fat. Optimal free testosterone levels for men should be in the range of 7.2 to 24 mcg/dl; total testosterone should fall between 241 to 827 mcg/dl. In women, low testosterone is damaging to bone density, a healthy libido and aspects of memory (especially task-oriented memory). If testosterone is too high (often associated with PCOS or insulin resistance), hair loss, acne, increased risk of breast cancer or infertility may occur.

- **Estradiol and estrone.** Estrogen values will vary in women depending on their age and point in the menstrual cycle. On day 3 of the menstrual cycle the optimal value for estrogen is 180 to 200 pg/ml for premenopausal women and 60 to 120 pg/ml for women in their late 40s and older. Men's estradiol should be less than 40 pg/ml. In both sexes, high estrogen encourages fat storage. Elevated levels of estrogen in men are typically found in cases of increased abdominal obesity because the fat cells here encourage the conversion of testosterone to estrogen. High levels of estrogen and low levels of testosterone set the stage for sexual dysfunction and prostate conditions and promote more weight gain in men. In women, excess estrogen is associated with PMS, weight gain around the hips, uterine fibroids and other gynecological conditions, as well as increased risk for certain types of cancers. Before menopause, estrogen is naturally highest in the first half of the menstrual cycle. After menopause, levels are normally consistent and much lower. As estrogen levels decline, more abdominal weight gain can arise, since estrogen affects insulin sensitivity. Lower levels of estrogen are also associated with a decrease in serotonin, which can lead to depression, anxiety, worrying and sleep disruption. Low estrogen can cause hot flashes, night sweats, urinary urgency and frequency, insomnia, depression, failing memory (especially when attempting to think of a word or name), hair texture and skin elasticity changes, a thickening waistline, vaginal dryness and a low libido. Low estrogen also increases the risk of inflammation, heart disease, diabetes, Alzheimer's disease and osteoporosis.

- **Progesterone.** Progesterone is naturally highest in the second half of the menstrual cycle, and normal values can range widely. Progesterone provides protection against anxiety, PMS, fibrocystic breast disease and water retention. It also encourages fat burning and is crucial for fertility. Progesterone protects the prostate gland in men and may help to restore low DHEA levels. In women, decreased levels are associated with infertility, amenorrhea, fetal death and toxemia in pregnancy.

- **TSH, Free T3, Free T4 and thyroid antibodies.** These four tests are required to accurately assess the function of the thyroid gland, our master gland of metabolism. TSH should be less than 2.0 to be optimal, not the currently accepted 4.7 reported by most labs. T3 and T4 should be in the middle of the laboratory reference range. Thyroid antithyroglobulin antibodies should be negative. Quite often I find elevated antibodies prior to abnormalities in TSH, T3 or T4, which may be an early signal of the development of thyroid disease. It's almost impossible to have low body fat along with an improperly diagnosed or managed case of hypothyroidism (underactive thyroid). Currently, it's estimated that 1 in 13 people suffers from hypothyroidism, with the majority of cases being missed because of improper testing or interpretation of the blood results. There is an increase in the risk of obesity, heart disease and blood sugar abnormalities in hypothyroid cases. Often, hypothyroid patients also have high levels of homocysteine and cholesterol. If you are attempting to conceive, thyroid antibody abnormalities should be addressed to improve your chances of conception.

- **25-hydroxy vitamin D3.** Vitamin D has proven immune-enhancing, cancer-protective, bone-building and insulin-regulating benefits. It is also important during pregnancy. Your levels should be over 50 ng/mL (125 nmolK). If your vitamin D is low, add 2,000 to 5,000 IU of vitamin D3 each day to your regimen, in addition to your multivitamin and calcium/magnesium supplement.
- **IGF-1.** This is a marker of growth hormone status. Because it remains constant in the blood longer than HGH (which tends to fluctuate in response to various stimuli), it is a more accurate indicator of HGH deficiency and is also more precise for monitoring HGH therapy than testing HGH directly. An optimal IGF-1 value will range between 200 and 300 ng/ml. Growth hormone is essential to maintaining healthy bones, skin and hair, as well as strong, lean muscle mass. It tends to naturally decrease as we age, but conditions such as sleep deprivation, diabetes, hypothyroidism, some cases of osteoporosis, anorexia and insulin resistance can cause levels to decline more rapidly.

In summary, the complete list of tests you can request from your doctor, in addition to the complete blood count, includes:

- RBC Magnesium
- Liver function tests for AST, ALT and bilirubin
- Copper
- Zinc

- Fasting glucose and insulin
- 2-hour postprandial (pp) glucose and insulin
- Fasting triglycerides
- Fasting cholesterol (total, HDL and LDL)
- HbA1c levels
- Uric acid
- Fasting homocysteine
- High-sensitivity C-reactive protein
- Ferritin
- Follicle-stimulating hormone (FSH) and luteinizing hormone (LH)
- DHEAs
- Cortisol
- Free and total testosterone
- Estradiol and estrone
- Progesterone
- TSH, Free T3, Free T4 and thyroid antibodies
- 25-hydroxy vitamin D3
- IGF-1

Some Notes about Completing Hormonal Health Assessments

Your hormones are usually best tested in the morning. In pre-menopausal women, the hormone tests (estradiol, progesterone, LH, FSH) should be completed on day 3 and/or 20 to 22 of your cycle (day 1 is your first day of bleeding). Day 3 assesses ovarian reserve and estrogen levels, while day 20 to 22 assesses progesterone levels. Both are important for fertility, insulin balance and prevention of PMS. If you are male or menopausal, you can have your blood tests completed on any day.

Note that you can also assess your hormones via saliva hormone analysis. This is argued to be a more accurate way to measure hormones because it looks at the free component of hormones rather than those bound to carrier proteins. When hormones are bound to other proteins, it blocks their effects in the body. It is the free component of hormones, therefore, that is biologically active. I use both saliva and blood testing in my clinical practice. I will complete a patient's blood tests at least once a year and saliva once a year as well, especially once the patient begins treatment with bioidentical hormones. Monitoring blood levels only can increase the risk of overdosing hormone replacement.

Instructions for the Blood Tests

Go to the lab after fasting for 10 to 12 hours. Premenopausal women should choose to go to the lab on the appropriate day of their cycle. Aim to be at the lab before 9 a.m. to 10 a.m., since your hormones fluctuate as the day goes on. Should you complete the 2-hour pp glucose and insulin tests, you will then return to the lab 2 hours later for a second blood draw after consuming a high-carb meal (e.g., pancakes/waffles, syrup and orange juice). During this 2-hour waiting period, do not eat anything else or exercise.

Once all your blood tests are completed, be sure to ask for a copy of all your results that you can keep for your records. That way, you and your health-care provider can keep a close eye on changes in your values from one year to the next.

The Underlying Imbalances of Metabolic Disruption: A Review of the Blood Tests for Each Imbalance

Should you wish to further understand these hormonal imbalances and their complications, I have summarized the tests and expected results that may confirm a diagnosis.

Excess Insulin/Insulin Resistance

TEST	RESULT INDICATING PRESENCE OF INSULIN RESISTANCE
Fasting glucose and insulin	Abnormally elevated fasting glucose and/or insulin. In general, both should be in the bottom third of the reference range.
2-hour pp glucose and insulin	Abnormally elevated fasting glucose and/or insulin. Again, both should be in the bottom third of the reference range.
Fasting cholesterol panel (total, HDL, LDL)	Elevated total and LDL; low HDL
Fasting triglycerides	Elevated
Uric acid	Elevated
Fasting homocysteine	Elevated (> 6.3)
Hs-CRP	High (> 0.8)
Free and total testosterone (saliva or blood)	Elevated in women; low in men
DHEA (blood or saliva)	Elevated in women; low in men
Estradiol (blood or saliva)	Elevated (premenopausal women and in men)
Ferritin	Elevated
Vitamin B12	Low (< 600)
RBC magnesium	Low
Folic acid	Low (< 1,000)
Liver function tests: AST, ALT, GGT	One or more liver enzymes may be abnormally elevated.
Zinc and copper	Copper tends to be high and zinc low in insulin-resistant patients.
25-hydroxy vitamin D3	Deficient in the majority of cases.

Excess Estrogen/Estrogen Dominance (Commonly Also Associated with Low Testosterone or Andropause in Men)

TEST	RESULT INDICATING PRESENCE OF ESTROGEN DOMINANCE/LOW TESTOSTERONE (MEN)
Fasting glucose and insulin	Normal or abnormally elevated fasting glucose and/or insulin (abnormal results are more likely in men with this condition)
2-hour pp glucose and insulin	Normal or abnormally elevated 2-hour pp glucose and/or insulin (abnormal results are more likely in men with this condition)
Hs-CRP	High (> 0.8)
Zinc and copper	Copper tends to be high and zinc low in cases of estrogen dominance, especially when caused by the use of the birth control pill
RBC magnesium	Low magnesium. (Since it is heavily involved in estrogen detoxification, levels are often low with estrogen dominance.)
Estradiol (blood or saliva)	Elevated
Estrone (blood or saliva)	Elevated
Estriol (blood or saliva)	Possibly low or normal
Progesterone (blood or saliva)	Often low
DHEA (blood or saliva)	Normal or low
Cortisol (blood or saliva)	Normal or elevated
Free and total testosterone (blood or saliva)	Women: normal; low with stress; elevated with insulin resistance Men: low
Specialized testing: urinary estrogen metabolite excretions from Metametrix Labs (the Estronex test) www.metametrix.com	Elevated levels of harmful estrogen metabolites in the urine

Inflammation

TEST	RESULT INDICATING THE PRESENCE OF INFLAMMATION
Fasting glucose and insulin	Abnormally elevated fasting glucose and/or insulin
2-hour pp glucose and insulin	Abnormally elevated 2-hour pp glucose and/or insulin
Hs-CRP	High (> 0.8)
Fasting homocysteine	High (> 6.3)
Vitamin B12 and folic acid	Often low B12 and folic acid
Fasting cholesterol panel (total, HDL, LDL)	Possibly elevated total and LDL; low or normal HDL
Uric acid	Often elevated
Ferritin	Can be high (> 110 in women; > 170 in men)
25-hydroxy vitamin D3	Often low
Liver function tests: AST, ALT, GGT	Normal or elevated
IgG food allergy testing	Often elevated
Antigliadin antibodies to rule out celiac disease	Normal or positive
ANA, rheumatoid factor (RF) and thyroid antibodies to assess risk of an autoimmune disease	Normal or positive

VEGETARIAN AND VEGAN SOURCES OF PROTEIN

The art of being wise is knowing what to overlook.

WILLIAM JAMES

FOOD	AMOUNT	PROTEIN(g)	CARBS (g)	FIBER (g)
Tempeh	1 cup	31	15.6	0
Seitan	3 ounces	11	10	1
Soybeans, cooked	½ cup	15	8	5
Lentils, cooked	½ cup	9	20	9
Black beans, cooked	½ cup	7	23	6
Kidney beans, cooked	½ cup	7	20	7
Veggie burger (may vary)	1 patty	10	9	3
Chickpeas, cooked	½ cup	6	27	5
Pinto beans, cooked	½ cup	7.7	22.4	8
Black-eyed peas, cooked	½ cup	6	16	4
Tofu, firm	½ cup	10	2	1
Lima beans, cooked	½ cup	6	18	6
Quinoa, cooked	½ cup	4	20	3
Textured vegetable protein (TVP), cooked	½ cup	24	14	8
Peanut butter (natural)	2 Tbsp	8	6	2
Veggie dog	1 link	11	6	1
Almonds	1 ounce	6	6	3.5
Soy milk, commercial, plain	1 cup	8	16	1.5

FOOD	AMOUNT	PROTEIN(g)	CARBS (g)	FIBER (g)
Bulgur, cooked	½ cup	3	8.5	2
Sunflower seeds	¼ cup	2.4	2.3	1
Cashews	1 ounce	5.2	8.5	1
Almond butter	2 Tbsp	6	6	1
Brown rice, cooked	½ cup	2.3	23	2
Spinach, cooked	2 cups	1.8	2.2	1.4
Broccoli, cooked	1 cup	4	11	5
Potato, cooked	1 medium	4.3	36	4

Note: Caloric breakdown may vary depending on the source and brand of certain products.

ACKNOWLEDGMENTS

Perseverance is not a long race;
it is many short races one after the other.

WALTER ELLIOT

The tight deadline and intense work schedule set around this book were a definite challenge, though I do feel a sense of excitement about it that is possibly even greater than with my previous projects. As always, a project of this nature is not possible without the help and support of many.

To my sweet husband, Tim: Your guidance with navigating the roles I seem to continually take on continues to be amazing—and to ensure my sanity. To my family: my sister and best friend, Maria; the Rivers (Uncle Bruce, Aunt Betty, and Mari); the Martins (Jeff, Kyle, Breeanne, and Maryann); and the Florians (Kelly Ann, Derck, Mark and Evan)—love you all. Thank you for putting up with the rigors of my work schedule and for understanding the missed weekends at the cottage or summer trips to Nova Scotia to see you, Mom, and your new deli (The Art of Eating)—brother Simon. To my friends Sandro, Lisa, BB, PB, Cynthia, Tony C. and Talie: I can't thank you enough for your care and support.

Gratitude to Tara Rose. We have an amazing propensity to brainstorm and similar working styles. Your suggestions, writing, editing and input made this book better (and fun to complete). Without your help, I am certain that it would never have been finished in this short time frame. Now project two is under our belts, and I look forward to our next! Thank you to Andrea Ritter and to Linda Pruessen for your editing skills and thoughtful ideas. Thank you to Trisha Calvo for your editorial assistance and for making the US version of this book perfect! You both make me sound better, keeping my message to the reader approachable and clear. Thank you to my agent, Rick Broadhead, for getting *The CSP* to publishers, for your fantastic attention to detail and exemplary work ethic. Thank you to Pamela Murray and Anne Collins of Random House Canada and Pam Krauss of Rodale for your enthusiasm about my writing (and for graciously agreeing to an extension when I needed it!). And, finally, a huge thank you to my PR team—Frances Bedford (Random House) and Karen Mazzotta (Rodale). Without your help, awareness of this book would be impossible.

I would also like to offer gratitude to Suzanne Somers for endorsing my work and for her continual efforts to bring preventive medicine to the forefront. Thank you Dr. William Davis, author of *Wheat Belly*, for also endorsing the CSP.

Thank you to Don Hunter for a lifetime of friendship and for creating the workouts in this book. You are exceptional at what you do. I am so lucky to have your input, as is everyone who has completed the exercise program. A big thank-you to Sam Gibbs, close friend and brilliant osteopath, who is also the multitasking genius who took the exercise photos in this book. Thank you to my colleague Dr. Adrienne Shulman and my friend Lorri MacDonald for reading the manuscript and offering feedback from the perspective of a health professional and informed health consumer, respectively.

Thank you to the team at Clear Medicine. I cannot begin to explain how blessed I feel to work in an environment that includes a team of such exceptional, experienced, passionate and caring professionals. Dr. Amy Tung, Dr. Adrienne Shulman, Dr. Cara MacMullan and Dr. Marika Berni (the Clear Medicine ND team); Rishi Angras and Sam Gibbs (the Clear Medicine Osteopathic team); Jill Hillhouse and Katie Hamilton (the Clear Medicine Nutrition team); Anthony Boudreau, Dr. Michelle Crispe, Reggie Reyes, Jacob Lay and

Dr. Marc Bubbs (the Clear Medicine Fitness Expert team); Dr. Fanny Ip (the Clear Medicine acupuncturist); Tara Rose, Jay Kelly, (the Clear Medicine management team); Liz, Jackie and Ange (the Clear Medicine administrative team)—you make all that I do, and so much more, possible. You truly do motivate and guide people to live healthier, balanced lives daily.

Thank you to my patients and to clients of Clear Medicine. We are incredibly lucky to work with clientele such as you.

Thank you, the reader, for picking up this book and for sharing your success stories on my Facebook pages or Web sites. You have not only made a difference in your own life but also have generously taken the time to provide the proof and necessary encouragement to so many others that change is possible and doable! And last, thank you for helping me to achieve my goal of inspiring others to take responsibility for their health and to live healthier lives.

RESOURCES

PRODUCT/RESOURCE	WEB SITE
HEAVY METAL DETOX	
Detoxamin EDTA suppositories	www.detoxamin.com
INFRARED SAUNA	
SaunaRay Far Infrared Saunas	www.saunaray.com
BODY-FAT/COMPOSITION ANALYZER	
Tanita: Home body-fat analyzer	www.tanita.com
NATURAL SKIN CARE AND MAKEUP	
Naturopathica: Environmental Defense Mask	www.naturopathica.com
Caudalie (Toxin-free skin care)	www.caudalie.com
Juice Beauty (Toxin-free skin care)	www.juicebeauty.com
John Masters (Toxin-free skin and hair care)	www.johnmasters.com
Burt's Bees (Natural skin care)	www.burtsbees.com
Alba Organics: Sugar Cane Body Polish Kukui Nut Organic Body Oil	www.albaorganics.com (Unlike the two products listed here, not all Alba products are free of harmful methylparabens and propylparabens.)
Dr. Hauschka Skin Care	www.drhauschka.com
Jane Iredale: Mineral makeup	www.janeiredale.com

PRODUCT/RESOURCE	WEB SITE
SUPPLEMENTS	
Wobenzym N: One of the top-selling natural anti-inflammatory enzyme formulas in the world	www.wobenzym-usa.com, www.thehormonediet.com or www.clearmedicine.com
All Clear Medicine Products, including those for detoxification, general health and hormonal concerns	www.carbsensitivity.com, www.clearmedicine.com or www.thehormonediet.com
Carlson Fish Oils	www.carlsonlabs.com
Nordic Natural Fish Oils	www.nordicnaturals.com
Ascenta (NutraSea) Fish Oils	www.ascentahealth.com
Jarrow	www.jarrow.com
Genuine Health (proteins +, all-natural whey protein isolate supplement, and greens +, green food supplements)	www.genuinehealth.com
New Chapter	www.newchapter.com
Dream Protein (all-natural whey protein supplement)	www.carbsensitivity.com, www.clearmedicine.com or www.thehormonediet.com
Pure Encapsulations (G.I. Fortify and Liver—G.I. Detox)	www.carbsensitivity.com, www.clearmedicine.com or www.thehormonediet.com
Glyci-Med Forte (Clear Medicine): Olive and avocado oil supplement to aid weight loss	www.carbsensitivity.com, www.clearmedicine.com or www.thehormonediet.com
Metagenics	www.metagenics.com, www.carbsensitivity.com, www.thehormonediet.com or www.clearmedicine.com
SPECIALTY FOODS	
Green and Black's: Organic chocolate	www.greenandblacks.com
NewTree: Fine Belgian dark chocolate	www.newtree.com
Camino: Organic fair-trade chocolate	www.cocoacamino.com

PRODUCT/RESOURCE	WEB SITE
SPECIALTY FOODS *(continued)*	
The Simply Bar: Gluten-free protein bar	www.carbsensitivity.com, www.thehormonediet.com or www.clearmedicine.com
Sambazon: Acai concentrate	www.sambazon.com
Navitas Naturals: Goji Power	www.navitasnaturals.com
Pom Wonderful: Pomegranate juice	www.pomwonderful.com
La Tortilla Factory: Pita, wraps and gluten-free products	www.latortillafactory.com
Muzi Teas: Green tea	www.muzitea.com
Organic Meadows: Organic pressed cottage cheese	www.organicmeadow.com
Fage: Greek yogurt	www.fageusa.com
Cabot: Reduced-fat cheese	www.cabotcheese.com
Kashi Company: GoLean high-protein, high-fiber cereal	www.kashi.com
Food for Life Baking Co.: Ezekiel breads	www.foodforlife.com
Bob's Red Mill Natural Foods: Gluten-free and other grain products	www.bobsredmill.com
So Nice: Unsweetened organic soy milk	www.sonice.ca
PROsnack Natural Foods: Elevate Me! (organic whole-food and protein bar)	www.prosnack.com
RELAXATION AIDS	
Somerset Entertainment: Sonic Aid (meditation and sleep CD series by Dr. Lee Bartel)	www.somersetent.com

PRODUCT/RESOURCE	WEB SITE
TOXIN-FREE HOUSEHOLD CLEANING PRODUCTS	
NatureClean	www.naturecleanliving.com
Attitude	www.labonneattitude.com
Seventh Generation	www.seventhgeneration.com
WATER FILTRATION SYSTEM	
Nimbus Water Systems	www.nimbuswatersystems.com
ORGANIC COTTON BEDDING AND MATTRESSES	
Guide to Less Toxic Products (provides numerous sources)	www.lesstoxicguide.ca
Essentia Natural Memory Foam Mattresses	www.myessentia.com
HEALTH INFORMATION RESOURCES	
Life Extension Foundation	www.lef.org
SeaChoice: Healthy seafood choices	www.seachoice.org
Harvard School of Public Health: The Nutrition Source	www.hsph.harvard.edu/nutritionsource/index.html
Whole Foods Market: Tasty soup recipes!	www.wholefoodsmarket.com/recipes
Environmental Working Group: Information about cosmetics, seafood safety, etc.	www.ewg.org
Calorie King: Nutrition information database	www.calorieking.com
Glycemic Index Foundation (University of Sydney; includes database)	www.glycemicindex.com
Internationl Table of GI Values	www.ajcn.org/cgi/content/full/76/1/5#SEC2
International Hormone Society	www.intlhormonesociety.org
SALIVA HORMONE TESTING—SPECIFICALLY 4-POINT CORTISOL	
Neuroscience Labs	www.neurorelief.com

GENERAL INDEX

Boldface page references indicate illustrations. <u>Underscored</u> references indicate tables or boxed text. See also the separate index of recipes.

Abdominal bloating, 41
Abs+, 269
Addiction. *See* Carb addiction
Adiponectin, 90, <u>122</u>, 289
Adrenaline, 84, 254
Aging
  appetite control loss with, 58
  carb sensitivity increase with, 4
  CoQ10 decrease with, <u>276</u>
  insulin resistance increase with, 16, 17, 39
Alarm clocks, 79–80
Alcohol, 89–90, 94, <u>240</u>
All Flora probiotics, 220, 269
Alpha lipoic acid (ALA), <u>276–77</u>
Alzheimer's disease, <u>49–51</u>
Androgen imbalance, 45–46, <u>52</u>
Anthocyanins, <u>124</u>
Antidepressant drugs, 67, 251
Anxiety, hormonal balance and, 66
Appetite
  aging and loss of control over, 58
  appetizers and, 90–91
  brain and sense of satiety, <u>63–64</u>
  carbs and loss of control over, 58
  carb sensitivity and increase in, 62–63
  cheat meals' effect on, 204
  eggs aiding control of, <u>123</u>
  emotional eating and, <u>85</u>, <u>86</u>
  excess insulin increasing, 42
  factors affecting, <u>59–60</u>, 74
  hormones controlling, <u>60–62</u>, 63
  hypothalamus gland and control of, 59
  leptin drop increasing, 35, 36
  sex and control of, 95–96
Appetizers, appetite control and, 90–91
Artificial coloring, avoiding, 111
Artificial sweeteners, 40, 88–89, 110
Ashwagandha, <u>81</u>, 103, 284
Avocados, <u>119–120</u>
Awakening from sleep, 77–78, 79–80

Beans, preventing gas from, 164
Berries, cravings curbed by, 117
Beta-sitosterol, <u>120</u>
Bio-K+ probiotics, 219, 268
Blender, portable, 347
Blood glucose or blood sugar
  carbs turned into, 25
  chromium and, <u>275</u>
  exercise improving, 290
  fasting blood sugar test, 44–45, 428
  "good" vs. "bad" carbs and, 25–26, **26**
  muscles' use of, 287
  net carbs and, 27–28, 29
  reduced by insulin, 31–32
  strength training vs. aerobic endurance training and, 288
  2-hour postprandial (pp) glucose and insulin test, 428
  uses in a healthy body, 30–31
  vitamin C and, <u>277</u>
  yoga improving, 292
Blood pressure, high, 48
Blood tests
  complete list of, 434–35
  copper, 427
  cortisol, 431–32
  DHEAs, 431
  estradiol and estrone, 432–33
  fasting cholesterol (total, HDL and LDL), 429
  fasting glucose and insulin, 428
  fasting homocysteine, 429–430
  fasting triglycerides test, 428–29
  ferritin, 430–31
  follicle-stimulating hormone (FSH), 431
  free and total testosterone, 432
  HbA1C levels, 429
  high-sensitivity C-reactive protein, 430
  IGF-1, 434
  instructions for, 436

liver function tests for AST, ALT, and bilirubin, 426–27
luteinizing hormone (LH), 431
notes about hormone tests, 435–36
progesterone, 433
RBC Magnesium, 426
saliva hormone analysis vs., 435–36
saving a copy of results, 425–26
TSH, Free T3, Free T4 and thyroid antibodies, 433–34
25-hydroxy vitamin D₃, 434
2-hour postprandial (pp) glucose and insulin, 428
uric acid, 429
zinc, 427–28
Blueberries, 118–19
Body fat. See Fat, body
Bombesin, 61
Bowel-cleansing formulas, 221–22
Bowel function, 247–49
Brain
   carb addiction and, 74–75
   glucose use by, 30–31
   insulin resistance in, 49–50, 63–64
   sense of satiety and, 63–64
Breakfast. See Meal plans
Breakfast, carbs at, 24, 109
B vitamins, 103

Caffeine, 111–12
Calcium, 273
Calories
   burned by muscle, 286
   checking on labels, 129
   excess insulin and consumption of, 42
   extreme restriction unsustainable, 203
   in fat loss equation, 9
   importance of sources of, 20
   metabolism lowered by reducing, 203
   percentage from carbs, 17
   stress hormones from restricting, 257
Cancer, 49, 241
Capsaicin, 138
Carb addiction. See also Cravings
   breaking with CSP, 71–72
   Carb Sensitivity Program breaking, 14
   cultural, 7, 8
   cycle of, 73
   digestive tract health reducing, 86–93
   dopamine and, 64–65, 67–68
   factors fueling, 73
   prevalence in overweight adults, 70
   questions for determining, 70–71

regular sex reducing, 95–96
serotonin and, 65–68
sleeping well reducing, 75–82
stress management reducing, 82–86
supplements reducing, 96–103
warmth and sunlight reducing, 93–95
withdrawal from, 64
"Carb coma," 42
Carbohydrates. See also Cheat meals
   American Diabetes Association recommendations, 7–8
   appetite control loss due to, 58
   balancing with fats and protein, 92–93, 130, 130
   benefits of reducing intake of, 17
   at breakfast, 24, 109
   checking on labels, 128–29
   cholesterol elevated by, 48–49
   cultural addiction to, 7, 8
   eliminating, ills of, 24–25
   "good" vs. "bad," 25–27, 26
   hidden sources of, 25
   hormonal effects of, 29–37
   individual tolerance variations for, 19–20
   insulin release triggered by, 9, 31
   intakes for women and men, 130
   low–GI, 26
   low-glycemic, insulin surge from, 10
   low-glycemic-load, 27
   net carbs, 27–29, 28
   never consuming alone, 109
   nutrient-poor, 40
   overeating and fat storage, 33
   percentage in hormonally-balanced diet, 16
   Phase One foods, 139, 147, 148
   Phase Two foods, 152, 159, 160
   Phase Three foods, 164, 172, 173
   Phase Four foods, 177, 185, 186
   Phase Five foods, 190, 198, 199
   Phase Six foods, 203, 213–14, 215
   problems with no-carb and low-carb diets, 18–19, 19
   serotonin released by, 66–67
   to avoid in Phase One, 149, 150
   to avoid in Phase Two, 161
   to avoid in Phase Three, 174, 175
   to avoid in Phase Four, 187, 188
   to avoid in Phase Five, 200, 201
   US dietary guidelines for, 7, 16–17
   varying with each CSP phase, 134–35

Carb sensitivity
  aging and increase in, 4
  appetite increase with, 62–63
  author's experience with, 1–2
  degrees of, 14
  importance of, 10
  inflammation linked to, 236
  insulin resistance circle with, 9–10
  in metabolic damage formula,
    233–34
  metabolic repair need with, 38
  metabolism impacted by, 14
  questions for determining, 14–15
  reversing, 55–56
  symptoms of, 1, 3
  unique to each person, 3
Carb Sensitivity Checklists
  about, 135
  Phase One, 150–51
  Phase Two, 162–63
  Phase Three, 175–76
  Phase Four, 188–89
  Phase Five, 201–2
Carb Sensitivity Program (CSP), 133. *See
  also specific phases*
  constipation during, 113–16
  cravings during, 112, 116–18
  described, 3, 13
  detoxification during, 111–12, 139
  dietary rules for all phases, 108–11
  dining out and, 113
  discovering your carb tolerance using,
    22, 107–8
  exercising while following, 112
  as extension of author's previous
    works, 3, 13
  feelings to expect on, 111–12
  general nutrition plan info, 134–36
  insulin reduced in body by, 18
  label reading during, 128–29
  metabolism repaired by, 10, 14
  pH balance and, 126–28
  quick summary of weekly meal guide,
    20–21
  shake ingredient options, 136–38
  snack options, 135–38
  supportive supplements,
    218–230
  weight loss on, 13
Carb Sensitivity Shakes. *See* Shakes
  and smoothies
Celtic sea salt, 281–82

Cheat meals
  benefits of, 203–4
  in Metabolic Repair Diet, 151, 163, 176,
    189, 202, 246, 261
  in Phase Six, 203–5
  quick guidelines for, 204–5
  water retention after, 205
Cherries, 123–24
Chia seed, 115, 120
Children, obesity in, 12, 52–53
Cholesterol
  blood tests for, 429
  improved by spices, 121
  lowered by beta-sitosterol, 120
  raised by carb consumption, 48–49
Cholestokinin (CCK), 60–61
Choline-Inositol supplement, 220
Chromium, 275
Cinnamon, 122–23
Circuit training, 296
CLA, 269
Clear Balance—Stress Modifying
  Formula, 80, 102
Clear Calm—GABA Enhancing Formula,
  97–98
Clear CLA, 269
Clear Detox—Digestive Health, 114,
  221–22
Clear Detox—Hormonal Health, 220
Clear Energy—Dopamine Support
  Formulla, 101
Clear Essentials—Morning and/
  or—Evening Pack, 266
Clear Fiber, 228, 272
Clear Flora, 115, 219, 268
Clear Metabolism, 283
Clear Mood—Serotonin Support
  Formula, 99
Clear Omega—Extra Strength Fish Oils,
  223, 268
Clear Recovery, 270
Clothing for sleep, 76–77
Coenzyme Q10 (CoQ10), 276
Coffee, 111–12
Conjugated linoleic acid (CLA), 269
Constipation, 113–16
Copper, blood test for, 427
Core, engaging during workouts, 301
Cortisol
  blood test for, 431–32
  caloric intake increased by, 68
  carb consumption fueled by, 74

effects of, 69
massage aiding breakdown of, 84
sleep deprivation and, 76
strenuous exercise increasing, 295
stress and, 68, 254
supplements reducing, 102–3
symptoms of excess, 101–2
Cravings, 116–18. *See also* Carb addiction
cessation during Phase One, 139
cheat meals' effect on, 204
coffee and, 112
preventing, 117–18
CSP. *See* Carb Sensitivity Program
CSP Flowcharts
Phase One, **151**
Phase Two, **163**
Phase Three, **176**
Phase Four, **189**
Phase Five, 202
CSP Metabolic Master Brew, 138
CSP Success Stories, 23, 37, 57, 72, 104,
133, 217, 230, 259, 285, 343

Dairy and substitutes
Phase One foods, 148
Phase Two foods, 160
Phase Three foods, 173
Phase Four foods, 186
Phase Five foods, 199
Phase Six foods, 215
to avoid in Phase One, 151
to avoid in Phase Two, 161
to avoid in Phase Three, 175
to avoid in Phase Four, 188
to avoid in Phase Five, 201
to avoid in Phase Six, 216
Depression, hormonal balance and, 66
Detoxification
during the CSP, 111–12, 139
supplements aiding, 220–22
DHA supplements, 222–24
DHEAs, blood test for, 431
Diabesity epidemic, 11–12
Diabetes
American Diabetes Association diet, 7–8
carb consumption related to, 8
diabesity epidemic, 11–12
fasting blood sugar test for, 44–45
health-care costs of, 12
intestinal bacteria and, 250
magnesium supplementation and, 272–73
medications and risk of, 251

nuts and nut butters preventing, 125
prevalence of, 11–12
projections for 2030, 12
spices as antidiabetic, 121
strength training improving, 288
type 2, reversing, 55–56
Dietary fats. *See* Fats, dietary
Diet diary, 108
Diets. *See also* Carb Sensitivity Program
(CSP)
confusion resulting from, 24
failure to lose weight on, 13–14
hormonally balanced, 16
low-fat, eating healthy fats vs., 16
medical disagreement about, 15
no-carb and low-carb, problems with,
18–19, **19**
yo-yo dieting, 257
Digestive tract health
alcohol and, 89–90
bowel function, 247–49
estrogen dominance and, 240
fiber supporting, 87–88
immune system and, 247
intestinal bacteria and, 249–250
olive oil aiding, 90
questions for determining, 248
supplements supporting, 86–87
timing of meals and, 91–92
Dining out, 113
Dinner. *See* Meal plans
Dopamine
carb addiction and, 64–65, 67–68, 74
sex increasing, 96
spike due to insulin, 42
supplements increasing, 100 101
symptoms of depletion, 100
Dream Protein, 225–26, 271
Drinks to avoid
Phase One, 151
Phase Two, 162
Phase Three, 175
Phase Four, 188
Phase Five, 201
Phase Six, 216
Drinks to enjoy
Phase One, 148
Phase Two, 160
Phase Three, 174
Phase Four, 187
Phase Five, 199–200
Phase Six, 215

Eating out, 113
Eggs, 123
Electromagnetic fields (EMFs), 78
Emotional eating, controlling, 85–86
Enterostatin, 61
EPA supplements, 222–24
Epigallocatechin gallate (EGCG), 278
Equipment for exercises, 298
Essential fatty acids
  brands recommended, 116
  constipation reduced by, 116
Estradiol, blood test for, 432–33
Estrogen
  blood tests for, 432–33
  effects of insulin resistance on, 45–46
Estrogen dominance, 239–241, 240
Estrone, blood test for, 432–33
Exercise. See also Metabolic Repair Workout
  blood sugar improved by, 290
  circuit training, 296
  during the CSP, 112
  estrogen dominance and lack of, 241
  overexercising, 295
  strength training vs. aerobic endurance
    training, 288–89
  walking, 112
Exercises
  Alternating Lateral Lunge with Single
    DB Front Raise, 307, 307
  Alternating Lunge Rotate Low to High,
    311, 311
  Alternating Lunge with Biceps Curl, 335,
    335
  Alternating T-bar Pushup, 310–11, 310
  Duck Squat with Front Shoulder Raise,
    328, 328
  Floor or Step Mountain Climbers, 339,
    339
  Hamstring Stretch LEFT Row/Twist/
    Press, 322, 322
  Hamstring Stretch RIGHT Row/Twist/
    Press, 319, 319
  Horizontal Up/Out, In/Down, 338, 338
  Isolated Squat with Concentration
    Biceps Curl LEFT, 325, 325
  Isolated Squat with Concentration
    Biceps Curl RIGHT, 321, 321
  Lying Chest Press with Leg Bicycle, 314,
    314
  Lying Triceps Extension with Bent
    Knees, 329, 329
  Plank with Leg Raise LEFT and Glute
    Flex, 313, 313

Plank with Leg Raise RIGHT and Glute
    Flex, 310, 310
  Prison Jacks, 326, 326
  SB Abdominal Reach, 306, 306
  SB Alternating Ab Crossover (hand to
    knee), 318, 318
  SB Alternating Back Row and Reverse
    Back Fly, 333, 333
  SB Alternating Chest Press, 317, 317
  SB Alternating Shoulder Press, 322,
    322
  SB Alternating Triceps Extension, 325,
    325
  SB Hamstring Curl, 306–7, 306
  SB Pushup Stance with Drawing Knees
    to Chest, 328, 328
  Side Plank LEFT with Lateral Arm
    Raise RIGHT, 334, 334
  Side Plank RIGHT with Lateral Arm
    Raise LEFT, 339, 339
  Split Leg Jump with Crossing Rotation,
    314, 314
  Standing Hammer Biceps Curl into
    90-degree Lateral Raise, 330, 330
  Standing Single Leg LEFT Balance with
    Single Arm Press LEFT, 337, 337
  Standing Single Leg RIGHT Balance
    with Single Arm Press RIGHT,
    332, 332
  Standing Squat/Press, 305, 305
  Three-Point Lunge LEFT, 321, 321
  Three-Point Lunge RIGHT, 316, 316
  Warmup for exercise, 302–3
  Weighted Stepup LEFT with High
    Knee RIGHT, 309, 309
  Weighted Stepup RIGHT with High
    Knee LEFT, 313, 313
  Wide Stance Alternating Shoulder
    Lateral/Front Raise, 324, 324

Fasting blood sugar test, 44–45
Fasting cholesterol (total, HDL and LDL)
    test, 429
Fasting glucose and insulin test, 428
Fasting homocysteine test, 429–430
Fasting triglycerides test, 428–29
Fat, body
  belly fat link to high insulin, 39
  fat loss equation, 9
  glucose storage as, 31
  insulin promoting storage of, 31, 32,
    38–39, 41–42, 107
  insulin resistance in, 45

interval cardio training for burning, 291–92
toxins accumulated in, 251
Fats, dietary. *See also specific kinds*
in all CSP phases, 134
in avocados, 119–120
balancing with protein and carbs, 92–93, 130, 130
checking on labels, 129
in chia seed, 120
consuming carbs with, 109
estrogen dominance due to, 240
healthy fats vs. low-fat diets, 16
intakes for women and men, 130
kinds to avoid or limit, 110
need for, 33
omega-3 fish oils, 222–24, 223
percentage in hormonally-balanced diet, 16
Phase One foods, 139, 147, 148
Phase Two foods, 159, 160
Phase Three foods, 173, 174
Phase Four foods, 185–86
Phase Five foods, 198, 199
Phase Six foods, 214, 215
right types for weight loss, 92
to avoid in Phase One, 149, 150
to avoid in Phase Two, 161–62
to avoid in Phase Three, 174, 175
to avoid in Phase Four, 187, 188
to avoid in Phase Five, 200, 201
types, sources, and risks/benefits, 131
Fatty liver disease, 51, 258
Feedback, sharing, 4
Feelings during the CSP, 111–12
Ferritin, blood test for, 430–31
Fiber
checking on labels, 129
constipation relieved by, 114, 115
cravings prevented by, 118
importance in diet, 87–88
supplements, 227–28, 272
FiberSMART, 222
Fiber-Tastic! 228, 272
Fiji brand water, 111
5-HTP, 81–82, 99
Flaxseed, 115, 120–21
Flowcharts. *See* CSP Flowcharts
Follicle-stimulating hormone (FSH) test, 431
Free T3 and Free T4 blood tests, 433–34
Fructose, avoiding, 110
Fruits, organic, 109

Fruits to avoid
Phase One, 149
Phase Two, 161
Phase Three, 174
Phase Four, 187
Phase Five, 200
Phase Six, 215–16
Fruits to enjoy
Phase One, 147
Phase Two, 159
Phase Three, 172
Phase Four, 185
Phase Five, 198
Phase Six foods, 213
FSH test, 431

Gamma-aminobutyric acid (GABA), 81, 97–98, 292–93
Gastin inhibitory peptide (GIP), 61
Genetics, lifestyle changes affecting, 55–56
Gentle Fibers, 228, 272
G.I. Fortify, 222
Glass containers, 348
Glutamine, cravings curbed by, 117
Gluten, 177
Glycemic index (GI)
described, 26
low–GI carbs, 26
net carbs and, 28–29
Glycemic load (GL)
described, 27
low-glycemic-load carbs, 27
Glyci-Med Forte, 90, 270–71
Glycogen, storage of, 30–31
Grains
gluten in, 177
limiting at breakfast, 109
not permitted in Phase One, 147, 149
not permitted in Phase Three, 172, 174
Phase Two foods, 159
Phase Four foods, 177, 185
Phase Five foods, 190, 198
Phase Six foods, 213
to avoid in Phase Two, 161
to avoid in Phase Four, 187
to avoid in Phase Five, 200
to avoid in Phase Six, 215
Green tea, 278

HbAIC levels test, 429
Health care
author's philosophy of, 4
three most important things for, 2

Heart disease, carbs and risk of, 48
Heart rate monitor (HRM), 293–94, 297
Herbal cleansing formulas, 220–21
High-sensitivity C-reactive protein
    (hs-CRP) test, 430
Homocysteine, blood test for, 429–430
Hormonal balance. *See also* Blood tests
    author's philosophy of, 13
    depression and anxiety and, 66
    diet for achieving, 16
    factors affecting, 29
    in fat loss equation, 9
    in healthy aging equation, 13
    high insuling disturbing, 17
    temperature and, 93
Hormones. *See also* Blood tests; *specific kinds*
    appetite controlling, 60–62
    calorie restriction and, 257
    carb elimination's effect on, 24–25
    carbs' effects on, 29–37
    nutrition habits causing imbalances,
      244–46
    saliva hormone analysis, 435–36
Hours for sleep, 77
HRM, 293–94, 297
Hs-CRP test, 430
Hunger. *See* Appetite
Hydration. *See* Drinks to enjoy; Water
Hypoglycemia, 41
Hypothalamus gland, 59
Hypothyroidism, 34–35, 282–83, 433–34

IGF-1 blood test, 434
Immune system, digestive tract health
    and, 247
Infants, obesity prevalence in, 12
Inflammation
    anti-inflammatory research, 235–36
    carb sensitivity linked to, 236
    chronic, 235
    menopause linked to, 237
    mental health linked to, 236
    metabolic damage and, 235–37
    PPAR imbalance and, 237
    signs and symptoms of, 237
    yoga reducing, 293
Inositol, 100
Insulin
    artificial sweeteners and, 88–89
    belly fat link to excess, 39
    benefits of correct amount, 30
    blood glucose reduced by, 31–32
    blood tests for, 428

calcium improving sensitivity to, 273
chromium and, 275
consequences of excess, 9–10
dopamine spike due to, 42
excess as root cause of diseases, 10
factors affecting, 243
factors leading to excess, 39–40
fat storage promoted by, 31, 32, 38–39,
    41–42, 107
functions of, 30–31
gender differences with excess, 45–46
hormones blocked by excess, 17
importance of balance in, 2
iodine and, 274
long-term impacts of excess, 43–46
magnesium enhancing function of, 34,
    272–73
means of balancing, 242
mineral levels and, 33–34
potassium and, 276
release triggered by carbs, 9
serotonin reduced by excess, 42
superfoods aiding sensitization, 109,
    118–125
super insulin-balancing nutrients,
    272–78
symptoms of excess, 40–42, 45–46
thyroid hormone affected by, 34–35
vitamin C and imbalance, 43
Insulin resistance. *See also* Metabolic
    syndrome
    aging and increase in, 16, 17, 39
    blood tests indicating, 428
    in the brain, 49–50, 63–64
    carb choices and degree of, 16
    carb sensitivity circle with, 9–10
    cellular progression of, 45, 238
    diagnosing, 47, 238
    diet's effect on, 32
    disagreement about diets for reducing, 15
    effects of, 43–44
    far-reaching effects of, **54**
    interval cardio training reducing, 290–91
    metabolic damage and, 237–38
    in metabolic damage formula, 233–34
    monounsaturated fats reducing, 122
    nicotine replacement therapy and, 54
    normal cell vs. resistant cell, **44**
    predisposition to, 9
    reversing, 55–56
    risks with, 31
    serotonin blocked by, 68
    strength training improving, 288

superfoods reducing, 118–125
vitamin D₃ reducing, 224
Interval, defined, 291
Interval cardio training
    benefits of, 290–92
    options for, 340–42
    rules for, 296–97
Intestinal bacteria, 249–250
Iodine, 274–75
Iron, blood test for, 430–31

Kidneys, glucose burned in, 30
Kitchen tips, time-saving, 347–49

Labels
    information for foods lacking, 130–31
    net carb calculation using, 28
    shopping tips using, 128–29
Laughter, stress reduced by, 85
Laxatives, avoiding if possible, 113–14
Legumes
    not permitted in Phase One, 147, 149
    not permitted in Phase Two, 159, 161
    not permitted in Phase Five, 198, 200
    Phase Three foods, 164, 172
    Phase Four foods, 185, 185
    Phase Six foods, 214
    preventing gas from beans, 164
    to avoid in Phase Three, 174
    to avoid in Phase Four, 187
Leptin
    appetite increase with drop in, 35, 36, 42
    artificial sweeteners and, 88–89
    benefits of correct amount, 36
    bodily "set" point and, 36–37
    metabolism affected by, 35–36
    serotonin's interaction with, 67
    thyroid hormone affected by, 36–37
Leptin resistance, 238–39
LH test, 431
Lifestyle
    genetics affected by changes in, 55–56
    supporting serotonin, 66
Light
    aiding sleep, 76, 78
    sun exposure, 95
Lignans, 121
Liquid Fish Oil, 224, 268
Live—G.I. Detox, 220
Live Probio+ 03mega probiotics, 220, 268
Liver
    estrogen dominance and, 240
    fatty liver disease, 51, 258

glycogen storage in, 30–31
insulin resistance in, 44–45
Liver function tests for AST, ALT, and
    bilirubin, 426–27
Low-glycemic carbs, insulin surge from, 10
L-Trepein, 220
L-tyrosine, 100–101, 284
Lunch. *See* Meal plans
Luteinizing hormone (LH) test, 431

Magnesium
    deficiency, 34
    insulin function enhanced by, 34, 272–73
    RBC Magnesium test, 426
Magnesium citrate, 115
Magnesium glycinate, 80–81, 115
Mannoheptulose, 120
Massage, stress reduced by, 84
Meal plans
    Metabolic Repair Diet after Phase One,
        263–64
    Phase One, 139–146
    Phase Two, 152–58
    Phase Three, 165–171
    Phase Four, 178–184
    Phase Five, 191–97
    Phase Six, 206–12
Medications, toxic, 250–51, 252
Meditation, stress reduced by, 83–84
MedOMEGA Liquid Fish Oil, 223, 268
Melanocortin, 95
Melatonin, 82, 94
Men
    estrogen dominance in, 239
    excess insulin and, 45
    protein, carb and fat intake for, 130
Menopause, inflammation and, 237
Mental health, inflammation and, 236
Metabolic damage
    conditions associated with, 234–35
    estrogen dominance and, 239–241
    factors causing, 242
    fatty liver disease causing, 258
    formula for, 233–34
    inflammation and, 235–37
    insulin resistance and, 237–38
    intestinal bacteria and, 249–250
    leptin resistance and, 238–39
    muscle lack or loss and, 255–56
    nutrient deficiencies, 255
    omega-3 fish oils restoring, 223
    repaired by Carb Sensitivity Program,
        10, 14

Metabolic damage *(cont.)*
    sleep deprivation causing, 256–57
    stress causing, 254
    toxins and medications causing, 250–52
    yo-yo dieting causing, 257
Metabolic profile assessment. *See* Blood
        tests
Metabolic Repair Diet. *See also* Carb
        Sensitivity Checklists; CSP
        Flowcharts
    carb sensitivity and need for, 38
    cheat meals in, 151, 163, 176, 189, 202,
        246, 261
    optional products, 270–72
    after Phase One, 151, 260–64
    after phases two through five, 163, 176,
        189, 202, 260–61
    super insulin-balancing nutrients,
        272–78
    supplements, 264–270
    time required for, 108
Metabolic Repair Pack, 265–66
Metabolic Repair Workout. *See also* Exercise
    daily routine, 299–300
    Day 1 Strength-Training Routine, 304–14
    Day 2 Strength-Training Routine,
        315–326
    Day 3 Strength-Training Routine, 327–339
    equipment for, 298
    general instructions for, 301–3
    heart rate monitor advantages, 293–94
    importance for insulin sensitivity,
        287–290
    increasing intensity of, 300
    interval cardio training, 290–92, 340–42
    poster displaying exercises, 300
    rules for, 296–97
    tips to keep on track, 340
    warmup for, 302–3
    weekly schedule, 298–99, 299
    yoga, 292–93, 297
Metabolic syndrome. *See also* Insulin
        resistance
    Alzheimer's disease and, 49–51
    androgen imbalance in women and, 52
    cancer risk and, 49
    childhood obesity and, 52–53
    cholesterol imbalance and, 48–49
    fatty liver disease and, 51
    heart disease risk and, 48
    high blood pressure and, 48
    iodine preventing, 274
    muscle tissue loss and, 51

osteoporosis risk and, 53
pregnancy complications and, 52
prevalence of, 46
reproductive abnormalities and, 51–52
risk factors for, 47
seasonal weight changes linked to, 50
skin abnormalities and, 51
stroke risk and, 49
Metabolism. *See also* Metabolic damage
    cheat meals' effect on, 203–4
    CSP Metabolic Master Brew, 138
    leptin and regulation of, 35–36
    lowered by reducing calories, 203
    vitamin C and, 277–78
Minerals, insulin and levels of, 33–34
Monounsaturated fats
    avocados providing, 119
    benefits of eating, 16
    nuts and nut butters providing, 125
    weight loss aided by, 122
Movies, funny, 85
MultiBiotic 4000 probiotics, 219, 268
Multivitamin, high-potency, 266–67
Muscles
    calories burned by, 286
    enhancing insulin sensitivity in,
        287–89
    glycogen storage in, 30–31
    insulin resistance and tissue loss, 51
    insulin resistance in, 45
    metabolic equation for, 255–56, 289
    strength training vs. aerobic endurance
        training and, 288–89

N et carbs, 27–29, **28**
Neuropeptide Y (NPY), 68–69, 74
Nicotine replacement therapy, 54
Nitrites, avoiding, 111
Norepinephrine, 74
Nusera lozenges, 117
Nutra Sea High Potency Capsules, 224, 268
Nutrient deficiencies, 240–41, 255
Nutrition labels. *See* Labels
Nuts and seeds
    insulin-sensitizing superfoods, 125
    peanuts, avoiding, 149, 161, 174, 187,
        200, 216
    Phase One foods, 147
    Phase Two foods, 159
    Phase Three foods, 172
    Phase Four foods, 185–86
    Phase Five foods, 198
    Phase Six foods, 214

Omega-3 extra strength, 223, 268
Obesity
  carb consumption related to, 8
  diabesity epidemic, 11–12
  prevalence in children and infants, 12
  prevalence in US and Canada, 46
  sun exposure reducing, 95
  vitamin D and, 95
Oils
  Phase One foods, 148
  Phase Two foods, 160
  Phase Three foods, 173
  Phase Four foods, 186
  Phase Five foods, 199
  Phase Six foods, 215
  to avoid in Phase One, 151
  to avoid in Phase Two, 162
  to avoid in Phase Three, 175
  to avoid in Phase Four, 188
  to avoid in Phase Five, 201
  to avoid in Phase Six, 216
Oligosaccharide, 164
Olive oil
  benefits of, 90
  as insulin-sensitizing superfood,
    121–22
Omega-3 fish oils, 222–24
Organic Clear Fiber, 228, 272
Osteoporosis, 53
Overexercising, 295
Oxyntomodulin (OXM), 61
Oxytocin, 96

Pcos, 1–2, 51–52
Peanuts
  avoiding in all phases, 149, 161, 174,
    187, 200, 216
  cautions for eating, 110
Peptide YY (PYY), 61
Phase One. See also Carb Sensitivity
    Program (CSP)
  additional assistance, 151
  Carb Sensitivity Checklist, 150–51
  constipation during, 114–16
  CSP Flowchart, 151
  detoxification during, 139
  foods to avoid, 149–150
  foods to enjoy, 147–48
  meal plan, 140–46
  Metabolic Repair Diet after, 151, 260–64
  overview, 139
  retrying after Metabolic Repair Diet,
    151, 261

Phase Two. See also Carb Sensitivity
    Program (CSP)
  additional assistance, 163
  Carb Sensitivity Checklist, 162–63
  CSP Flowchart, 163
  foods to avoid, 161–62
  foods to enjoy, 159–160
  meal plan, 152–58
  Metabolic Repair Diet after, 163, 260–61
  overview, 152
  retrying after Metabolic Repair Diet,
    163, 261
Phase Three. See also Carb Sensitivity
    Program (CSP)
  additional assistance, 176
  Carb Sensitivity Checklist, 175–76
  CSP Flowchart, 176
  foods to avoid, 174–75
  foods to enjoy, 172–74
  meal plan, 165–171
  Metabolic Repair Diet after, 176, 260–61
  overview, 164
  retrying after Metabolic Repair Diet,
    176, 261
Phase Four. See also Carb Sensitivity
    Program (CSP)
  additional assistance, 189
  Carb Sensitivity Checklist, 188–89
  CSP Flowchart, 189
  foods to avoid, 187–88
  foods to enjoy, 185–87
  meal plan, 178–184
  Metabolic Repair Diet after, 189, 260–61
  overview, 177
  retrying after Metabolic Repair Diet,
    189, 261
Phase Five. See also Carb Sensitivity
    Program (CSP)
  additional assistance, 202
  Carb Sensitivity Checklist, 201–2
  CSP Flowchart, 202
  foods to avoid, 200–201
  foods to enjoy, 198–200
  meal plan, 191–97
  Metabolic Repair Diet after, 202, 260–61
  overview, 190
  retrying after Metabolic Repair Diet,
    202, 261
Phase Six. See also Carb Sensitivity
    Program (CSP)
  cheat meals in, 203–5
  foods to avoid, 215–16
  foods to enjoy, 213–15

Phase Six *(cont.)*
   meal plan, 206–12
   overview, 203
pH balance, 126–28
Phosphatidylserine (PS), 103
Polycystic ovarian symdrome (PCOS),
   1–2, <u>51–52</u>
Potassium, <u>226–27</u>, <u>275–76</u>
Pregnancy, metabolic syndrome and, <u>52</u>
Preservatives, avoiding, 111
ProbioMax Daily DF probiotics, 269
ProbioMax Daily probiotics, 220
Probiotic supplements, 114–15, 219–220,
   268–69
ProDHA Capsules, 223, 268
Produce. *See* Fruits to avoid; Fruits to
   enjoy; Vegetables, nonstarchy;
   Vegetables, starchy
ProEFA, 223, 268
Progesterone, blood test for, 433
Proliferator-activated receptors (PPARs), 237
Protein
   in all CSP phases, 134
   balancing with fats and carbs, 92–93,
      130, <u>130</u>
   checking on labels, 129
   consuming carbs with, 109
   cooking in batches, twice weekly, 348–49
   cravings prevented by, 117
   intakes for women and men, <u>130</u>
   need for, 33
   percentage in hormonally-balanced
      diet, 16
   Phase One foods, 139, 147–48
   Phase Two foods, 159–160
   Phase Three foods, 173, 174
   Phase Four foods, 185–86
   Phase Five foods, 198–99
   Phase Six foods, 214–15
   to avoid in Phase One, 149–150
   to avoid in Phase Two, 161
   to avoid in Phase Three, 174–75
   to avoid in Phase Four, 187–88
   to avoid in Phase Five, 200–201
   to avoid in Phase Six, 216
Protein bars, <u>148</u>, <u>160</u>, <u>173</u>, <u>186</u>, <u>199</u>, <u>215</u>
Proteins +, 226, 271
PS, 103
PYY, <u>61</u>

RBC Magnesium test, 426
Relora, 102
Reproductive abnormalities, <u>51–52</u>

Resistance training. *See* Metabolic Repair
   Workout
Restaurants, eating at, 113
Resveratrol, 271
Rhodiola, 102–3

Saliva hormone analysis, 435–36
Saliva test for pH balance, 127
Salmon, avoiding farmed, 111
Salt or sodium, 34, 129, <u>226</u>, <u>281–82</u>
Seasonal weight changes, <u>50</u>, 65
Serotonin
   appetite control and, <u>61–62</u>, 63
   carb addiction and, 65–68, 74
   carb intake releasing, 66–67
   insulin resistance blocking, 68
   leptin's interaction with, 67
   lifestyle supporting, 66
   reduced by excess insulin, 42
   seasonal weight changes and, 65
   supplements increasing, 99–100
   symptoms of depletion, 66, 98–99
Serving sizes
   on nutrition labels, 128
   Phase One foods, 147–48, <u>147</u>
   Phase Two foods, 159–160, <u>159</u>
   Phase Three foods, 172–73, <u>172</u>, <u>173</u>
   Phase Four foods, 185–86, <u>185</u>, <u>186</u>
   Phase Five foods, 198–99, <u>198</u>, <u>199</u>
   Phase Six foods, 213–14, <u>213</u>, <u>214</u>
"Set" point, leptin and, 36–37
Sex, appetite control and, 95–96
Shaker cup, 348
Shakes and smoothies
   options for ingredients, 136–38
   recipes using superfoods, <u>125</u>
   as snacks, 135
Skin abnormalities, <u>51</u>
Skin care products, <u>252–53</u>
Skipping meals, avoiding, 91–92
Sleep
   amount needed, 77
   awakening from, 77–78, 79–80
   carb consumption and, 94
   natural sleep aids, <u>80–82</u>
   rules for healthy rest, 76–80
Sleep deprivation
   cravings with, 118
   estrogen dominance with, <u>241</u>
   ills of, 75–76
   leptin depletion with, 35–36
   metabolic damage due to, 256–57
Smooth Food 2 probiotics, 220, 269

Smoothies. *See* Shakes and smoothies
Snacks. *See also* Meal plans
    approved options, 135–38
    cravings prevented by, 117
    in Phase One menu plan, 139
    preparing in bulk, 348
    shakes for, 135, 136–38
    before and after workouts, 297
Sodium or salt, 34, 129, 226, 281–82
Space for sleeping, 78–79
Spices, as insulin-sensitizing superfoods, 121
Spices and condiments to avoid
    Phase One, 151
    Phase Two, 162
    Phase Three, 175
    Phase Four, 188
    Phase Five, 201
    Phase Six, 216
Spices and condiments to enjoy
    Phase One, 148
    Phase Two, 160
    Phase Three, 173
    Phase Four, 186–87
    Phase Five, 199
    Phase Six, 215
Strength training. *See* Metabolic Repair
        Workout
Stress
    calorie restriction and, 257
    cortisol released by, 68, 254
    managing, 82–86
    metabolic damage due to, 254
    prolonged, 69–70
    reducing cravings due to, 117
    serotonin depleted by, 66
    stress-related eating, 82
    yoga relieving, 292
Stretching after workouts, 303
Stroke, 49
Success stories. *See* CSP Success Stories
Sugars. *See also* Blood glucose or blood
        sugar; carbs
    avoiding to prevent cravings, 117
    hidden sources of, 117
    insulin release triggered by, 31
    uses in a healthy body, 30–31
Sulfites, avoiding, 111
Sun exposure, 95
Super DHA Capsules, 223, 268
Superfoods, insulin-sensitizing, 118–125
    avocados, 119–120
    blueberries, 118–19
    cherries, 123–24

chia seed, 120
cinnamon, 122–23
eggs, 123
flaxseed, 120–21
nuts and nut butters, 125
olive oil, 121–22
selecting often, 109
shake recipes using, 125
spices, 121
vinegar, 124
whey protein isolate, 119
Supplements
    benefits of, 218
    bowel-cleansing formulas, 221–22
    conjugated linoleic acid, 269
    constipation relieving, 114–16
    cortisol reducing, 102–3
    CSP Kit, 219, 228
    CSP Metabolic Repair Kit, 280–81
    daily prescription for CSP, 229–230
    for digestive tract health, 86–87
    dopamine enhancing, 100–101
    dosing chart for Metabolic Repair, 279–280
    fiber, 227–28, 272
    GABA enhancing, 97–98
    Glyci-Med Forte, 90
    herbal cleansing formulas, 220–21
    high-potency multivitamin, 266–67
    Metabolic Repair, 264–270, 278, 279–281
    Metabolic Repair Pack, 265–66
    omega-3 fish oils, 222–24, 267
    optional products, 270–72
    probiotic, 114–15, 219–220, 268–69
    serotonin enhancing, 99–100
    sleep aids, 80–82
    super insulin-balancing nutrients, 272–78
    supportive for all phases, 218–230
    thyroid supporting, 283–84
    vitamin D$_3$, 224, 269–270
    whey protein isolate, 119, 225–26, 271

Taurine, 98
Tea, herbal, for curbing cravings, 117
Temperature for sleeping, 79, 93–94
Testosterone
    blood tests for, 432
    effects of insulin resistance on, 45–46, 52
Thyroid antibodies blood test, 433–34
Thyroid hormone
    blood tests for, 433–34
    cheat meals increasing, 203
    hypothyroidism, 34–35, 282–83, 433–34
    insulin's effect on, 34–35

Thyroid hormone *(cont.)*
    iodine and, 274–75
    leptin's effect on, 36–37
    strenuous exercise reducing, 295
    thyroid-supporting supplements, 283–84
Timing of meals, 91–92, 110, 139
Toxin exposure, 40
Toxins
    metabolism disrupting, 250–52
    in skin care products, 252–53
Trans fatty acids, avoiding, 110
Triglycerides, 33, 428–29
TSH blood test, 433–34
25-hydroxy vitamin D$_3$, blood test for, 434
2-hour postprandial (pp) glucose and
        insulin test, 428

Ultra CLA, 269
Uric acid, blood test for, 429
Urine test for pH balance, 127

Vegetables, nonstarchy
    Phase One foods, 147
    Phase Two foods, 159
    Phase Three foods, 172
    Phase Four foods, 185
    Phase Five foods, 198
    Phase Six foods, 214
Vegetables, organic, 109
Vegetables, starchy
    limiting at breakfast, 109
    not permitted in Phase One, 147, 149
    not permitted in Phase Three, 172, 174
    Phase Two foods, 159
    Phase Four foods, 185
    Phase Five foods, 198
    Phase Six foods, 213
    to avoid in Phase Two, 161
    to avoid in Phase Four, 187
    to avoid in Phase Five, 200
    to avoid in Phase Six, 216
Vinegar, 124
Vitamin C
    chewable, cravings curbed by, 117
    constipation relieved by, 115
    insulin imbalance and, 43
    as super insulin-balancing nutrient,
        277–78
    taking during the CSP, 111
Vitamin D
    D$_3$ supplements, 224, 269–270
    obesity and, 95
    25-hydroxy vitamin D$_3$ test, 434

Walking, benefits of, 112
Water, 111, 115. *See also* Drinks to avoid;
        Drinks to enjoy
Water retention, 41, 205
Websites
    additional assistance for phases, 151,
        163, 176, 189, 202
    Book Extras on, 139, 278
    nutritional values info, 130–31
    ordering products, 115, 219, 228, 280
    poster of workout exercises, 300
    sharing feedback, 4
    skin care product info, 252, 253
    warmup and cooldown routine, 303
Weighing yourself, 108–9
Weight gain
    from antidepressant drugs, 67
    artificial sweeteners causing, 88–89
    sleep deprivation and, 76
Weight loss
    calcium improving, 273
    on Carb Sensitivity Program, 13
    dietary fats and, 92
    diets failing to produce, 13–14
    intestinal bacteria and, 249–250
    monounsaturated fats aiding, 122
    sleeping well aiding, 76
    strength training vs. aerobic endurance
        training and, 288–89
    vitamin D$_3$ aiding, 224
Whey protein isolate, 119, 225–26, 271
Withdrawal from carb addiction, 64
Women
    excess insulin and, 45–46
    premenopausal, blood test instructions
        for, 435, 436
    premenopausal, estrogen dominance
        in, 239
    protein, carb and fat intake for, 130

Yoga, 292–93, 297
Yo-yo dieting, 257

Zinc
    blood test for, 427
    as super insulin-balancing nutrient,
        273–74
    supplements, 427–28

RECIPE INDEX

Recipes are suitable for all phases unless otherwise noted.

Almond butter
  Coconut Almond Butter Protein Bars
    (Phase Five), 423
Almond flour
  Wasabi Whitefish with Almond Crust,
    380
Almond milk
  Berries and Oats Breakfast Smoothie
    (Phase Five), 409
  Berrylicious Iron-booster Smoothie, 351
  Chocolate Hazelnut Coffee Smoothie,
    350
  Cinnamon Apple Smoothie, 355
  Cinnamon Roll Smoothie, 355
  Skinny Banana Split Smoothie, 353
  Strawberry Shortcake Smoothie, 352
  Sweet Apple Pie Smoothie, 359
  Wild Berry Breakfast, 354
Apples
  Apple, Arugula and Chicken Salad
    (Phase Four), 405
  Cinnamon Apple Smoothie, 355
  Cinnamon Roll Smoothie, 355
  Coconut Almond Butter Protein Bars
    (Phase Five), 423
  Crispy Chicken and Lettuce Wraps,
    379
  Not So Devilish Eggs, 421
  Portobello Mushroom Omelette, 361
  Salmon and Dill Omelette, 362
  Selenium-boosting Shrimp and Salsa,
    376
  Sweet Apple Cinnamon Delight (Phase
    Five), 412
  Sweet Apple Pie Smoothie, 359
  Tuna Waldorf Salad, 383
Apricots
  Apricot-glazed Chicken and Kale, 372
  Apricot Yogurt Smoothie, 350

Arugula
  Apple, Arugula and Chicken Salad
    (Phase Four), 405
Asparagus
  Garlic Chicken and Asparagus, 370
  Red Potato and Asparagus Casserole
    (Phase Five), 418
Avocados
  Awesome Avocado and Egg Breakfast,
    360
  Miso Salad, 368

Bacon. *See* Turkey bacon
Bananas
  Alkalizing Breakfast Smoothie, 358
  Banana Bread Smoothie (Phase Five),
    410
  Berrylicious Iron-booster Smoothie, 351
  Chocolate Banana Smoothie, 351
  Coco-Vanilla Smoothie, 356
  Mint Chocolate Smoothie, 352
  Orange Vanilla Shake, 353
  Perfect Balance Banana Bread, 424
  Piña Colada Smoothie, 357
  Skinny Banana Split Smoothie, 353
Barley
  Barley and Spinach-stuffed Bell
    Peppers (Phase Five), 411–12
Beans. *See also* Green beans
  Beautiful Bean and Protein Salad
    (Phase Three), 396
  Bison Chili and Beans (Phase Three),
    398
  Fresh Mint Chickpea Salad (Phase
    Three), 397
  Halibut and Rapini in Portobello
    Mushroom Sauce (Phase Three),
    394
  Turkey Bacon Scallops (Phase Four), 402

Beef
    Feta Cheese Meatballs with Grilled
        Vegetables, 371
Beets
    Chilled Dill and Beet Salad (Phase
        Two), 386
    Warm Beet and Goat Cheese Salad
        (Phase Two), 389
Bell peppers
    Baby Bok Choy and Chicken, 375
    Barley and Spinach-stuffed Bell
        Peppers (Phase Five), 411–12
    Beautiful Bean and Protein Salad
        (Phase Three), 396
    Bison Chili and Beans (Phase Three),
        398
    Crispy Chicken and Lettuce Wraps,
        379
    Curry Chicken Soup, 377
    Fresh Mint Chickpea Salad (Phase
        Three), 397
    Pepper and Spinach Omelette, 363
    Selenium-boosting Shrimp and Salsa,
        376
    Spicy Pepper Salmon with Pear Salsa,
        384
Berries
    Berries and Oats Breakfast Smoothie
        (Phase Five), 409
    Berrylicious Iron-booster Smoothie, 351
    Cheesecake Smoothie, 358
    Choco-Berry Breakfast (Phase Five),
        410
    Chocolate Hazelnut Coffee Smoothie,
        350
    Quick Cinnamon Quinoa (Phase Four),
        403
    Root Beer Float Smoothie, 356
    Salmon with Spinach and Strawberry
        Salsa, 381
    Strawberry Shortcake Smoothie, 352
    Wild Berry Breakfast, 354
Bison
    Bison Chili and Beans (Phase Three),
        398
Black beans. See Beans
Blueberries
    Blueberry Chicken Salad, 365
    Wild Berry Breakfast, 354
Bok choy
    Apricot-glazed Chicken and Kale, 372
    Baby Bok Choy and Chicken, 375

Broccoli
    Baby Bok Choy and Chicken, 375
    Curry Chicken Soup, 377
    Halibut and Rapini in Portobello
        Mushroom Sauce (Phase Three),
        394
Bulgur
    Chicken with Bulgur and Mushrooms
        (Phase Four), 407

Carrots
    Carrot and Ginger Soup (Phase Two),
        387
    Spicy Lentil Burgers (Phase Three),
        399
Cauliflower
    Cauliflower and Kale Soup, 382
    Curry Chicken Soup, 377
Celery
    Celery with Tuna Salad, 419
    Fresh Mint Chickpea Salad (Phase
        Three), 397
    Scrumptious Edamame Salad (Phase
        Two), 385
    Tuna Waldorf Salad, 383
Cereal
    Breakfast Cereal Smoothie (Phase
        Four), 400
Cheese. See also Cottage cheese
    Barley and Spinach-stuffed Bell
        Peppers (Phase Five), 411–12
    Blueberry Chicken Salad, 365
    Garlic Chicken and Asparagus, 370
    Grilled Mediterranean Salad, 369
    Mini Turkey Lettuce Wraps, 422
    Portobello Mushroom Caps, 420
    Spicy Pepper Poppers, 424
    Summer Tomato Lentils (Phase Three),
        395
    Warm Beet and Goat Cheese Salad
        (Phase Two), 389
    Weightless Wasa Crackers (Phase
        Four), 422
Chicken. See also Turkey; Turkey Bacon
    Apple, Arugula and Chicken Salad
        (Phase Four), 405
    Apricot-glazed Chicken and Kale,
        372
    Baby Bok Choy and Chicken, 375
    Blueberry Chicken Salad, 365
    Carrot and Ginger Soup (Phase Two),
        387

Chicken with Bulgur and Mushrooms
(Phase Four), 407
Crispy Chicken and Lettuce Wraps, 379
Curry Chicken Soup, 377
Ezekial Crumb-coated Chicken (Phase
Four), 406
Garlic Chicken and Asparagus, 370
Grilled Chicken Skewer Wraps (Phase
Four), 408
Honey Chicken and Sweet Potatoes
(Phase Five), 413
Immunity-boosting Ginger Chicken,
374
Mini Turkey Lettuce Wraps, 422
Scrumptious Edamame Salad (Phase
Two), 385
Spicy Turkey Muffins (Phase Five), 416
Summerlicious Squash with Yogurt
Chicken (Phase Two), 391
Summer Squash and Sesame Chicken
(Phase Two), 388
Chickpeas
Beautiful Bean and Protein Salad
(Phase Three), 396
Fresh Mint Chickpea Salad (Phase
Three), 397
Turkey Bacon Scallops (Phase Four), 402
Chocolate
Chocolate Banana Smoothie, 351
Chocolate Hazelnut Coffee Smoothie,
350
Mint Chocolate Smoothie, 352
Coconut water
Piña Colada Smoothie, 357
Coffee
Chocolate Hazelnut Coffee Smoothie,
350
Cottage cheese
Cheesecake Smoothie, 358
Cucumber and Cottage Cheese Salad,
373
Mint Chocolate Smoothie, 352
Quick Cinnamon Quinoa (Phase Four),
403
Crackers
Weightless Wasa Crackers (Phase
Four), 422
Cucumbers
Ahi Tuna Steak and Salad, 367
Crispy Chicken and Lettuce Wraps, 379
Cucumber and Cottage Cheese Salad,
373

Immunity-boosting Ginger Chicken,
374
Miso Salad, 368
Rosemary Salmon Steaks (Phase Five),
415
Salmon with Spinach and Strawberry
Salsa, 381
Scrumptious Edamame Salad (Phase
Two), 385
Tuna Waldorf Salad, 383

Desserts
Sweet Apple Cinnamon Delight (Phase
Five), 412
Dill
Chilled Dill and Beet Salad (Phase
Two), 386
Salmon and Dill Omelette, 362

Edamame
Scrumptious Edamame Salad (Phase
Two), 385
Eggplant
Grilled Mediterranean Salad, 369
Mexican Summer Salad, 366
Eggs
Awesome Avocado and Egg Breakfast,
360
Breakfast Salsa Dish, 364
Choco-Berry Breakfast (Phase Five), 410
Cinnamon Sweet Potato Pancakes
(Phase Five), 414
Coconut Almond Butter Protein Bars
(Phase Five), 423
Not So Devilish Eggs, 421
Pepper and Spinach Omelette, 363
Perfect Balance Banana Bread, 424
Portobello Mushroom Omelette, 361
Red Potato and Asparagus Casserole
(Phase Five), 418
Salmon and Dill Omelette, 362
Spicy Lentil Burgers (Phase Three),
399
Spicy Turkey Muffins (Phase Five), 416
Wasabi Whitefish with Almond Crust,
380
Entrées
Ahi Tuna Steak and Salad, 367
Apricot-glazed Chicken and Kale, 372
Baby Bok Choy and Chicken, 375
Barley and Spinach-stuffed Bell
Peppers (Phase Five), 411–12

Entrées *(cont.)*

    Bison Chili and Beans (Phase Three), 398

    Blueberry Chicken Salad, 365

    Cherry Tomato Salmon in Wine Broth (Phase Four), 404

    Chicken with Bulgur and Mushrooms (Phase Four), 407

    Crispy Chicken and Lettuce Wraps, 379

    Curried Pumpkin and Green Beans (Phase Two), 390

    Curried Red Lentils with Shrimp or Tofu (Phase Three), 392

    Ezekial Crumb-coated Chicken (Phase Four), 406

    Feta Cheese Meatballs with Grilled Vegetables, 371

    Garlic Chicken and Asparagus, 370

    Grilled Chicken Skewer Wraps (Phase Four), 408

    Halibut and Rapini in Portobello Mushroom Sauce (Phase Three), 394

    Honey Chicken and Sweet Potatoes (Phase Five), 413

    Immunity-boosting Ginger Chicken, 374

    Lovely Lemongrass Tofu (Phase Three), 393

    Perfect Peppercorn Fish, 378

    Quick Cinnamon Quinoa (Phase Four), 403

    Rosemary Salmon Steaks (Phase Five), 415

    Salmon with Spinach and Strawberry Salsa, 381

    Sautéed Shrimp and Green Beans, 373

    Selenium-boosting Shrimp and Salsa, 376

    Spicy Lentil Burgers (Phase Three), 399

    Spicy Pepper Salmon with Pear Salsa, 384

    Spicy Turkey Muffins (Phase Five), 416

    Summerlicious Squash with Yogurt Chicken (Phase Two), 391

    Summer Squash and Sesame Chicken (Phase Two), 388

    Summer Tomato Lentils (Phase Three), 395

    Sweet Tooth–Satisfying Salmon (Phase Five), 417

    Turkey Bacon Scallops (Phase Four), 402

    Wasabi Whitefish with Almond Crust, 380

Ezekial breads

    Ezekial Crumb-coated Chicken (Phase Four), 406

    Grilled Chicken Skewer Wraps (Phase Four), 408

Fish and seafood

    Ahi Tuna Steak and Salad, 367

    Cherry Tomato Salmon in Wine Broth (Phase Four), 404

    Halibut and Rapini in Portobello Mushroom Sauce (Phase Three), 394

    Perfect Peppercorn Fish, 378

    Rosemary Salmon Steaks (Phase Five), 415

    Salmon and Dill Omelette, 362

    Salmon with Spinach and Strawberry Salsa, 381

    Sautéed Shrimp and Green Beans, 373

    Scrumptious Edamame Salad (Phase Two), 385

    Selenium-boosting Shrimp and Salsa, 376

    Spicy Pepper Salmon with Pear Salsa, 384

    Sweet Tooth–Satisfying Salmon (Phase Five), 417

    Tuna Waldorf Salad, 383

    Turkey Bacon Scallops (Phase Four), 402

    Wasabi Whitefish with Almond Crust, 380

Fruits

    Alkalizing Breakfast Smoothie, 358

    Apple, Arugula and Chicken Salad (Phase Four), 405

    Apricot Yogurt Smoothie, 350

    Berrylicious Iron-booster Smoothie, 351

    Breakfast Cooler Smoothie, 354

    Cheesecake Smoothie, 358

    Chocolate Banana Smoothie, 351

    Chocolate Hazelnut Coffee Smoothie, 350

    Cinnamon Apple Smoothie, 355

    Cinnamon Roll Smoothie, 355

    Coconut Almond Butter Protein Bars (Phase Five), 423

Crispy Chicken and Lettuce Wraps, 379
Jelly Sandwich Smoothie, 357
Mint Chocolate Smoothie, 352
Orange Vanilla Shake, 353
Perfect Balance Banana Bread, 424
Perfect Peppercorn Fish, 378
Piña Colada Smoothie, 357
Portobello Mushroom Omelette, 361
Quick Cinnamon Quinoa (Phase Four), 403
Quinoa Salad with Orange, Walnuts and Mint (Phase Four), 401
Root Beer Float Smoothie, 356
Salmon and Dill Omelette, 362
Salmon with Spinach and Strawberry Salsa, 381
Selenium-boosting Shrimp and Salsa, 376
Skinny Banana Split Smoothie, 353
Strawberry Shortcake Smoothie, 352
Sweet Apple Pie Smoothie, 359
Tuna Waldorf Salad, 383
Wild Berry Breakfast, 354

Grains
Banana Bread Smoothie (Phase Five), 410
Barley and Spinach-stuffed Bell Peppers (Phase Five), 411–12
Berries and Oats Breakfast Smoothie (Phase Five), 409
Cherry Tomato Salmon in Wine Broth (Phase Four), 404
Chicken with Bulgur and Mushrooms (Phase Four), 407
Choco-Berry Breakfast (Phase Five), 410
Ezekial Crumb-coated Chicken (Phase Four), 406
Grilled Chicken Skewer Wraps (Phase Four), 408
Quick Cinnamon Quinoa (Phase Four), 403
Quinoa Salad with Orange, Walnuts and Mint (Phase Four), 401
Rosemary Salmon Steaks (Phase Five), 415
Spicy Turkey Muffins (Phase Five), 416
Turkey Bacon Scallops (Phase Four), 402
Weightless Wasa Crackers (Phase Four), 422

Green beans
Beautiful Bean and Protein Salad (Phase Three), 396
Curried Pumpkin and Green Beans (Phase Two), 390
Sautéed Shrimp and Green Beans, 373
Greens, salad
Ahi Tuna Steak and Salad, 367
Apple, Arugula and Chicken Salad (Phase Four), 405
Grilled Chicken Skewer Wraps (Phase Four), 408
Rosemary Salmon Steaks (Phase Five), 415
Spicy Lentil Burgers (Phase Three), 399
Spicy Turkey Muffins (Phase Five), 416
Tuna Waldorf Salad, 383
Warm Beet and Goat Cheese Salad (Phase Two), 389

Halibut
Halibut and Rapini in Portobello Mushroom Sauce (Phase Three), 394

Jalapeño peppers
Spicy Pepper Poppers, 424

Kale
Apricot-glazed Chicken and Kale, 372
Cauliflower and Kale Soup, 382
Kasha
Turkey Bacon Scallops (Phase Four), 402
Kidney beans. See Beans
Kiwi
Salmon with Spinach and Strawberry Salsa, 381

Lamb
Feta Cheese Meatballs with Grilled Vegetables, 371
Lemongrass
Lovely Lemongrass Tofu (Phase Three), 393
Lentils
Curried Red Lentils with Shrimp or Tofu (Phase Three), 392
Lovely Lemongrass Tofu (Phase Three), 393
Spicy Lentil Burgers (Phase Three), 399

Lentils *(cont.)*
  Summer Tomato Lentils (Phase Three), 395
Lettuce. *See also* Greens, salad
  Crispy Chicken and Lettuce Wraps, 379
  Grilled Chicken Skewer Wraps (Phase Four), 408
  Mini Turkey Lettuce Wraps, 422
  Summer Tomato Lentils (Phase Three), 395

Meats. *See also* Chicken; Turkey
  Bison Chili and Beans (Phase Three), 398
  Feta Cheese Meatballs with Grilled Vegetables, 371
Mint
  Fresh Mint Chickpea Salad (Phase Three), 397
  Mint Chocolate Smoothie, 352
  Quinoa Salad with Orange, Walnuts and Mint (Phase Four), 401
Miso
  Miso Salad, 368
Mushrooms
  Chicken with Bulgur and Mushrooms (Phase Four), 407
  Halibut and Rapini in Portobello Mushroom Sauce (Phase Three), 394
  Portobello Mushroom Caps, 420
  Portobello Mushroom Omelette, 361

Oats
  Banana Bread Smoothie (Phase Five), 410
  Berries and Oats Breakfast Smoothie (Phase Five), 409
  Choco-Berry Breakfast (Phase Five), 410
  Coconut Almond Butter Protein Bars (Phase Five), 423
  Spicy Turkey Muffins (Phase Five), 416
Onions
  Apricot-glazed Chicken and Kale, 372
  Awesome Avocado and Egg Breakfast, 360
  Carrot and Ginger Soup (Phase Two), 387
  Cauliflower and Kale Soup, 382
  Chilled Dill and Beet Salad (Phase Two), 386
  Crispy Chicken and Lettuce Wraps, 379

Curried Pumpkin and Green Beans (Phase Two), 390
  Curried Red Lentils with Shrimp or Tofu (Phase Three), 392
  Grilled Mediterranean Salad, 369
  Honey Chicken and Sweet Potatoes (Phase Five), 413
  Immunity-boosting Ginger Chicken, 374
  Perfect Peppercorn Fish, 378
  Red Potato and Asparagus Casserole (Phase Five), 418
  Sautéed Shrimp and Green Beans, 373
  Selenium-boosting Shrimp and Salsa, 376
  Spicy Pepper Salmon with Pear Salsa, 384
  Summerlicious Squash with Yogurt Chicken (Phase Two), 391
  Sweet Tooth–Satisfying Salmon (Phase Five), 417
Onions, green
  Awesome Avocado and Egg Breakfast, 360
  Baby Bok Choy and Chicken, 375
  Chicken with Bulgur and Mushrooms (Phase Four), 407
  Fresh Mint Chickpea Salad (Phase Three), 397
  Lovely Lemongrass Tofu (Phase Three), 393
  Scrumptious Edamame Salad (Phase Two), 385
  Spicy Turkey Muffins (Phase Five), 416
Oranges
  Orange Vanilla Shake, 353
  Perfect Peppercorn Fish, 378
  Portobello Mushroom Omelette, 361
  Quinoa Salad with Orange, Walnuts and Mint (Phase Four), 401

Pears
  Salmon and Dill Omelette, 362
  Spicy Pepper Salmon with Pear Salsa, 384
Peppers, jalapeño
  Spicy Pepper Poppers, 424
Peppers, sweet. *See* Bell peppers
Phase Two recipes, 385–391
Phase Three recipes, 392–99
Phase Four recipes, 400–408, 422
Phase Five recipe, 423

Pineapple
Piña Colada Smoothie, 357
Plums
Breakfast Cooler Smoothie, 354
Potatoes. *See also* Sweet potatoes
Red Potato and Asparagus Casserole
(Phase Five), 418
Protein bars
Coconut Almond Butter Protein Bars
(Phase Five), 423
Pumpkin
Curried Pumpkin and Green Beans
(Phase Two), 390

Quinoa
Cherry Tomato Salmon in Wine Broth
(Phase Four), 404
Quick Cinnamon Quinoa (Phase Four),
403
Quinoa Salad with Orange, Walnuts
and Mint (Phase Four), 401

Radishes
Scrumptious Edamame Salad (Phase
Two), 385
Rapini
Halibut and Rapini in Portobello
Mushroom Sauce (Phase Three),
394
Raspberries
Cheesecake Smoothie, 358
Wild Berry Breakfast, 354
Rice, brown
Rosemary Salmon Steaks (Phase Five),
415
Root beer
Root Beer Float Smoothie, 356

Salads
Ahi Tuna Steak and Salad, 367
Apple, Arugula and Chicken Salad
(Phase Four), 405
Beautiful Bean and Protein Salad
(Phase Three), 396
Blueberry Chicken Salad, 365
Celery with Tuna Salad, 419
Chilled Dill and Beet Salad (Phase
Two), 386
Cucumber and Cottage Cheese Salad,
373
Fresh Mint Chickpea Salad (Phase
Three), 397

Grilled Mediterranean Salad, 369
Mexican Summer Salad, 366
Miso Salad, 368
Quinoa Salad with Orange, Walnuts
and Mint (Phase Four), 401
Scrumptious Edamame Salad (Phase
Two), 385
Tuna Waldorf Salad, 383
Warm Beet and Goat Cheese Salad
(Phase Two), 389
Salmon
Cherry Tomato Salmon in Wine Broth
(Phase Four), 404
Rosemary Salmon Steaks (Phase Five),
415
Salmon and Dill Omelette, 362
Salmon with Spinach and Strawberry
Salsa, 381
Spicy Pepper Salmon with Pear Salsa,
384
Sweet Tooth–Satisfying Salmon (Phase
Five), 417
Salsa
Breakfast Salsa Dish, 364
Salmon with Spinach and Strawberry
Salsa, 381
Selenium-boosting Shrimp and Salsa,
376
Spicy Pepper Salmon with Pear Salsa,
384
Scallops
Turkey Bacon Scallops (Phase Four),
402
Seafood. *See* Fish and seafood
Shrimp
Curried Red Lentils with Shrimp or
Tofu (Phase Three), 392
Sautéed Shrimp and Green Beans, 373
Selenium-boosting Shrimp and Salsa,
376
Soups
Bison Chili and Beans (Phase Three),
398
Carrot and Ginger Soup (Phase Two),
387
Cauliflower and Kale Soup, 382
Curry Chicken Soup, 377
Soy milk
Chocolate Banana Smoothie, 351
Cinnamon Apple Smoothie, 355
Strawberry Shortcake Smoothie, 352
Wild Berry Breakfast, 354

Spinach
  Alkalizing Breakfast Smoothie, 358
  Awesome Avocado and Egg Breakfast, 360
  Barley and Spinach-stuffed Bell Peppers (Phase Five), 411–12
  Berrylicious Iron-booster Smoothie, 351
  Blueberry Chicken Salad, 365
  Miso Salad, 368
  Pepper and Spinach Omelette, 363
  Salmon and Dill Omelette, 362
  Salmon with Spinach and Strawberry Salsa, 381
Strawberries
  Cheesecake Smoothie, 358
  Jelly Sandwich Smoothie, 357
  Orange Vanilla Shake, 353
  Salmon with Spinach and Strawberry Salsa, 381
  Strawberry Shortcake Smoothie, 352
  Weightless Wasa Crackers (Phase Four), 422
Summer squash
  Summerlicious Squash with Yogurt Chicken (Phase Two), 391
  Summer Squash and Sesame Chicken (Phase Two), 388
Sweet potatoes
  Cinnamon Sweet Potato Pancakes (Phase Five), 414
  Honey Chicken and Sweet Potatoes (Phase Five), 413
  Sweet–Tooth–Satisfying Salmon (Phase Five), 417

Tofu
  Curried Red Lentils with Shrimp or Tofu (Phase Three), 392
  Lovely Lemongrass Tofu (Phase Three), 393
Tomatoes
  Ahi Tuna Steak and Salad, 367
  Awesome Avocado and Egg Breakfast, 360
  Bison Chili and Beans (Phase Three), 398
  Cherry Tomato Salmon in Wine Broth (Phase Four), 404
  Cucumber and Cottage Cheese Salad, 373
  Garlic Chicken and Asparagus, 370

  Immunity-boosting Ginger Chicken, 374
  Mexican Summer Salad, 366
  Miso Salad, 368
  Perfect Peppercorn Fish, 378
  Summer Tomato Lentils (Phase Three), 395
Trout
  Spicy Pepper Salmon with Pear Salsa, 384
Tuna
  Ahi Tuna Steak and Salad, 367
  Celery with Tuna Salad, 419
  Tuna Waldorf Salad, 383
Turkey. *See also* Chicken; Turkey Bacon
  Chicken with Bulgur and Mushrooms (Phase Four), 407
  Mini Turkey Lettuce Wraps, 422
  Spicy Turkey Muffins (Phase Five), 416
Turkey bacon
  Breakfast Salsa Dish, 364
  Turkey Bacon Scallops (Phase Four), 402

Vegetables. *See also* Salads; *specific kinds*
  Apricot-glazed Chicken and Kale, 372
  Awesome Avocado and Egg Breakfast, 360
  Baby Bok Choy and Chicken, 375
  Barley and Spinach-stuffed Bell Peppers (Phase Five), 411–12
  Cauliflower and Kale Soup, 382
  Crispy Chicken and Lettuce Wraps, 379
  Curried Pumpkin and Green Beans (Phase Two), 390
  Curry Chicken Soup, 377
  Ezekial Crumb-coated Chicken (Phase Four), 406
  Feta Cheese Meatballs with Grilled Vegetables, 371
  Grilled Chicken Skewer Wraps (Phase Four), 408
  Halibut and Rapini in Portobello Mushroom Sauce (Phase Three), 394
  Honey Chicken and Sweet Potatoes (Phase Five), 413
  Immunity-boosting Ginger Chicken, 374

Pepper and Spinach Omelette, 363
Perfect Peppercorn Fish, 378
Red Potato and Asparagus Casserole
    (Phase Five), 418
Sautéed Shrimp and Green Beans, 373
Summerlicious Squash with Yogurt
    Chicken (Phase Two), 391
Summer Squash and Sesame Chicken
    (Phase Two), 388

Walnuts
    Quinoa Salad with Orange, Walnuts
        and Mint (Phase Four), 401
Wasa crackers
    Weightless Wasa Crackers (Phase
        Four), 422
Whey protein isolate
    Alkalizing Breakfast Smoothie, 358
    Apricot Yogurt Smoothie, 350
    Banana Bread Smoothie (Phase Five),
        410
    Berries and Oats Breakfast Smoothie
        (Phase Five), 409
    Berrylicious Iron-booster Smoothie, 351
    Breakfast Cereal Smoothie (Phase
        Four), 400
    Breakfast Cooler Smoothie, 354
    Carb Sensitivity Shake, 419
    Cheesecake Smoothie, 358
    Choco-Berry Breakfast (Phase Five),
        410
    Chocolate Banana Smoothie, 351
    Chocolate Hazelnut Coffee Smoothie,
        350

Cinnamon Apple Smoothie, 355
Cinnamon Roll Smoothie, 355
Coconut Almond Butter Protein Bars
    (Phase Five), 423
Coco-Vanilla Smoothie, 356
Jelly Sandwich Smoothie, 357
Mint Chocolate Smoothie, 352
Orange Vanilla Shake, 353
Piña Colada Smoothie, 357
Root Beer Float Smoothie, 356
Skinny Banana Split Smoothie, 353
Strawberry Shortcake Smoothie, 352
Sweet Apple Cinnamon Delight (Phase
    Five), 412
Sweet Apple Pie Smoothie, 359
Wild Berry Breakfast, 354

Yogurt
    Alkalizing Breakfast Smoothie, 358
    Apricot Yogurt Smoothie, 350
    Coco-Vanilla Smoothie, 356
    Crispy Chicken and Lettuce Wraps, 379
    Perfect Balance Banana Bread, 424
    Strawberry Shortcake Smoothie, 352
    Summerlicious Squash with Yogurt
        Chicken (Phase Two), 391

Zucchini
    Grilled Mediterranean Salad, 369
    Mexican Summer Salad, 366
    Perfect Peppercorn Fish, 378
    Summerlicious Squash with Yogurt
        Chicken (Phase Two), 391

ABOUT THE AUTHOR

NATASHA TURNER, N.D., is a leading naturopathic doctor and founder of Clear Medicine, a Canadian-based wellness boutique that provides integrated health care. She is also the author of two international bestselling books, *The Hormone Diet* and *The Supercharged Hormone Diet*. She lives in Toronto with her husband.

www.carbsensitivity.com